# AIDS and STDs in Africa

# AIDS and STDs in Africa

## Bridging the Gap Between Traditional Healing and Modern Medicine

Edward C. Green

Routledge
Taylor & Francis Group
NEW YORK AND LONDON

First published 1994 by Westview Press

Published 2018
by Routledge
605 Third Avenue, New York, NY 10158

and by Routledge
4 Park Square, Milton Park, Abingdon, Oxon OX14 4RN

*Routledge is an imprint of the Taylor & Francis Group, an informa business*



**A CIP catalog record for this book is available from the Library of Congress.**

ISBN: 978-0-367-01405-6 (hbk)

# Contents

# Tables

# Acknowledgments

Some of the ethnomedical data from Swaziland presented in this paper was collected while I was working for the Academy for Educational Development under contract no. 465-0087 with the Agency for International Development (AID). Subsequent research in Nigeria, Liberia, Mozambique, South Africa, and Tanzania was funded by AID (SOMARC, HEALTHCOM, and AIDSCAP projects), sometimes with additional funds from the Population Crisis Committee (now Population Action International), the Pathfinder Fund, and the European Community. Among donor agencies, AID has been especially open to supporting programs involving traditional healers since the late 1970s. AID has supported several training programs for African healers by providing direct funding as well as technical support from medical anthropologists and others.

The views and opinions expressed in the book are my own and are not necessarily shared by any sponsoring organization or agency. I would like to thank the following colleagues for their valuable help in research and interpretation of findings: Joseph Phinias Mangcuzu Gama, Elias Nyoni, Lydia Makhubu, Petros Gama, Ernest Mnisi, and Wellington Mbele in Swaziland; Annemarie Jurg, Taju Tomas, and Armando Djedje in Mozambique; Mike Egboh and Esther Onuaguluchi in Nigeria; Harold Monger in Liberia; Bongie Zokwe and J. D. Dupree in South Africa; Anne Outwater, George Lwihula, Lucy Nkya, Hawa Nyamichwo, and Salina Mkony in Tanzania; and Sue McLaughlin in connection with all countries. I also want to thank D. Michael Warren, Charles Good, Patrick Oseweri, and Joop deJong for their critical readings of the manuscript and H. Russel Bernard for guiding me toward applied anthropology.

*Edward C. Green*

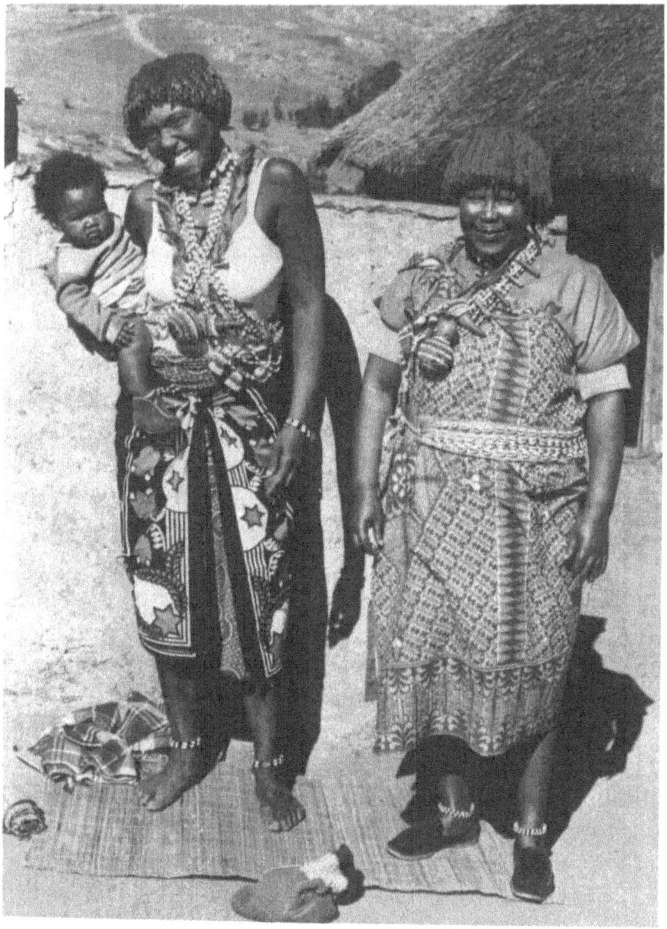

# Introduction

The war against AIDS in Africa is not going well ("Africa" denotes sub-Saharan Africa throughout this book). In his opening address to the 8th International Conference on AIDS (1992), Jonathan Mann admitted, "The old public health vision has become a straightjacket" confining planners to approaches to the prevention of AIDS that are not succeeding. In an interview with *Africa Report* (1992), Dr. Peter Lamptey, director of USAID's $168 million global project to control AIDS, observes that with only a very few exceptions, even the most successful condom promotion programs in Africa have "failed to make a dent in the epidemic." I agree with these assessments. I believe that the two-pronged approach that has dominated AIDS control programs thus far—namely, the promotion of condom use and restricting one's number of sexual partners (and there may be a mixed message right there)—has merit but is too little, too late for Africa.

For all their major emphasis in AIDS control programs in Africa (and elsewhere), in actual use condoms may only have a 50 percent effectiveness rate in reducing most sexually transmitted diseases. This is due to incorrect usage and to available products being of poor quality, partly because of inadequate storage and transportation under tropical conditions. These reasons are quite apart from problems of availability and acceptability in Africa. Millions of dollars have been spent on promotion and millions of condoms have been distributed in Uganda, the African nation with the greatest number of AIDS cases, yet the percentage of men regularly using condoms was about 3 percent in early 1993. How much programmatic emphasis on condoms is justified if at best we can hope to increase condom prevalence from 3 percent to perhaps twice that in the next two to three years? Note also that by African standards, condoms are reasonably accessible and AIDS awareness is high in Uganda. In view of all these problems, where else should there be programmatic emphasis?

AIDS is primarily a heterosexually transmitted disease in sub-Saharan Africa, unlike the pattern found in the industrialized West. Heterosexual intercourse, in fact, accounts for over 80 percent of African HIV cases. A major contributing factor appears to be the prevalence of other untreated or improperly treated sexually transmitted diseases (STDs) that facilitates the transmission of HIV. Most sub-Saharan countries of Africa suffer inordinately from STDs, compared with both industrialized countries and other less-developed parts of the world, even apart from the recent pandemic of AIDS. Because of the link between the presence of STDs and the heterosexual transmission of AIDS, there is now an additional and urgent reason to treat and prevent STDs—to curtail the spread of HIV infection.

Unlike AIDS, most standard or nonviral STDs are curable as well as preventable. Yet there have been surprisingly few financial or other resources thus far devoted to STD control programs. Another problem is how actually to lower the incidence of STDs. Most STD cases in Africa appear not to be presented at biomedical health facilities (biomedical will be used as a short-hand way of denoting Western-style, scientifically based, allopathic medicine); they are taken to traditional healers. True, traditional healers provide most of the health services of whatever sort in Africa (de Zalduondo, Msamanga, and Chen 1989). But beyond that, STDs are often regarded as an area of particular competence by African healers, as evidence presented in this book will show. The clients of traditional healers—the majority of Africans—also seem to believe that traditional medicines are especially effective in treating STDs. This means that for better or worse, traditional healers see and treat most of the cases of STDs in Africa. It also means that it would be more difficult to persuade millions of Africans to seek biomedical treatment for STDs than, say, for tuberculosis or cholera—even if African health ministries were in a position to launch an effective mass-treatment program for STDs, which they are not.

I believe these facts must be accepted if we are to seriously impact the high incidence and prevalence of STDs and therefore HIV infection rates in Africa. Yet what I term facts are not as yet acknowledged or accepted by most of what can justifiably be called the AIDS establishment. Only the odd anthropologist or health educator seems to argue for a role for traditional healers in AIDS control and prevention, and even their arguments rarely focus on STDs. In fact, those few who argue for a role for traditional healers in AIDS prevention tend not to mention STDs, while those who argue for preventing AIDS by controlling STDs tend not to mention traditional healers.

In Family Health International's otherwise useful and authoritative *Handbook for AIDS Prevention in Africa* (1990), there is a chapter titled the "Control and Prevention of Sexually Transmitted Diseases," which outlines a variety of intervention strategies. There is no mention of traditional healers; plans for Africa are discussed as if traditional healers did not exist. There is another chapter in the same book called "Counseling and AIDS." Again there is no mention of traditional healers even as potential lay counselors, even though virtually every other possible community-based human resource is described. In Chapter 7 of the present book, traditional healers themselves provide some description and discussion of their role as counselors in AIDS and STD prevention, as well as in related areas. Some of these South African healers are actively addressing AIDS risk factors that are scarcely even being discussed in most official AIDS prevention programs. In Chapter 9, healers in Dar es Salaam provide glimpses of the type of counseling they offer HIV-positive clients, aimed at improving the body's ability to fight infection as well as overcoming a defeatest attitude.

A recent, well-reasoned book with the promising title *AIDS in Africa* (Barnett and Blaikie 1992) stresses the need to analyze the social and epidemiological contexts of HIV transmission. Yet there is no listing in the index of indigenous or traditional healers; nor, for that matter, of sexually transmitted diseases, the male circumcision factor in HIV transmission, or spermicides that seem to protect against both STDs and AIDS. In the last chapter, the authors report without endorsement or other comment that several countries in Southern Africa plan to involve traditional healers in national AIDS campaigns.

The present book will emphasize factors in the spread and control of AIDS that have thus far received insufficient (or no) attention in the literature or the international AIDS conferences, let alone in the AIDS control programs funded by high-resource donors. This will not fill in the last few missing pieces of an otherwise nearly complete puzzle. Some of the puzzle may be put together in the wrong way. The risk factors and strategies for control of HIV infection that form the focus of this book are central, not marginal, in the understanding and control of AIDS, and I will draw upon empirical evidence from several disciplines to back this assertion. I believe much of the generally acknowledged failure of AIDS control programs in Africa to date stems from the failure to recognize and address some of the central facts of the epidemiology of AIDS in Africa.

I argue in this book that some sort of collaborative action program involving traditional healers is necessary if we wish to significantly impact the spread of AIDS and other STDs in Africa. AIDS programs need the active cooperation of traditional healers in order to treat and prevent standard STDs such as gonorrhea, syphilis, and chlamydia. Traditional healers can also do much to help promote condom and spermicide use, safer sex practices, and restriction of the number of sexual partners. I hope to help answer the complex policy and program questions of exactly how viable collaborative programs involving traditional healers can be developed.

It has always made public health sense for African ministries of health to work cooperatively rather than competitively with traditional healers, but never more so than in the midst of the current AIDS pandemic. Africa is already unable to pay for adequate health care services. High birth rates, poor economic prospects for at least the short term, and now the staggering direct and indirect costs associated with AIDS in many countries make the situation significantly worse. In the face of these realities, cooperation between the "modern" or biomedical and "traditional" health sectors (these terms are loaded and inadequate, yet they are widely used) seems unavoidable as well as logical and desirable. Yet more than fifteen years after joint WHO/UNICEF resolutions calling for use of indigenous health practitioners in Third World government-sponsored health programs, there are only a handful of active programs of intersectoral collaboration in all of Africa.

I also argue that the role of STDs in transmitting the AIDS virus has been given insufficient attention in AIDS prevention programs. For example, for some years a diagram purporting to show which sexual practices are most unsafe has been used for the purpose of AIDS education in many parts of Africa, courtesy of an influential U.S.-funded AIDS prevention project. Sexual practices are, in fact, ranked along a continuum ranging from unsafe to relatively safe. However, there is nothing at all about sexual intercourse with STD-infected partners anywhere on the chart. Intercourse with an STD-infected partner is probably the surest way of getting AIDS in Africa, yet there will be no preventive education on this if the risk chart is followed. Again, a peer education manual currently used in Tanzania, which starts with a section specifically on STDs, likewise makes no mention of the risks of intercourse with a partner known or likely to have an STD—or even of a causal relationship between STDs and AIDS.

In presenting the issues and arguments, I will draw upon my own research and project experience in Swaziland, Mozambique, Liberia, Nigeria, South Africa, and Tanzania. In spite of its focus on AIDS and STDs, the book should also be of value to the reader not particularly interested in AIDS or STDs—or to the related area of child spacing/family planning—but interested in the broader public health role of traditional healers and to questions of collaboration with such healers. Most of the principles, issues, and lessons that relate to AIDS/STDs also apply to other areas of potential public health collaboration.

Most chapters provide original ethnographic data, therefore it seemed best to arrange them by country. By doing so, the findings are chronologically presented, starting with the first country of my data collecting.[1] The alternative would have been to organize by topic or issue, with only brief or passing reference to the culture, society, and time period, and with findings introduced selectively to buttress one position or another. I saw two disadvantages to this. First, we would end up with fragmented findings devoid of social or cultural context. Second, my opportunities for data gathering relating to STDs and AIDS cover a twelve-year period (1981 to 1992), and by focusing on one country or cultural area at a time, differences related to time—to how much was known at the time both by myself, by others in the scientific community and by healers themselves—is at least partially preserved. As the ethnographic chapters progress chronologically, I am learning more about AIDS and STDs in Africa and so are other researchers, program planners, educators and campaigners, project implementers, and the like. Scientific information about AIDS and HIV is also disseminating to traditional healers over the same period, so that healers from whatever country tend to become more knowledgeable about the new disease over time.

It is also the case that in 1981, there was less accumulated experience with African health programs involving collaboration with traditional healers. As my work relating to traditional healers took me from one country to another (with unrelated assignments in between), my own knowledge of how best to collaborate with healers—and how to avoid various pitfalls—expanded along with that of other researchers and program planners in the field.

## Notes

1. With the exception of Nigeria, due to change of topic.

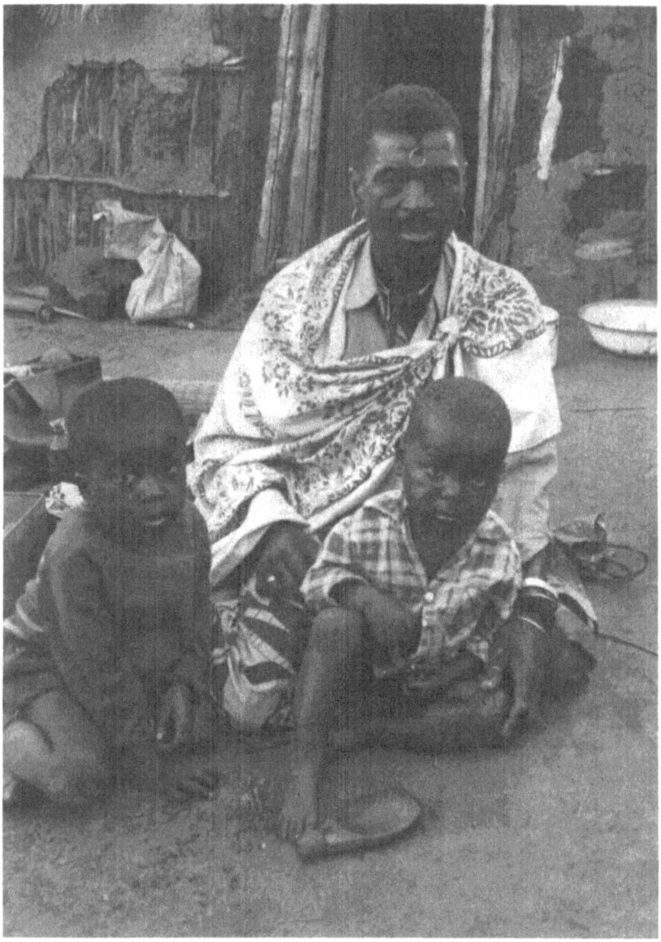

# 1

# The Intriguing Epidemiology of AIDS in Africa[1]

In industrialized countries where AIDS is well established, HIV transmission has occurred primarily through male homosexual intercourse and blood-to-blood contact among IV drug abusers (Pattern I transmission, in UN/WHO parlance.) In sub-Saharan Africa, HIV is transmitted primarily through heterosexual intercourse, infecting women as often as men (Pattern II)(UN 1990:162–163). It is not coincidental that Pattern II countries are also characterized by high incidence and prevalence of standard sexually transmitted diseases (STDs) such as gonorrhea, syphilis, chlamydia, and chancroid. STDs, particularly those associated with genital ulceration, enhance the efficiency of HIV transmission (Greenblatt et al. 1988; Pepin et al. 1989; Mhalu 1990; Piot and Tezzo 1990; WHO 1990; Prual, Chacko, and Koch-Weser 1991; Wasserheit 1992; Laga et al. 1993). In the words of Wasserheit (1992:61), "The interrelationships between human immunodeficiency virus (HIV) infection and other sexually transmitted diseases (STDs) are unique, complex, and intriguing. They probably explain, in part, the heterogenous faces of the HIV epidemic around the globe. . . ." Efforts to limit the heterosexual transmission of HIV in Africa must therefore address the high prevalence of other, standard STDs.

Compared with both industrialized countries and other less developed parts of the world, most sub-Saharan African countries suffer inordinately from sexually transmitted disease (STDs). They have higher prevalence rates of traditional STDs, such as gonorrhea and syphilis, higher proportions of antimicrobial-resistant organisms and higher levels of complications from STDs including pelvic inflammatory disease, infertility, ectopic pregnancies, spontaneous abortion, stillbirth, cervical cancer, congenital syphilis, chlamydial pneumonia, and infant blindness (UN 1990; Althaus 1991). The incidence of standard STDs, along with associated complications, rose markedly during the 1980s in Africa (Meheus and De Schryver 1991:202). Since STD-infected women are more likely than men to be asymptomatic and therefore to go untreated, and since the complications associated with STDs affect women (and their children) more than men, STDs place an even greater burden on women.

Prevalence figures for specific STDs are often unreliable or totally lacking, because a country may lack a functioning STD control system, many STD victims do not know they are infected, and STDs are often treated outside the orthodox health care system. In either case victims often do not enter into official health care systems and statistics (Prual, Chacko and Koch-Weser 1991; Piot and Hira 1990:85–86). However, screening of pregnant women in many parts of Africa has yielded syphilis prevalence rates of 10 percent to over 30 percent, and gonorrhea prevalence rates of 10 percent to nearly 20 percent in some areas (Greenblatt et al. 1988; Georges et al. 1990; Mhalu 1990; Piot and Hira 1990:86; Piot and Tezzo 1990). Although gonorrhea, syphilis, and chlamydia are the most common STDs in Africa, other diseases such as chancroid, papillomavirus, and lymphogranuloma venereum have also become significant health problems (Georges et al. 1990; Meheus and De Schryver 1991). Together, various STDs account for a high percentage of morbidity in many parts of Africa. According to a recent review, "STDs are among the top five causes of consultation at health services in many African countries" and ranking would be even higher for fifteen to forty year olds (Meheus and De Schryver 1991:20). For example, in Zambia STDs are second only to malaria in recorded number of cases, and it has been suggested that many cases of STDs in that country are not recorded because they are treated by "traditional doctors" and because the diseases are regarded as shameful in that their presence reflects "loose morals" (Sajiwandani and Baboo 1987).

More than 80 percent of all cases of HIV infection in Africa have been found to be heterosexually transmitted, through penile-vaginal intercourse. Up to 10 percent seem to be due to blood transfusions, resulting from contaminated blood supplies, although the proportion may be up to 25 percent in children. Perinatal mother-to-child transmission, resulting in pediatric AIDS, accounts for most of the remaining cases. The role of injections or anal intercourse in HIV transmission appear to be "small or very small" (Piot and Harris 1990:10–15). This contrasts with the United States, Western Europe, Australia, and New Zealand where most HIV infections result from male homosexual intercourse or parenteral (skin piercing) transmission (Pattern I). In the United Kingdom, only 6 percent of all AIDS deaths between 1982 and the end of 1991 are believed to have been transmitted heterosexually. If we control for the risk factors such as a partner being an IV drug user, a male bisexual, or someone from a Pattern II country, we are left with 19 heterosexually transmitted cases out of 3,156 in 10 years, or about one-half of one percent (CDSC 1992:9).

AIDS statistics from South Africa between 1982 and February 1993 show the emergence of Pattern I and II side by side in a single country. There were a total of 438 cases among whites of which 97 percent were male; 89 percent of these were sexually transmitted male-to-male. Only 5 percent were transmitted heterosexually and the role of other risk factors among these cases is not known. There were no pediatric cases. Among blacks there were 1,305 cases, half among males and half among females. Only .005 percent of total cases were sexually transmitted male-to-male; 70 percent were transmitted heterosexually and 28 percent were pediatric. The sizable Asian population had only 5 male cases, of which 4 were sexually transmitted male-to-male (*Epidemiological Comments* 1993:50).

Why are patterns of heterosexual transmission so strikingly different between Pattern I and II populations? Possible factors that have been hypothesized include the high prevalence of other STDs in Africa, compromised or activated immune systems stemming from the abundance of microbes present in Africa; the noncircumcision of males; variations in the amount of virus that people have in vaginal or semen secretions, and use of vaginal tightening agents, abrasives or irritants in some areas of Africa. The first of these has the most empirical support to date. A pattern of having multiple sexual partners has also been postulated and is discussed below and in Chapter 4, *Sexual Behavior.*

## STDs and HIV Infection

The presence in Africa of other sexually transmitted diseases, especially those such as syphilis and chancroid which are characterized by genital ulceration, assists the heterosexual transmission of the AIDS-causing human immunodeficiency virus. Stated succinctly:

> The reason why in Africa heterosexual transmission of HIV seems rather efficient and bi-directional probably lies in the high prevalence of other sexually transmitted diseases: diseases such as gonorrhea, chancroid or syphilis cause mucosal or squamous epithelial discontinuity in the genitalia and may thus facilitate transmission of HIV during genital intercourse (van der Graff and Diepersloot 1986:206. See also Nsubuga et al. 1990).

There appear to be reasons other than lesions or ulceration that account for the heterosexual transmission of HIV in the presence of other STDs. It is known for example that gonorrhea provokes a lymphocyte response which might increase the amount of virus transmitted from an HIV infected person (Biggar 1986). The gonorrheal pus discharge or other "unresolved urethral infection" may help carry HIV-infected fluids ". . . into the man's urethra and engage the white blood cells trying to resolve the urethral infection. . . ." (Dupree 1992). It seems that any type of STD infection attracts to the area of infection T lymphocytes or macrophages which are then available for invasion by HIV (Wasserheit 1992:69). Whatever the causal mechanisms, statistical evidence accumulates suggesting that nonulcerative STDs also facilitate the transmission of HIV, and this is of great significance because in most populations chlamydia, gonorrhea, and trichomoniasis are far more prevalent than ulcerative diseases such as syphilis (Wasserheit 1992:64).

There is growing evidence that HIV infection has a reciprocal relationship with other STDs: an HIV-infected person may be more susceptible to STD infection; the STD (especially the ulcerative type) may be characterized by more pronounced and more persistent symptoms; and treatment failure may be more common due in part to altered, atypical symptoms (Wasserheit 1992:71).

There are some who argue that the role of standard STDs as major cofactors in the heterosexual spread of HIV infection still is not well-understood, particularly those STDs that do not involve lesions or ulceration. Yet while it may be premature to conclude that the incidence of a particular STD must be reduced by some predictable amount if the spread of AIDS is to be curtailed in Africa, it makes public health sense to proceed as if all STDs play a significant role in the spread of AIDS and to renew efforts to reduce their incidence in Africa—especially since the reduction of STDs is a worthy public health goal in itself.

The question might arise, if STDs are so important in HIV transmission in Africa, why are HIV (HIV-I) prevalence rates relatively low in West Africa which also has high STD prevalence? Factors accounting for significant geographic differences in HIV infection rates have not been adequately established but they may include the practice of male circumcision, timing of the onset of the epidemic, and variations in sexual behavior (Bongaarts et al. 1989:373; Piot and Harris 1990:12). Much importance is ascribed to sexual practices, although we have little reliable data on these. This has not prevented arriving at conclusions prematurely. For example, Huband (1991) quotes WHO statistics showing the Ivory Coast to be "the sixth worst affected country in Africa for cases of AIDS," and based on no more than his selective observations, attributes this to the "busy red light districts" in the capital city. The head of the largest global AIDS assistance project in the United States recently speculated that in addition to STD variations and historical factors, the great differences in seroprevalence within Africa is probably due to "multiple sexual partners in some countries" (Lamptey 1992:29). I have seen no evidence to suggest that West Africans differ significantly from Central, Southern, or East Africans in practices related to multiple sexual partners.

A geographic relationship between migratory labor systems and prevalence rates of both HIV and standard STDs has also been suggested, presumably because migratory labor results in "long absences, increased family breakdown, and increased numbers of sexual partners" (Hunt 1989:353). However recent studies have shown that "infection in partners of HIV-infected persons is not determined solely by numbers of sexual encounters," but rather by multiple biologic factors, of which "genital ulcerative disease" is probably a major determinant (Holmberg et al. 1990. See also Chapter 4, *Sexual Behavior,* below).

Rather than looking to presumed exotic sexual practices or "promiscuity," the causes of Africa's relatively high STD rates are to be found more in poverty and its consequences such as chronic shortage of funds and personnel for STD prevention and treatment that constrain virtually all health programs in Africa, reluctance on the part of STD sufferers to consult medically trained personnel, inappropriate self-medication, growing antimicrobial resistance to standard antibiotics such as penicillin, low condom user rates, and probably ineffective treatment from traditional healers, among other factors (Van Der Geest 1982; FHI 1986; Msamango and Pallangyo 1987; Piot and Tezzo 1990; Meheus and De Schryver 1991; Caldwell et al. 1993).

Another explanation is also beginning to gain some credence. Bongaarts and his colleagues found a strong statistical correlation between lack of male circumcision and HIV seroprevalence in the capitals of thirty-seven African countries, including thirteen in West Africa (Bongaarts et al. 1989:373–375). Although most geographically localized studies of risk factors have not even considered circumcision, some that have have also discovered positive associations between lack of male circumcision and either HIV-1 infection (Greenblatt et al. 1988; Cameron et al. 1989; Marx 1989; Jessamine et al. 1990; Serwadda et al. 1992) or HIV-2 infection (Pepin et al. 1992). (HIV-2 is a virus similar to HIV-1 but it leads to a less serious form of immunosuppression, one that advances more slowly. It is more prevalent in West Africa than HIV-1.) Some researchers (but certainly no policymakers) have even proposed the possibility of advocating male circumcision as a method for controlling the spread of HIV (Plummer, Moses, and Ndinya-Achola 1991).

It is not known what the causal connection is here but Barton (1989:13) notes that "post-coital abrasions in the foreskin are common in uncircumcised males," and Fink (1987:1546) tells us that such men ". . . in general are predisposed to preputial inflammation" which itself might facilitate HIV transmission. Plummer, Moses, and Ndinya-Achola (1991:6) hypothesize that "the area underneath the foreskin provides a warm, moist environment in which the virus can survive, and which is more susceptible to infection." It may also be that HIV entry to the blood stream is facilitated by the presence of dendritic leukocytes of the Langerhans/dendritic cell lineage, which are abundant in the foreskin and are easliy invaded by HIV (Langhoff and Haseltine 1993; Fink 1987). Oates (1987:1546) believes the problem is not in the foreskin but in the frenum or the frenal area where microlacerations can result from sexual activity.

It may be that the relationship, if established, is indirect: circumcision may provide males some protection against standard STDs, which themselves assist in the sexual transmission of HIV. Yet there are findings suggesting a more direct link. In a prospective study of seronegative men in Kenya, the authors found that "uncircumcised men had an increased risk of seroconversion which was independent of their risk of genital ulcer disease. Over 95 percent of attributable risk in men with sexually transmitted diseases was either genital ulceration or the presence of foreskin" (Jessamine et al. 1990:81).

It should be noted that some studies refute the lack of circumcision-STD/HIV susceptibility hypothesis. However some traditional healers in South Africa have made their own observations and developed their own opinions on this subject, it would seem independently of epidemiological polemics. Some have begun to advise clients to become circumcised in order to prevent at least standard STDs, noting that their repeat STD patients tend to have rashes, "dirt," or infections under their foreskins (See Chapter 7, *The Circumcision Factor*).

## Impacting STD Incidence

Curtailing the spread of STDs promises to be a greater task than it might appear at first. As Barton (1989:11) notes, there are no "facile or straight-forward" measures of effective STD control in Africa, the claims of several authors notwithstanding. The problem is not simply one of paying for more standard antibiotics and then ensuring that these reach clinics and hospitals, although funding and logistics remain part of the problem. Prior to the AIDS outbreak, donor organizations and ministries of health contributed relatively little to the control or even the understanding of STDs in Africa, certainly when compared with common diseases of childhood, nutrition, family planning, or other endemic, infectious diseases such as malaria and schistosomiasis. Perhaps this is because STDs are not as "respectable" as the more publicized health concerns of mothers and children, and possibly African governments do not wish to publicize the extent of STD prevalence in their countries. If the major justification for diverting funds to maternal and child health is that conditions that would be more difficult and expensive to treat at a later stage are thereby prevented, surely the same argument can now be made for treating STDs in order to limit the spread of AIDS in Africa.

Furthermore, many Africans suffering from an STD do not seek orthodox medical treatment. They may treat themselves with ineffective medicines or with antibiotics. Widespread misuse of antibiotics has led to the emergence of new strains of gonorrhea that are resistant to penicillin, therefore difficult and expensive to treat (FHI 1986:4; Masango and Pallangyo 1987; Meheus and De Schryver 1991). However, in my experience, self-treatment and home remedies are less common than reliance upon traditional healers for treatment of STDs. This premise lies at the root of most of the AIDS-related arguments and policy or program recommendations presented in this book, therefore let us look more closely at the premise and at supporting evidence.

## STDs: The Domain of Traditional African Medicine

Ethnomedical studies in Africa have shown that both healers and their clients tend to recognize the efficacy of Western-style biomedical treatment for certain illnesses or conditions. I have conducted surveys in Swaziland, Nigeria, and South Africa in which traditional healers were asked which illnesses or conditions are more amenable to traditional treatment and which are more amenable to biomedical treatment. A survey containing a similar set of questions was conducted independently in Mathare, Kenya (Good 1987:306).

Healers in all four countries conceded that there are conditions for which Western biomedical treatment is superior to traditional treatment. However, conditions characterized by symptoms such as pain in urination and pus discharge from the penis were in all cases thought to be treated more effectively by traditional medicine. As can be seen in Table 1.1, various STDs—usually described by indigenous names—are ranked first in Swaziland[2] and South Africa, sixth in Nigeria, and fifth in Kenya[3] as a condition believed better treated by African medicine.

It might be argued that the above conditions are cited simply because they are all prevalent in Africa, therefore healers are called upon to treat STDs whatever particular efficacy they or their clients attribute to traditional treatment. However, the question asked was not, "Which conditions do you treat most often?" In Swaziland, Nigeria, and South Africa the question was, "Do you believe traditional medicine can be more successful than modern medicine in treating certain types of disease?" If the answer was yes, then "Which conditions and why is it so?" The phrasing of the question in Kenya seems to have been very similar. In any case, we

TABLE 1.1 Conditions Believed Better Dealt with by Traditional Versus Biomedical Practitioners (ranked in order of frequency cited by healers)

| *Swaziland* (N=144) | *Nigeria* (N=399) | *South Africa* (N=28) | *Kenya* (N=45) |
|---|---|---|---|
| gonorrhea, various STDs, genital sores | madness | various STDs | witchcraft |
| *umklwebho* (a type of sorcery) | childbirth | mental illness | madness |
| children's illnesses | fractures and bonesetting | epilepsy | abdominal pains |
| migraines | bewitchments | high blood pressure | edemas |
| evil spirits | gonorrhea and other STDs | midwifery | gastro-enteritis; |
| various bewitchments | sterility and impotence; | witchcraft and sorcery | infertility |
| | malaria and fevers | fertility | epilepsy |
| | diarrhea | heart failure | STDs |

see different conditions cited when we ask healers to specify cases in which modern medicine can be more successful than traditional medicine, as summarized in Table 1.2. It should be remembered that biomedical diagnostic categories, when referred to by traditional healers, may be imprecise to say the least.

Although "VD or drop" is ranked fifth in frequency of citation in Swaziland, there were only twelve citations here versus eighty-four citations asserting that these conditions were treated more effectively by traditional medicine—all from the same 144 healers. STDs did not make the list in Nigeria or South Africa, although in Kenya they were ranked sixth (compared to fifth in Table 1.1). To generalize from these findings in West, East and Southern Africa, traditional healers see the strength of biomedical treatment lying in certain diseases like tuberculosis, and in its mysterious technology and surgical procedures. A major strength of traditional medicine is believed to lie in treatment of STDs.

These findings concerning STDs—particularly gonorrhea—do not seem to be at odds with those from other sub-Saharan societies, (e.g. Orubuloye, Caldwell, and Caldwell (1991). A report from the Vane-Avatime area of Ghana on the Nazareth Healing Complex, a church-sponsored holistic healing center that combines traditional herbal medicine with modern biomedicine and Christian faith healing, describes a natural division of labor between the three healing systems (Western biomedical, African traditional, and Christian) and lists gonorrhea as a condition that comes under the "Traditional and Herbal Department" (Baku 1988:3). And a small study in two peri-urban neighborhoods of Maputo, Mozambique, found "STDs" to be the fourth most common condition to

TABLE 1.2 Conditions Believed Better Dealt with by Biomedical Versus Traditional Practitioners (ranked in order of frequency cited by healers)

| *Swaziland* (N=144) | *Nigeria* (N=399) | *South Africa* (N=28) | *Kenya* (N=45) |
|---|---|---|---|
| cholera | whenever traditional treatment fails | TB | TB |
| TB or chest | operations, IV drip | X-rays | surgical problems |
| blood transfusion or curing "lack of blood" | blood transfusion, sutures, etc. | "shortage of blood" requiring transfusion | malaria |
| headache (malaria?) | | "shortage of water," dehydration | transfusions, infusions |
| VD or drop | | | fractures |
| heart attacks | | | STDs |
| stomach | | | pneumonia |
| anything requiring surgery or other medical technology | | | anemia |
| | | | epilepsy |
| | | | orthopedic surgery |

be treated by traditional healers, even when biomedical treatment was easily accessible (Jurg, Tomas, and de Jong 1991).

Are indigenous African medicines in fact successfully treating STDs? Although there has been little ethnopharmacological or other biomedical research in this area, I suspect indigenous STD treatments are probably for the most part biomedically ineffective—or insufficient (Sajiwandani and Baboo 1987). This topic is explored somewhat in Chapter 5. I have also found some evidence of the concurrent use by healers of antibiotics and herbal medicines for STD treatment (see Chapters 3 and 7), which raises a number of important public health issues.

Although in their discussion of nosology in traditional medicine in Zaire, Bibeau et al. (1980:13) cite "venereal disease" as "precisely differentiated" from other disease categories, I and several other researchers have not found this to be the case. I have found that other illnesses and conditions not classified as sexually transmitted in biomedical nosology may be locally regarded as such by African healers and their clients. For example, in Swaziland, the locally recognized symptom of "blood-in-urine" (*umthundungati*), the Swazi term for which is a common designation for urinary schistosomiasis, is believed by some to result from *likhubalo*, an STD; therefore some regard schistosomiasis as a sexually transmitted disease. In my studies in both Swaziland and central Mozambique, I found that certain types of sexual relations were thought to cause the symptoms of tuberculosis. In another study of pulmonary TB in Inhambane Province, Mozambique, researchers found that TB is believed to be a sexually transmitted disease by most surveyed and that (therefore?) most patients seek traditional therapy in these cases. Specific mention was made that it was the violation of sexual taboos, such as intercourse with widows or with women who have recently had an abortion, that caused symptoms (Pateguane 1983).

## Notes

1. Some of the material in this chapter has appeared in Green, E. C., "Sexually Transmitted Disease, Ethnomedicine and AIDS in Africa." *Social Science and Medicine* Vol. 35, No. 2, 1992, pp. 121–130.

2. I previously published a table (Green 1992:124) which showed gonorrhea ranked third as a claimed specialty by Swazi healers. Since then, I re-examined the original tallies from the 1982 questionnaires. There were 40 citations of *likhubalo,* a locally-recognized STD. There were additionally 27 citations of penis sores, "VD," or "drop," the last-mentioned closely resembling gonorrhea. Citations relating to *all* STDs total 67, 25 more than the next most frequent citation, *umklwebho.*

3. Since, according to the author, there were some ties in earlier rankings (Good 1987:306).

# 2

# Issues in the Development of Collaborative Programs[1]

## African Healers

It is always dangerous to make generalizations about the people and cultures of sub-Saharan Africa, yet it is necessary to engage in some of this for our purposes. Most of the generalizations attributed to Africa that follow in fact pertain to the Niger-Congo ethnolinguistic group (Green 1980:490–491). This is the numerically largest and geographically most widespread group in Africa, covering most of sub-Saharan Africa except for the Horn and central portions of the Sudan. The Niger-Congo grouping relates the Bantu-speaking peoples of the Congo basin and southeast Africa historically and culturally to the dense population of West Africa, from which area the former group migrated, beginning a few centuries before Christ. Noting the common heritage, historian E. Murphy observes, "The Bantu-speaking peoples share with their West African cousins common fundamental attitudes about God, religion, kinship, the nature of the world, and life" (1972:179).

With this in mind, there are several types and subtypes of indigenous healers that have been identified throughout sub-Saharan Africa and described in the anthropological literature. The most common distinction among *traditional* healers[2] is that between herbalist and diviner-medium. In ideal-typical terms, the former tends to work primarily with natural *materia medica* while the latter has additionally cultivated a relationship with ancestor and other spirits believed to assist in divination and healing. In recent generations, two other types of healer have emerged that may be termed indigenous but nontraditional, namely the religious faith healer and the alternative healer. I have attempted a somewhat arbitrary taxonomy of these in Table 2.1.

Conventional wisdom has it that herbalists are somewhat more likely than other broad categories of healers to be interested in cooperating with modern health personnel, although this may be because governments have made more overtures to herbalists. However it should be

TABLE 2.1 Taxonomy of Indigenous African Healers

| *Class* | *Sub-class* | *Specialists within Sub-Class* |
|---|---|---|
| Diviner-medium | diviner-medium<br>shaman, priest<br>witch identifier | oracle<br>spirit medium<br>ceremonial specialist |
| Herbalist | herbalist | childrens' disease specialist<br>bonesetter<br>infertility or impotence specialist<br>traditional birth attendant |
| Alternative healer | "black-bagger" injectionist | |
| Religious faith healer | Christian faith healer ("Cherubim," "Zionist," "Jerico")<br>Muslim faith healer ("Marabout," etc.) | |

recognized that: (1) distinctions between categories of healers may be vague, and the same individual might qualify as two or three types of healer simultaneously; (2) diviner-mediums have shown great interest in learning about Western biomedicine, and some have proven to be among the most enthusiastic training participants; and (3) diviner-mediums are often attributed higher status than herbalists, meaning that—among other considerations—it may be politically unwise to exclude diviners from collaborative programs.

In selecting indigenous healers for inclusion in HIV/AIDS prevention programs, it is probably best to find out who is currently being consulted for STDs and/or AIDS, however they are classified by themselves or others. Specialists in treating various locally recognized sexually transmitted diseases are found throughout Africa, since STDs are epidemic in many or most regions and since—as discussed in Chapter 1—STDs are widely regarded as conditions highly responsive to traditional treatment. Another category of likely candidates for HIV/AIDS prevention programs might be traditional healers who specialize in delaying pregnancy, since such healers may already have some knowledge and experience with contraceptives. Such specialists are probably less common than those who treat STDs. Specialists in delaying pregnancy seem to increase with urbanization and cash-dependency (and the monetary cost of rearing children), and they may be drawn from the ranks of specialists in midwifery and/or gynecological problems. It may be useful to investigate the differences between males and females within the same category of healer with regard to their involvement in treating STDs or AIDS, or in delaying pregnancy.

Experience suggests that it is preferable to collaborate with traditional as distinct from alternative healers. The problems associated with collaborating with traditional healers, discussed below, are increased severalfold when it comes to injectionists and others untrained in either the traditional or biomedical sector who set themselves up as purveyors of allopathic biomedicine. Some of the negative reputation and "bad press" associated with traditional healers is actually due to harm caused by alternative healers. Of course, news writers and critics from medical circles may not appreciate the difference between the two types of healers.

Among other advantages, traditional healers have numerical superiority over all other healers including biomedical. There have been healer-to-population ratio estimates based on specialized censuses taken in several African countries. We see a ratio of 1:287 for Uganda (Hogel et al. 1991:29); 1:234, 1:575, or 1:260 for Zimbabwe (Gelfand et al. 1985; Chavunduka 1986); 1:200 for Lagos state, Nigeria (Green 1989); 1:100 for rural and urban Swaziland (Green and Makhubu 1984: 1073); 1:407 (rural) or 1:280 (urban) for Ghana (Wondergem, Senah, and Glover 1988:24); roughly 1:200 for two periurban areas of Mozambique (Maputo and Manica provinces) (Jurg, Tomas and de Jong 1991); "conservative estimates" of 1:375 and 1:454 for two Dar es Salaam neighborhoods (Swantz 1990:13) and 1:60 for periurban Senegal (Fassin and Fassin 1988:354).

The *physician*-to-population ratio in a country like Mozambique is about 1:50,000, with some 52 percent of doctors concentrated in the capital city and most of the rest practicing in the next largest cities. The nurse-to-population ratio is 1:5,300, meaning that traditional healers easily outnumber the combined biomedically trained health force in countries like Mozambique. Throughout Africa we see a similar pattern of inadequate numbers of doctors and concentration of these in the largest cities. Africa's high birth rates and general economic downturn—resulting in decreases in Ministry of Health operating budgets—mean that even greater proportions of the population remain unserved by biomedical health personnel. Traditional healers are the acknowledged de facto primary health care providers in rural areas, and this is not only by default. High concentrations of healers in periurban areas suggests that they are still frequently consulted even when hospitals and clinics are available.

Before proceeding it may be useful to make a distinction between cooperation and another term preferred by some, integration. Cooperation implies a better working relationship between the traditional and allopathic health sectors whereby appropriate referrals between the two sectors are developed and become more routine, certain of the traditional healer's skills are upgraded, and the cultural sensitivity of allopathic health workers is increased—to the point of learning about the more effective traditional healing practices and even integrating these in their practice. "Collaboration" appears to be used somewhat synonymously with cooperation, but the term further implies that cooperation is between somewhat equal partners.

"Integration" implies a fundamental alteration in both healing systems and in the roles of the respective practitioners, although in practice it is the traditional healer who is expected to change. The danger here is that the traditional healer may become a second-rate paramedical worker and thereby cease to carry out his or her important function in the local community—a function that has social, psychological, and spiritual as well as bodily health dimensions. Such an outcome could be disruptive in multiple ways, including the undermining of a community's capacity to solve its own health problems (Taylor 1979; Green and Makhubu 1984:1077). I have come to prefer use of the term collaboration because it seems more active and dynamic than cooperation, and because it implies cooperation between equal partners.

Use of the term training also deserves comment. Training is a somewhat derogatory or at least condescending word because it implies that traditional healers are somehow deficient, but once they are trained (as if remedially) by some method only we can recommend, they can be enlightened and their practice improved. This of course is presumptuous, paternalistic, and arrogant, and it ignores the great extent to which "they" can educate "us." However, programs related to collaboration with African healers often rely on monies earmarked as training funds, therefore use of the term may be unavoidable at least when communicating with donor agencies and government ministries.

## Indigenous Knowledge Systems

In addition to indigenous healers and their role in providing health care, indigenous knowledge systems are important in their own right. Indigenous knowledge systems (IKS) refers to that body of accumulated wisdom that has "... evolved from years of experience and trial-and-error problem solving by groups of people working to meet the challenges they face in their local environments, drawing upon the resources they have at hand." (McClure 1989:1). That the abbreviation IKS is now used in some development circles[3] suggests there is recognition—however belated—of the value of a people's existing or traditional ways of understanding their own world.

Development assistance programs typically introduce a "modern" or "scientific" technology based on a knowledge system deemed superior to a preexisting knowledge system that will hopefully be supplanted. In this way, development assistance resembles colonialism and imperialism. The implicit or explicit assumption is that the traditional or indigenous knowledge system is irrational and disfunctional, that it is based on myths or superstitions, and that in any case it remains an obstacle in the way of realizing the benefits of the new technologies of the donor group (Compton 1989; Warren et al. 1989).

While it may be true that nations in a position to provide development assistance are in general technologically superior to recipient nations, it does not follow that all forms of the recipient country's indigenous knowledge are inferior. That country may not have developed sophisticated weapons systems but it may have developed a way of growing maize under conditions of uncertain rainfall that are well-suited to local conditions. Or it may have discovered natural medicines that relieve the symptoms of high blood pressure or headaches. In any case, a society's creativity and genius is embodied in its IKS. IKS forms the basis for local decision making in health as in other domains. An understanding of health-related indigenous knowledge is also essential for health planners and program implementers, if plans and programs are to be culturally appropriate and therefore effective. And such knowledge is accessible to planners, implementors, and others through approaches that involve the cooperation of traditional healers, if only through research.

## The Policy Background of Collaborative Programs

In 1977 the World Health Assembly of the World Health Organization passed a resolution promoting the development of training and research related to traditional medicine, both the medicines themselves and indigenous practitioners. The following year in Alma Ata, WHO and UNICEF issued additional resolutions supporting the use of indigenous health practitioners in government-sponsored health programs.

In 1984 the WHO *Global Medium-term Programme* on traditional medicine offered further observations and direction regarding traditional healers, suggesting that upgrading the skills of indigenous healers makes more sense than creating new cadres such as village health workers: "Some countries tend to create new community health workers rather than incorporate practitioners of traditional medicine into their health delivery systems, especially at the primary health care level" (WHO 1984:3). This document lists the option to "upgrade the skills and knowledge of traditional practitioners and to incorporate useful practices into the training programmes of other health workers." It notes that some countries try to make use of traditional healers without proper orientation or training for either the healers or the modern health workers with whom they are to work (WHO 1984:4). Section 4c. specifically calls for training of traditional healers and traditional birth attendants in countries where these practitioners "provide services to otherwise underserved segments of the population. . . ." Elements of traditional medicine should also be incorporated in the training curricula for modern health workers.

WHO recommends that training of healers be preceded by the establishment of an official government policy regarding healers. Furthermore, elaborating a legal framework for the practice of traditional medicine "may be indicated" under certain circumstances, although these are not specified (WHO 1984:5). The document goes on to say traditional healers must be involved at all stages in planning involving themselves ". . . to facilitate the ready acceptance by their peers of suggestions for change including the assumption of new responsibilities, for example, in the field of health education." Programs involving healers should be carried out in a way that does not "destroy their individuality" (WHO 1984:5–6). And in countries "where little has been done, initial efforts will concentrate on studies aimed at identifying traditional practices" and there will be support from WHO for medicinal plant studies with a view toward reducing drug budgets and promotion of self-reliance (WHO 1984:5).

On May 13, 1988, the 41st Health Assembly passed a resolution on "Traditional Medicine and Medicinal Plants." The reference and justification makes no mention of primary health care, but rather couches it in terms of conservation, ". . . realizing that, as a consequence of the loss of plant diversity around the world, many of the plants that provide traditional and modern drugs are threatened with extinction." Still, the 42nd World Health Assembly of WHO, Agenda Item 1.(5) (1989), "urges member states . . . to explore ways in which traditional practitioners may be used to extend the coverage of primary health care."

In reviewing the response of African governments, collaborative programs were initially directed at traditional birth attendants (TBAs) as distinct from traditional healers. WHO (1979:7) defines a TBA as a person who assists the mother at childbirth and who initially acquires the necessary skills by working with other TBAs or is self-trained, a definition that has been adopted by other researchers, e.g., Lewis, Janowitz, and Potts (1985). TBAs often perform their services without cash compensation, their activities are usually limited to childbirth and events immediately surrounding it, and their prestige does not typically rival that of doctors or nurses. They do not compete directly with formally trained health-service providers and this may explain why there have been more collaborative programs involving TBAs than those involving traditional healers, throughout Africa (Bannerman et al. 1983).

The first well-documented collaborative program involving traditional healers in Africa predated the resolutions (having started in 1954) and focused on psychiatric care (Lambo 1973, 1967). More recent programs have focused on primary health care, especially on the "appropriate health technologies" of child survival such as oral rehydration therapy. Others have been restricted to screening and referral of patients to government clinics (MacCormack 1986:157). However, official, national-level collaborative programs of any sort are still rare in Africa.

Nearly ten years after Alma Ata, Murray Last identified a remarkably diverse coalition of interests that have with varying degrees of advocacy promoted or supported collaboration between indigenous practitioners and African health professionals:

> Governments (whether parties, bureaucracies, or military men) who need both to cut costs and maintain popular support; WHO (or a section within it) urging these governments on with ideas and international pressure; psychiatrists puzzled by solutions to patients' problems in other cultures and pharmacologists on the look-out for new compounds; idealists seeking to develop a truly national medicine and skeptics weary of the medical profession, its claims and its drug companies; radicals of varying persuasion, backing for example the countryside against the town or the "folk" against the bourgeoisie; or realists who simply remark that "primary health care" is already, de facto, the province of traditional medicine and therefore want local knowledge and skills recognized for what they are. (Last 1986:1).

To this could be added a number of Western anthropologists, public health professionals, and assorted scholars. Fassin and Fassin (1988:355) offer a cynical, caustic view of motives of some who champion collaborative programs, suggesting that those who promote the legitimacy of healers are themselves seeking legitimacy and exposure to the limelight within their own relatively noninfluential academic disciplines. Anthropologists, health educators, and even poorly trained peripheral health workers may seek a kind of celebrity status, especially on the international level of publications. The authors suggest the expatriate advocate of collaboration gets an ego boost upon being adopted as "a true African" by traditional healers. "He appears simultaneously as a scientist of modern medicine and a savior of traditional medicine. . . ." The authors conclude that as the debate about traditional healers intensifies, we should look at all the actors involved and see what each has to gain or lose in the debate (Fassin and Fassin 1988:355).

Mention should also be made of the group of ethnobotanists, ethnopharmacologists, phytochemists and various allies who are interested in promoting or resurrecting the use of indigenous, herbal medicines in national health programs. For example, the Centre International des Civilizations Bantu (CICIBA) puts out the "Bulletin de Liaison" to a wide variety of (largely Francophone) scholars of African traditional medicine who are interested in both studying and conserving medicinal plants. However, such groups do not necessarily favor programs of collaboration with traditional healers. Some prefer to exploit traditional medicinal plants while bypassing healers altogether—as if healers were not worthy of the knowledge they have safegarded for centuries. For example, one team (not necessarily connected with CICIBA) which worked in Ghana offered the opinion that traditional healers seem to be on the decline, moreover their role in health care delivery is inadequately researched, therefore "At present, it is not clear that traditional healers are the most appropriate intermediaries to improve and reinforce the utilization of herbal medicines" (le Grand and Wondergem 1990:28–29. For an opposing ethnobotanical view see Matthe (1989).

In order that we not be diverted now from concern with the practitioners of traditional medicine, I have postponed detailed discussion of African traditional medicine itself and its public health value to a later section in this chapter.

## The Emergence and Reemergence of Collaborative Programs

Supporters of collaborative programs involving traditional healers constitute a diverse and vocal group, yet by the latter 1980s, collaborative health care programs "sanctioned at the national level" appeared limited to Nigeria, Ghana, and Swaziland, at least according to the published literature (Good 1987:302; WHO 1990b). Of these programs, T. A. Lambo's pioneer Aro project was no longer functioning. Another program in Araromi, Nigeria appeared to be in either the planning or the earliest implementation stage. Programs I initiated in Benue and Lagos states, Nigeria were implemented in the late 1980s and seem to be no longer functioning, at least with foreign donor funding. And the well-documented PRHETIH project in Ghana and oral rehydration project in Swaziland was stalled in the late 1980s but was revived later (Ventevogel 1992). Two district-level projects were spawned by PRHETIH in Dormaa and Berekum, Ghana, and appeared to be functioning by the late 1980s (Warren 1987). Yet a 1990 assessment of the situation in Ghana claimed to find declining interest in "cooperation" on the part of the government due to "limited results achieved in training healers and in research in medicinal plants" (le Grand and Wondergem 1990:21).

There are and were other collaborative programs unknown outside (and no doubt within) their respective countries because nothing about them has appeared in the published literature. For example, there was a workshop in Zambia in 1977 intended to inaugurate collaboration between biomedical and traditional practitioners in the areas of children's diseases and maternal health including child spacing (Hall 1977). Any resulting collaboration seems not to have lasted more than a few years (WHO 1990b:12–13). There also have been some small-scale, local-level collaborative programs sponsored by church organizations, such as the Nazareth Healing Complex in the Vane-Avatime area of Ghana (Baku 1988:3).

In sum, by the end of the 1980s there was not much to show in Africa a decade and a half after the Alma Ata resolution. Evidently, there are some powerful counter-forces at work. It seemed there had been little progress—especially in Africa—since an assessment made earlier in the decade by an advocate of collaboration that:

> . . . little progress has been made in actually utilizing indigenous practitioners, especially healers, in these national systems. It appears in fact that in the entire developing world there are only one or two countries in which traditional healers have actually been incorporated, as traditional healers, in the national health care system (Pillsbury 1982:1825).

Pillsbury went on to ask why, in the presence of policy support from WHO as well as many national governments and international donor organizations for incorporating indigenous health practitioners, there had been so little progress in implementing such policy. There certainly had not been the degree of progress that some had envisioned soon after Alma Ata.

However, with the transition into the 1990s there is evidence that the spread of AIDS has prompted African ministries of health and donors to look anew at the collaboration issue, and specifically to consider ways they might collaborate with traditional healers in AIDS control efforts. In fact, there had been recommendations in the 1980s from anthropologists and others calling specifically for intersectoral collaboration in the area of AIDS and STDs (Good 1988; Green 1988). By the end of 1992, collaborative AIDS programs had actually begun in Mozambique (Green, Jurg, and Dgedge 1991), Swaziland (Nhlengethwa and Perez, 1991), Zambia (Chirwa and Sivile 1989a, 1989b), Zimbabwe (Musara 1991; Chavanduga 1991), South Africa (Mathe 1989; Green, Zokwe, and Dupree 1992), Tanzania (Ulrich, Waziri, Nesja, and Scheinman 1991), Uganda (where the Uganda AIDS Commission has started a program), and no doubt elsewhere. With the exception of Mozambique (described in Chapter 5) and

Tanzania, the major objective of these programs seems to be to develop healers as condom promoters, to prevent HIV infection through sterilization of healers' instruments that come into contact with bodily fluids, to modify healers' practices that put them at risk themselves for HIV infection, to encourage referrals of healers clients to hospitals and social welfare centers, and to counsel healers' clients on the prevention of both HIV infection and other STDs (e.g., Nhlengethwa and Perez 1991).

Such programs are still very experimental and it may be some time before a model emerges that can be recommended to African health ministries and donors for replication. There seem to be few precedents to suggest detailed ways to involve African healers in programs whose primary aim it is to control common STDs other than AIDS. However, before turning attention to the AIDS question, the constraints to collaborative programs that have emerged between Alma Ata and the end of the 1980s ought to be considered, because these constraints still impede and shape AIDS-related and other collaborative programs.

## Constraints to Collaborative Programs

One factor constraining collaborative programs is the logical development of health programs over time. It is understandable that government officials and their foreign advisors would begin with the development of humanpower that is immediately available and supervisable, namely government employees. It would be unrealistic to expect that indigenous practitioners—even if they outnumber Western-trained health personnel by hundreds to one and offer far better rural outreach—would be developed as health service providers before Western-trained personnel in either the public or private sectors. However, if this were a significant constraining factor, there should be evidence that governments are now turning increasingly to traditional health practitioners, evidence that is difficult to find (Pillsbury 1982; Janzen 1986; MacCormack 1986).

A more basic factor may be "cultural distance" between indigenous practitioners and medically educated Africans and their expatriate advisers: the two groups embrace distinct and perhaps intrinsically incompatible worldviews or paradigms of illness. In the words of one observer, traditional healing practice is "frequently premised on supernatural and other belief systems that are distinctly alien to and not easily comprehended by modern-sector practitioners" (Pillsbury, 1982:1827). Resistance to, or rejection of, magico-religious belief systems has been particularly strong in Africa because health care has largely been in the hands of missionary groups which offer competing religious belief systems quite apart from the scientific paradigm.

Still, there seem to be areas of at least potential congruence. As Janzen puts it:

> . . . the point of greatest convergence between African medicine and allopathic medicine is between the collective, community-oriented movements of the former, and the community-oriented primary health care programs of the latter. From the former there come health precepts such as balance, rhythm, coolness, purity, and plenitude, and from the latter essential prerequisites of these states such as adequate and clean water, infant care, sewage facilities, adequate nutrition, and good housing, all organized within local communities (Janzen, 1987:50).

Another important factor inadequately documented in the literature seems to be economic and prestige competition between the two sectors. Such competition began with the introduction of Western medicine in Africa. When the first missionaries came to Africa, they ". . . recognized in western medicine an instrument for extending their influence among the people," therefore they actively sought patients at the presumed expense of indigenous healers (Furnivall 1948:357). Orley (1980:127) suggests that Western medicine began to be accepted because it was effective and ". . . it provided some hope to people for whom all other traditional methods had failed," and it may have been cheaper than traditional medicine because it was usually heavily subsidized by the church or state. Yet Africans have continued to consult traditional healers, even when biomedical practitioners are available and cheaper—or free.

It should also be noted that economic development, like culture contact and labor migration, has itself led to a deterioration of health. Furnivall (1948: 355–356) made this point and cited as probable causes centralization of populations, often in overcrowded villages or in slums; a decline in subsistence agriculture in favor of cash crops; a decline in nutrition for the last reason as well as increasing reliance on cash and therefore cheap, less-nutritious foods; and a "deterioration of native medical practice."

I would take issue only with the last point. Many contemporary healers have developed financially lucrative practices, some of which are located in urban areas where Western-style medicine is available. Such healers may take patients away from physicians, as can be seen in Lagos where a number of healers have earned enough cash to build multi-bed hospitals with modern equipment and to own one or more expensive cars. The wealthy, successful traditional healer stands as a rebuke to the biomedically trained physician who practices in the same neighborhood.

Resentment of indigenous practitioners by African medical professionals has probably grown in recent years due to the development among African healers of what can only be called professionalization. In this context, the term refers to the institutionalization of more standardized, empirically based indigenous training of healers; the (usually self-initiated) adoption of aspects of Western medicine or other nonindigenous medicine such as homeopathy; and, especially, the formation of professional associations of traditional healers.

According to a 1985 WHO report, there were healers' associations operating under official auspices, at either national or district levels, in at least twenty-three African countries: Ghana, Nigeria, Zimbabwe, Swaziland, Zambia, Benin, Central African Republic, Congo, Guinea, Ivory Coast, Madagascar, Niger, Rwanda, Cameroon, Togo, Senegal, Mali, Liberia, Zaire, Uganda, Kenya, Tanzania, and Burkina Faso (WHO 1985). There are also healers' associations that may or may not be operating officially in countries such as Malawi, Botswana, South Africa, Mozambique, and doubtless elsewhere. National associations of traditional healers often boast memberships in the thousands and they sometimes have "modern sector" titular heads or advisors such as physicians, university professors or civil servants (cf. Chavunduka 1986:48). The inclusion of such advisors can be seen as a survival strategy: associations supported or led by a professor or doctor are harder for governments to dismiss as backward or inconsequential.

A characteristic of the healers that comprise these associations is that they are especially interested in learning more about modern/Western health care, they want to work in cooperation with the modern sector through involvement with ministries of health, they want to change the popular image of traditional healers as "primitive witchdoctors," and they want to become as respectable among government officials as they typically are in their own communities.

In 1990, the Southern African Traditional Healers Council (SATHC) claimed over 220,000 members in South Africa and neighboring countries. It claimed 135 constituent or affiliated traditional healer organizations, and it estimated each member healer has "60–100 clients or patients" (SATHC nd). If an average client load of 80 is multiplied by 220,000, some 17,600,000 people would appear to be reachable through the SATHC. (Since 1992, the SATHC has been reorganized as the Traditional Healers Organization of South Africa, retaining its earlier president.) Even allowing for considerable exaggeration of numbers, it seems clear that healer associations have at least the potential to reach large numbers of people at the "grassroots," especially in health and spiritual matters.

In this regard, the SATHC puts out a bimonthly newsletter in English and several Bantu languages, in which a number of recent issues have discussed AIDS. Sound, basic preventive advice is given, such as remaining faithful to one's partner, "following traditional values of keeping your virginity until marriage," and "... if your strength (to refrain from sex) falters, a condom or acceptable premarital safe sex (practice) such as '*ukusoma*' [thigh sex] can keep you from getting the disease" (*Siyavuma* 1990:7, paren. mine).

Murray Last (1986:10–11) has discussed the rise in professionalism among African healers as a reaction to the postcolonial development of the biomedical professions. African physicians, whose own rise of professionalism has meant to them decolonization, Africanization of jobs, and meeting the European on equal terms, have tended to regard traditional healers as something of an anachronism, as a throwback to a time when Europeans may have believed that "second-best" was good enough for Africans. In short, traditional healers have been regarded by African physicians as a threat to their own professionalism. Therefore they have often opposed initiatives that would result in official recognition of, or increased power among, indigenous healers.

> As a result, what we are now seeing is a kind of "second generation" of traditional healers who have adapted their methods to meet the competition, and organized themselves to defend their right to practice against criticism from an expanding medical profession. The prize is recognition from the government, and ultimately a share in the salaries, supplies, and buildings provided by government (Last 1986:11).

Other observers present quite a different view of healers' associations. Wondergem and Glover (1990:110) assert that traditional healers in Ghana compete with each other for money and prestige and therefore "have little interest in becoming organized. They use their organization primarily to act against other interest groups and not to exchange views or experiences." The authors cite "serious conflicts within ... various healers associations" as the major reason that "implementation of policy (of cooperation) has come to a standstill." (Wondergem and Glover 1990:21, paren. mine). However, one wonders about the reliability of these observations and conclusions. For example, the authors report that Ghanaian healers do not use very many medicinal plants and that they "hardly ever treat sick children," assertions at variance with the literature on Ghanaian ethnomedicine (Warren 1974).

MacCormack (1986:153) also holds a distinct view of healers' associations. In fact, she regards "requiring that practitioners form an association and present themselves with a well-organized hierarchy of officers where there is no cultural tradition for doing so" as one of several "tactics used to exclude traditional practitioners from primary health care training." She further observes that healers' associations might simply become organizations of "junior professionals," subordinate to the medical professions, that might be legislated against at any time. While there may be truth in this, at least regarding the motives of some physicians and government functionaries, it has been my observation that healers who join and participate in an association tend to feel that strength in numbers offers them genuine political power and prestige in the wider society. They also join these associations voluntarily, not because of government enticement or coercion. Still, I have found evidence of problems with formal healer associations, especially in South Africa (Chapter 8).

There are reasons beside professional elitism and fear of economic and status competition that help explain why the medical establishment may resist opportunities to cooperate with or extend recognition to indigenous practitioners. These include misunderstanding about the nature of traditional health beliefs and practices and a genuine concern that indigenous practitioners practice in ways that may be harmful to patients. When I was involved in advocating for and designing a collaborative program for healers in Swaziland—one focusing on diarrheal disease and ORT—we had to face the issue that a number of healers gave herbal enemas to children with infectious diarrhea, thereby exacerbating dehydration. The counter to critics of our would-be program took the form of a question: If healers are engaged in practices detrimental to public health, don't health and government officials have a public health responsibility to try to change these practices, rather than ignore them? Eventually workshops focusing on child diarrheal disease were conducted with traditional healers, and a year later there was evidence that "trained" healers were abandoning enemas and adopting ORT in cases of child diarrhea (Green 1986; Hoff and Maseko 1986).

For their part, African government officials tend to regard indigenous practitioners as a somewhat embarrassing anachronism, especially when dealing with donor organization officials or other outsiders. Traditional healers project an image of the backward, the primitive, the heathen, even of the illegal. It should be remembered that most colonial regimes supported medical missionary efforts to illegalize or severely curtail the practices of "witchdoctors." Today, Western-educated African elites would prefer to pretend that "witchdoctors" are a thing of the past rather than a genuine force to be reckoned with.

Political ideology may also bias government officials against indigenous practitioners. As Last (1986:13) notes, Marxist governments such as those of Mozambique and Tanzania may oppose healers ". . . on the grounds that healers were, and potentially still are, part of the old 'feudal' system, unproductive, giving support to chiefs, furthering 'superstition' and liable to exploit the poor in their need." Traditional healers, as guardians of the traditional moral and religious order, may also be viewed by Marxists as reactionary purveyors of "the opium of the people." As described in more detail in Chapter 5, healers were suppressed and even actively persecuted in Mozambique as promoters of "obscurantism" during the earlier years of Marxist FRELIMO party rule.

In fact, traditional healers tend to be conservative by nature if not by definition. Healers in South Africa describe their role in terms of "securing the stability of the country"; guarding the culture and traditions of the people, and mystically empowering a variety of existing leaders in the region of whatever political persuasion, from Hastings Banda to Nelson Mandela and Robert Mugabe (Molakeng 1991:21–22; SATHC nd.).

Whatever the reigning political ideology, physician attitudes and biases influence government policy. As Good observes,

> . . . the biomedical establishment is powerfully represented in African health ministries. It often disassociates itself from popular and progressive initiatives, and is always powerful enough to determine what changes and programs are acceptable. Furthermore, if a proposal to promote cooperation between biomedicine and traditional medicine comes from a foreign (non-African) source it can easily be dismissed on the grounds that "they don't know our problems," or "they want us to be satisfied with second-class health care" (Good 1987a).

In fact foreign donors, planners, and administrators usually have little or no understanding of, or access to, African healers or the worldview they represent. Access to healers may well be subject to the approval of ministries of health that represent local medical establishment views. For example, a high-ranking Ministry of Health official in West Africa told me that he did not believe traditional healers still practiced in his country, except perhaps in remote rural areas. His office was next door to one of a number of prominently advertised clinics run by traditional healers. This same urban neighborhood also had an active branch of a national-level traditional healers association.

It should be stressed that some African Ministry of Health officials dedicate much time and energy to arguing the case for collaboration with healers and to establishing pilot programs to demonstrate that collaboration can work. Unfortunately, rapid personnel turnover and the common practice of shuffling individuals within and between ministries has the effect of diminishing the influence of officials whose continuing support and involvement may be crucial to sustaining collaborative programs. The same can be said of foreign researchers and advisers involved in establishing and supporting such programs, since they seldom stay in the same country for more than two to four years.

Finally, Western development planners and other professionals (including some Africans) tend to think of traditional systems—whether relating to health care, land tenure, communal ownership, kinship obligations, or ancestor veneration—as archaic and dysfunctional, as a way of life to be overcome if there is to be progress and development. What such a view fails to recognize is that traditional systems may be well suited to the social, psychological, and other needs of participants in these systems; that traditional systems may be a great source of comfort to Africans undergoing rapid culture change, providing security and continuity in an unpredictable, changing world; and that traditional systems tend to be genuine functioning systems whereas the same cannot as yet be said of the modern-urban alternative.

In fact, many African healers who are themselves successfully adapting to rapid culture change serve as what might be called change brokers, guiding and reassuring Africans who are "torn by the conflicting expectations of their changing worlds," as Ulin (1974:129) put it in connection with Botswana. In Swaziland, healers broker change by preparing magical medicines that help school children pass O-level examinations, that help adults succeed in business, and that help influence judges favorably in civil court cases. In Dar es Salaam, healers provide medicines for business success, job opportunities, favorable legal judgments, passing school examinations, and the success of soccer teams (Swantz 1990). Some of this shift of emphasis in client demand in rapidly changing societies is due to a tendency of people to resort to magic (or sorcery) in order to influence events in unfamiliar domains over which they believe they have no control (Malinowski 1948). These examples also illustrate the dynamic and adaptive, rather than static, nature of "traditional" medicine.

Until recently, some health planners and others believed traditional healers were a dying breed in Africa, that in a generation or two they would all but disappear. Indeed this seems to be a popular view of the traditional healer, outside of Africa. In a *New York Times* article "Shamans and Their Lore May Vanish with Forests" (June 11, 1991, p. C1), Daniel Goleman asserts: ". . . the shamans are a dying breed. Like a bellwether species whose decline signals that an entire ecosystem is in peril, the dwindling number of shamans is a sign of the demise of their cultures."

I have seen no evidence that healers either become relatively fewer in numbers as Africans migrate to cities, or—as recently averred by two researchers in Ghana—that their practices become more biomedical in nature and "spiritual elements of treatment are abandoned" (le Grand and Wondergem 1990:28). My observations and survey findings in Swaziland and Nigeria conform more to the survey findings of Bibeau et al. (1980:8) in Zaire who report:

> . . . the proportion of herbalists practicing divination in the urban areas (74–79 percent) was higher than in rural areas (52 percent). Perhaps urban

> healers have to compete more often with modern medicine, which is essentially naturalist, and need to distinguish themselves from it. Likewise, they are probably oriented toward divination because their clients request it to clarify the unfamiliar problems facing them in the urban environment.

Swantz (1990: 79) likewise reports that the urban Zaramo healer in Dar es Salaam has been adept at proposing solutions to new problems associated with urban tensions, thereby "showing adaptation to social change and thus successfully preserving his role in Zaramo society."

Fassin and Fassin (1988:354) found a healer-to-population ration of 1:60 in their census of a periurban area of Dakar, Senegal, the highest such ratio I have seen for Africa. It is possible that healers may actually be growing in number as Africa urbanizes. In any case it appears that healers are adapting and adjusting to conditions associated with rapid culture change and that they are meeting the changing needs of rural and urban Africans currently and in the foreseeable future. Healers also adapt to changing economic and demographic changes. During a trip to Nigeria in 1985, I found Yoruba healers using both traditional and non-traditional, improvised methods to meet a recent surge in demand for preventing unwanted pregnancies, a demand probably influenced by accelerated urbanization and cash-dependency in an economy crippled by depressed oil prices. The Planned Parenthood Federation of Nigeria (PPFN) was aware of at least twenty distinct methods of fertility regulation used by Yoruba herbalists, some of them relying on Western-manufactured products (Green 1986).

## An Outline of the Continuing Policy Debate

It may be useful at this stage to summarize in outline form the arguments for and against intersectoral collaboration. Some of these points have already been discussed or alluded to above. (TM will stand for traditional medicine and TH for traditional healer.)

### *Points Against Collaboration*

- Some traditional practices are harmful, e.g., giving enemas for child diarrhea; drinking urine or rubbing urine in eyes for conjunctivitis; douching with bleach for contraception; or making incisions with unsterilized razors.
- Traditional treatment may be ineffective and even if harmless, serve to prevent or delay patients from receiving appropriate treatment (Imperato 1974; Katz and Katz 1981; Good 1987:305).
- Some Africans charge that outsiders advocate a "double standard of

health care," with "second-class medicine for the rural masses" while Western medicine is reserved for urban elite.

- Those who favor collaboration with African healers have a pessimistic, defeatist attitude that the masses cannot be educated to change their tradition-bound thinking and behavior. They are said to advocate "giving up" on the problems of modern sector health manpower and service delivery.
- Traditional healing is a hinderance to progress, development, and "enlightenment." Specifically, it impedes acceptance of scientific thinking and perpetuates magical thinking (Asuni 1979; Velimirovic 1981). In the recent words of one African doctor, "Most of it (traditional medicine) is based on superstition, meaningless pseudo-psychological mumbo-jumbo, which is positively harmful." (Motlana, quoted in Freeman and Motsei 1990:7).
- Traditional medicine and its practitioners reinforce and perpetuate "superstitions" and belief in witchcraft, along with "irrational" and unnecessary fears and anxieties—not to mention witchcraft accusations and reprisals against innocent victims of such accusations.
- Patients may undergo traditional and modern treatment simultaneously, posing risk of overdosing or at least of counteracting the effects of Western medicine.
- Traditional medical thinking and behavior holds little or no place for fallibility. Healers must project and protect their image of omnipotence, and therefore make exaggerated and unrealistic claims. Healers seldom admit failure or an inability to understand or treat any problem.
- Dosages of herbal medicines are seldom standardized. Such medicines may be of widely varying potencies due to differences in storage and other factors.
- Traditional psychotherapy does not increase patient's self-awareness or lead to personality maturation (cf. Asuni 1979).
- Extending recognition to traditional healers and initiating any kind of collaboration or training raises expectations and even demands among healers. It's a kind of Pandora's box: today it's oral rehydration salts, tomorrow they'll want antibiotics and a wing of the government hospital. At the very least, demand to participate in government-sponsored training sessions will outstrip government's ability or willingness to provide training. Since the government and local medical associations are not prepared to go very far, does it make sense to go down the collaboration path at all?
- Extending recognition and initiating any sort of collaboration also extends at least tacit legitimacy and a measure of government approval to traditional healing practices and practitioners—which

doctors and nurses by their training generally do not approve of and do not want to legitimize. Collaboration may also increase patient confidence in traditional healers, causing patients to make even more useless expenditure on ineffective medicines and therapies.

- One reason modern medicine seems to be losing in its competition with traditional medicine is that patients often consult traditional healers first. By the time the healer or the patient gives up on traditional therapies, the patient may be beyond help. When such patients are finally treated at modern medical facilities, they may die—which then reflects badly on the efficacy of modern medicine.
- Traditional healers tend to be nonliterate and therefore not to keep written patient records; this makes collaboration difficult. (But note that this is changing; healers often have young assistants or schoolchildren who read, write and even keep records for them.) THs who join professional associations may be better educated, but skeptics have argued that THs who join such associations are more likely to lack "traditional legitimacy" in their communities (Fassin and Fassin 1988). Others assert that THs'competitiveness prevents their associations from functioning effectively (Wondergem and Glover 1990).
- There are some priority areas of promotive health care that African healers, by their training, beliefs and orientation, would never promote, for example child spacing or contraception.

Some who have joined the debate appear to have reserved their misgivings for Africa and Africans. For example, Velimirovic and Velimirovic (1978:182–183) make an implicit distinction between African and Asian healing systems including healers. Unlike their Asian counterparts, African healers do not belong to a "formalized medical system" or a healing system based on knowledge that is shared through writing. Because of this, "The practitioners of non-formalized traditional medicine are not linked by any dogma or theory, and cooperation between them is rare—in most cases they actually compete among themselves. . . . Their knowledge is transmitted from person to person, not taught in special institutions." The authors go on to suggest that such healers cannot be trained.

Of course, it does not follow that because medical knowledge is not recorded in books or "taught in special institutions," indigenous practitioners do not share a common system of beliefs and practices. The evidence presented in this book refutes such a conclusion—in fact there seems to be considerable cultural continuity and homogeneity in African ethnomedical systems from geographically diverse societies, attesting to the strength, durability and viability of these systems.

***Points in Favor of Collaboration***

- Whatever biomedical health professionals think of TM, it is largely to THs that people turn in time of illness. THs are generally respected health care providers and opinion leaders in their communities.
- National health services in developing countries lack adequate numbers of personnel, and these are unevenly distributed, with nearly all doctors in the major cities. The resulting rural outreach is poor. THs may outnumber doctors 100 to 1 or more. THs are the de facto providers of primary health care in Africa.
- THs provide client-centered, personalized health care that is culturally appropriate, holistic, and tailored to meet the needs and expectations of the patient. THs share the cognitive understandings and cultural values of those they treat.
- If traditional healers engage in harmful practices, there is a public health responsibility to try to change those practices and try to substitute safer practices. This can only be accomplished if there is dialogue, and some degree of cooperation, with traditional healers. There is also evidence that healers will modify or abandon practices if they are shown that such practices are harmful.
- At the local or village level, traditional healers do not compete directly with physicians, but with village health workers or assistant nurses, whose training and competence may well amount to less than the traditional healer. Almost certainly, the TH enjoys greater prestige and credibility in health and spiritual matters.
- Traditional healers cannot be wished away or legislated out of existence. This has been tried by both colonial and postindependence governments, and all attempts have failed. THs occupy a critically important role in African societies. They perform a function broader and more complex than that of their medical counterparts in the modern sector. Traditional healers are priests, religious ritual specialists, family and community therapists, moral and social philosophers, teachers, visionaries, empirical scientists, and perhaps political leaders in addition to being healers in the more restricted, Western sense. Their existence and durability stand as evidence that they meet important social needs, and these needs are in no way diminished as the clients they serve urbanize and undergo rapid sociocultural change. If anything, the needs increase. Rapid sociocultural change has been shown to lead to a variety of psychosocial problems, and healers who have experienced these problems themselves may be especially adept at helping people who are "torn by the conflicting expectations of their changing worlds."
- Surveys and limited program experience in Africa have shown that traditional healers are highly motivated to learn about Western

medicine, to attend training workshops, and to cooperate with modern health sector personnel. As concluded at a conference on traditional medicine, "Traditional medical systems are open, not closed, to techniques and concepts characteristic of cosmopolitan medicine" (Rubel and Sargent 1979). There is a parallel between African healing and the broader, indigenous religious (or "magico-religious") belief systems from which it developed. Neither are rigid, orthodox, exclusive or purist; instead both are open and easily incorporate and integrate new beliefs, ideas and practices.

- Since healers have been organizing themselves in recent years, governments and donor organizations can now communicate with healer organizations through professional associations of traditional healers. Healers who belong to—and who occupy leadership roles in—professional organizations tend to be especially eager to collaborate with the modern sector and to learn about Western medicine. They tend to be especially open about new ideas and practices.
- Any efforts toward cooperation seem to improve relations between the two health sectors, which results in earlier and more frequent referrals from traditional healers to clinics. The healer can perform a "triage" function by treating the less seriously ill and only sending the more serious cases on to the clinic or hospital (cf. J. Westermeyer, 1976).
- Any efforts that promote cooperation seem to improve communication between the two health sectors, allowing access to the beliefs and practices found among healers and presumably their clients. This, in turn, allows for the development of creative, culturally appropriate, and effective health education strategies. It also facilitates interventions aimed at discouraging practices proved to be harmful.
- Freedom of religion and other fundamental rights are often trampled when there are attempts to directly or indirectly legislate against traditional healers. The rise of faith healers associated with Christianity or Islam only makes the problem more complex.
- An efficient, cost-effective training-of-trainers approach is possible by focusing public health training efforts on leaders of healer associations and on senior healers under whom novice healers apprentice. Members—and especially leaders—of traditional healer associations may be especially open to new ideas. In some countries (e.g., Swaziland and Nigeria), the "traditional" training of healers has become more formalized, empirically oriented, institutionalized, and influenced by rise of biomedical professionalism in Africa. A great and unprecedented opportunity now exists for adding public health ideas and methods into the "traditional curriculum" of healer training.

Note that there may well be two or more sides to each of these arguments. For example, the image of traditional healer omnipotence can be beneficial since a patient's expectations can influence his recovery. Or if patients are consulting both a healer and a doctor simultaneously and are taking two types of medicines at once, does it not make more sense for the healer and doctor to be aware of this and to be talking to each other and collaborating in treating the patient, rather than pretending that the other doesn't exist?

Space does not permit point-by-point discussion of each argument; in fact, I find a few of the arguments against collaboration difficult to refute. However, I come down on the side of *trying* collaboration because I find these arguments more compelling and more realistic.

In addition to their change-brokering skills, indigenous practitioners have several other important advantages over Western-trained health care personnel. These advantages have been pointed out by anthropologists and others so often that they will only be outlined here. African healers are accessible, affordable, and culturally appropriate and acceptable, thereby fulfilling the major criteria for effective service delivery (Ademuwagun 1979; Asuni 1979:33; Pillsbury 1979; Lorenzelli 1985). They have credibility as well as respect and prestige in local African communities, otherwise people would not seek their advice and pay for their services. African healers make little distinction between body, mind, and spirit in therapy; the whole person is treated. The holistic perspective of African healers has led to considerable insight and success in treating a wide variety of illnesses that have a psychosomatic component. While there is a movement in modern medicine toward recognizing the psychosomatic component in *all* illness, most physicians are ill equipped to deal with a patient's psychosocial problems (Green 1980:493).

It is clearly advantageous to develop collaborative health care programs with health practitioners who have their own sources of income rather than with "locally chosen volunteers" that often lack any sort of health care interest or background, regular cash income, or prestige or at least credibility as health advisors in their own communities. In any case, the morale problems associated with cash income and community acceptance that often plague the usual type of community health worker (cf. Jancloes 1984) seem unlikely to cripple programs involving traditional healers.

Perhaps the most powerful argument is that public health goals probably cannot be realized in Africa without some type of collaboration involving indigenous healers. The numbers simply are not there: the number and geographic distribution of Western-trained medical personnel, the number of clinics and hospitals in rural areas, and the amount of money available to ministries of health are all inadequate to meet existing needs. If anything, numbers work in the other direction: sub-Saharan African populations are growing at a rate of between 2.5 percent and 4.0 percent annually, requiring corresponding increases in medical personnel and facilities just to maintain current inadequate levels of service. Furthermore, the recent scourge of AIDS promises to tax health budgets and personnel to an unprecedented degree. Economic and manpower arguments in favor of collaboration can only become stronger in the foreseeable future.

In view of all these factors, it would seem that if the cooperation of indigenous practitioners can be enlisted in public health programs, there can be no more potent impetus for improvement in the public health. Although actual collaborative programs have been few and far between, surveys of African healer attitudes and limited programmatic experience have consistently shown willingness on the part of the healers to learn more about Western medicine and to cooperate and collaborate with Western-trained practitioners (Messing 1976; Osborne et al. 1977; Rubel and Sargent 1979; Green and Makhubu 1984; Chiquzie et al. 1987; Good 1987a). Prestige and recognition appear to be fundamental incentives underlying healers' willingness to cooperate. Healers may well enjoy prestige in their local communities, but collaboration with physicians or government officials bestows a respectability and recognition in the modern/urban sector that indigenous practitioners have come to value. This prestige, along with any skills acquired in Western medicine as a result of contact with Western-trained practitioners, enables a healer to attract more clients and expand his or her practice. It is understandable why the relatively few healers who have participated in government-sponsored training courses prominently display any certificates or diplomas that testify to their training, something I have seen in Swaziland and Nigeria. Fassin and Fassin (1988) cite cases from their fieldwork of urban traditional healers whose business multiplied after displaying a notice that they have official government recognition, or that they belong to a traditional healers' association. The authors claim highly respected healers do not need this. This may be, but they might still *want* such recognition.

Another incentive to healers is the possibility of earning money through sale of commodities such as condoms or oral rehydration salts which are promoted by health ministries or donor groups. However, collaborative programs for healers in Africa seem to have thus far limited commodity sales to very inexpensive items with little potential for profit margin—or as skeptics have commented, for profiteering.

A survey of Swazi healers showed that if they were to choose which aspects of Western medicine they could learn about, they would choose X-ray technology, blood transfusions, and antibiotics injections (Green and Makhubu 1984:1073). Instead of these mysteries of modern medical science, healers who participated in government-sponsored workshops learned about mixing sugar-salt solution to rehydrate children with diarrhea. A plan to develop healers as promoters and distributors of packaged oral rehydration salts was defeated by physicians who felt traditional healers could not be trusted with modern "medicine."

This anecdote is not meant to demean the importance of inexpensive child survival technologies but rather to illustrate the eagerness of traditional healers to have contact with government health programs at any level and the extreme reluctance on the part of many African physicians and government officials to share power. MacCormack (1986:153) has made a similar observation, noting that medical techniques and the use of drugs "... are the very skills physicians are least likely to relinquish if they perceive themselves as being in competition for patients and general social status."

## Should Healers Be Salaried by African Governments?

If traditional healers are already providing most of Africa's health care, should some of the public money spent on health somehow go to healers—if not money raised by taxes, at least a proportion of the donor assistance to the health sector that is contributed annually? While this sounds reasonable, we run into a number of problems when we consider how this actually might be accomplished. For example, it has been argued that healers should be put on some sort of salary by ministries of health. If assistant nurses and even minimally trained village health workers receive compensation, why shouldn't traditional healers? There are a number of reasons arguing for caution here.

First, if healers became salaried, they would have to fit in somewhere in the existing medical hierarchy. They would be assigned a civil service classification and rank. In view of biomedical attitudes toward practitioners regarded as not medically trained or medically competent, it is highly doubtful that healers would be ranked or salaried at anywhere near the level of doctors or even full nurses. Instead they probably would be ranked low on the scale, closer to village health workers. This raises the possibility that traditional healers would not be willing to work for a health ministry under such circumstances. Healers already enjoy considerable status and they tend to be at least relatively well off in their own communities. For a healer to become something like a village health worker, he or she would risk a loss of status if not wealth. This seems to be one reason that village health worker programs have not attracted more traditional healers to their ranks. It seems safe to say that there at least would be great potential for status and role confusion and conflict if traditional healers were to be incorporated in health or other ministries.

Orley (1980:128) makes a blunt point about the question of trying to recruit healers into biomedical systems:

> Before considering this further, we should perhaps ask ourselves whether it is not being presumptuous to assume that traditional healers would want to be recruited into Western medical practice. They probably get more money in their practice of traditional medicine, and they might find it a much more satisfying way to practice the healing art.

Indeed, he makes the point that one of the reasons for the acceptance of Western biomedicine during the colonial period was its lesser expense "... compared with that provided by traditional healers, which often required sacrifices of several animals and fees for the healer, who was not subsidized by the Church or State" (Orley 1980:127). There is even evidence today that clinic use can drop off measurably when low clinic fees are raised slightly (Yoder 1989), suggesting that "demand" for biomedicine is still weak, at least in the form in which it is currently offered.

There is some disagreement about the fees or in-kind compensation healers receive in contemporary Africa. Some entertain the romantic notion that in-kind fees amount to little more than token or symbolic payment. This has not been my own experience in the countries where I have worked. Payment in cows, goats, or even chickens represents a considerable sacrifice for most Africans, whether they are peasant farmers or employed townsmen. In any case, the trend is toward cash rather than in-kind payment and while more reliable data on healer fees is much needed to settle the question, my experience has been that healers often charge higher patient fees than government- or church-run hospitals or clinics. This is not surprising since most health care in Africa has been heavily subsidized by government and church up to now, and patient fees have been kept artificially and unusually low.

A more serious issue perhaps is what the effects on traditional medicine might be if its practitioners were salaried by governments. With incorporation into the civil service would come control and probably manipulation. This might appeal to some biomedical planners and administrators whose thought might be: if there are countless thousands of "untrained" healers "practicing medicine without a license," why not bring them into the ministry, train them, and control their practice? Would that not serve the public health, at least by cutting back harmful practices?

The question we must ask is what else would be changed, transformed, or distorted? Biomedicine as practiced in Africa and the United

States is similar in that power is highly concentrated in the hands of doctors and administrators. U.S. physicians have spent a good deal of time and energy guarding their power prerogatives against incursions from nurses and other auxiliary health care personnel (Kotelchuck 1976). This tendency—found in Africa as well—coupled often with arrogant, disapproving physician attitudes toward traditional healers, not to mention ignorance of traditional medicine as it actually is practiced, strongly suggests that biomedically trained ministry personnel in charge would attempt to transform healers into something they are not—and would probably not want to be.

Carl Taylor, summarizing a symposium on traditional healing, noted:

> We have learned how to identify community resources from community development experts. As we found the natural leaders, the health system tended to co-opt them so that they were no longer really community representatives. This could also happen to indigenous practitioners where a process of synthesis is attempted. While this strengthens the health system at low cost—especially if sufficient seduction can be exercised to get them to work as volunteers—it may well weaken the communities' capacity to solve their own health problems (Taylor 1979:84).

It may be noted that the African National Congress is studying ways the ANC might cooperate with traditional healers under a new, majority-rule regime in South Africa. During a 1992 conference, an ANC spokesman said he ". . . did not think that traditional healers should become part of formal health services . . . (because) there was resistance to incorporation from both the formal and traditional health workers" (Wilson 1992:38).

Incorporation and government salaries could "professionalize" healers in the negative sense: governments would assume the responsibility of issuing formal credentials to healers; there might be restrictive licensing and increased costs to consumers (in the private sector); service would become increasingly impersonal; record keeping might become an end in itself; and the authority of physicians could be extended and their monopoly in health care further consolidated with a vast new "cadre" of underlings to supervise. At least one African medical professional has already suggested that traditional medicine not be legally available in Africa without a prescription from a physician—while at the same time admitting that medical professionals know nothing of the contents of traditional medicines (Adikwu 1992:122).

My feeling is that meddling with traditional medicine is fraught with unforseen and possible negative outcomes. One does not have to be an anthropologist to recognize that healers play a complex role and carry out complex, interrelated functions in their communities. We know from the written and archaeological human record that healing is one of the first roles—if not the very first—to become specialized in human societies. Healers have only become scientifically trained allopaths in the very recent historic period, and they are still outnumbered by indigenous, traditional healers in most of the world. A majority of Africans vote with their feet and their pocketbooks by choosing the services of the latter, even when the former are available and perhaps cheaper. Clearly there is a need for the type of service indigenous healers provide.

I believe that the only real justification for interfering with traditional health systems at all is in the cause of improving public health. Considering that it is not always clear how best to accomplish this, as well as factors relating to African cultures and traditional healing itself, we should proceed with great caution. Given two or more alternatives involving interventions with traditional medicine, we should choose the option that is least intrusive and potentially disruptive to that system.

In any case, what is the political or economic plausibility of the incorporation option? Given present conditions, it seems extremely unlikely that health ministries would be able or willing to pay for thousands of new employees. The first argument doubtless would be that with the small allocations of public funds devoted to health services, ministries cannot presently pay for adequate numbers of existing, *trained* health-care personnel. How can they then multiply personnel ranks by several hundred percent to accommodate "untrained" health staff? And if some traditional healers were invited to join government ranks, wouldn't all healers demand the option to join?

This last consideration would probably end the argument for a great many health planners and administrators in Africa; there would be no need to raise the other points we have been discussing. Any health-related plan seems doomed to defeat if local medical establishments oppose it. Such bodies are politically influential and persuasive in their arguments about "proper medical care" for Africans.

Some might argue that when facing a deadly epidemic such as AIDS, the above considerations lose some of their relevance or merit. I think they do not. Africa has faced and still faces other diseases of epidemic proportion, several of which account for more morbidity and mortality than AIDS. This does not alter the problems associated with attempting to transform healers into government-salaried paraprofessionals.

There are other ways indigenous healers might share or benefit from some of the financial resources for AIDS being channeled into Africa. For example, resources could be directed to national associations of traditional healers. True, there may be more than one association claiming to represent most or even all of a nation's healers. The solution would then be to find a way to fairly and equitably allocate resources among truly representative associations.

If the resources are money, we still face the problem of possible manipulation, co-optation or subordination of healer associations by governments, a point made by MacCormack (1986:153). Perhaps there would be less likelihood for this if the resources were nonmonetary, for example medical supplies. Assuming government willingness to "transfer" certain "technology" to traditional healers, health care related products could then be given—or sold at discounted wholesale prices—to organizations of healers in some type of social marketing or community-based distribution (CBD) program in which healers could earn a profit when they used such products in the care of their clients.

## The Question of Medicinal Plants

Traditional African medicine consists of *materia medica* as well as practitioners. There is little emphasis in this book on the former because I believe research or policy development relating to medicinal plants and other natural materials may hold comparatively little potential for public health impact, at least in the short term. Research related to the medicinal value of plants may be justified in several ways: (1) achieving community or national self-reliance in health by promoting locally available and already accepted herbal medicines; (2) developing an indigenous pharmaceuticals industry, based on local plants, that reduces national dependence on expensive, imported drugs; (3) promoting natural health care and reducing the iatrogenic effects of modern medicine; (4) finding out what traditional healers are using and if medicines are found to be dangerous and highly toxic, trying to persuade healers to substitute safer plants or at least reduce dosages; or (5) finding an effective-seeming indigenous medicine for the symptoms of a high-priority illness such as child diarrhea, then finding ways to promote more widespread use of the medicine.

All of these ideas sound promising at first glance and all have been tried in Africa, yet there has been little progress toward the realization of these goals; there are also serious problems of economic justification in every case. For example, research aimed at the pharmaceutical industry as the target—with the idea of earning money or at least being able to promote an indigenous herbal medicine—seems seldom if ever to fulfill its promise. My colleagues in the Department of Traditional Medicine, in the Mozambique Ministry of Health had direct experience in this. For some time they had investigated popular medicines used to treat malarial symptoms. Through discussions with traditional healers in a community near Maputo, as well as monitoring progress of their malarial clients, they narrowed their interest to two plants that seemed to reduce malarial symptoms. One in particular, known as *munangati* in the Tsonga language (*ngati* means blood in Nguni languages), was laboratory tested with blood culture, and it indeed reduced parasitic load in the blood (Jurg, Tomas, and Pividal 1991).

The problem was what to do with findings of this sort. My colleagues soon came up against a harsh reality: the large pharmaceutical companies have hundreds of such "promising" plants lined up to be tested, including many with demonstrable antiparasitic action against *P. falciparum*. However, testing is slow, expensive, and laborious. The cost of testing in fact averages about $231 million per plant and takes about twelve years to develop a new drug (WRI 1993:16). Companies need to get a return on their investment, yet the people who suffer from tropical diseases tend to be poor. In the case of *munangati*, the international pharmaceutical industry was not interested in analyzing the Mozambican plant, even though malaria is the most endemic, prevalent disease of the tropics. Minor irritations of the wealthy nations such as postnasal drip may actually have more potential for profit than tropical diseases such as oncho- or schisto- or trypanosomiasis.

Farnsworth (quoted in Bailey 1986) observed that in the early 1980s, there were only two U.S. pharmaceutical companies supporting research to investigate new drugs from plant sources.[4] This research cost about $200,000 and represents a negligible part of a prescription drug industry, which was over $8 billion annually. In addition to the costs of developing drugs from plant sources, Bailey (1986) suggests additional reasons for corporate reluctance to support applied phytochemistry. One is a bias against traditional and natural substances in favor of synthetic chemicals. Another is a desire to maintain control over the production and sale of medically useful compounds. It appears to be easier to control synthetic compounds; anyone might pick up and use organic compounds; and herbs cannot be patented. However, this fear may be unjustified since natural compounds rarely occur in optimal form for medicinal use; they usually must be modified synthetically or related compounds must be synthetically manufactured. Even if the industry had been interested in exploring a potential antimalarial, any resulting manufactured medicine would be largely out of physical and financial reach of the mass of Mozambicans. If our target is the rural "masses," we always run up against the problem of expensive testing before a government is willing to risk formally promoting an herbal medicine. If we talk about reinforcing community self-reliance on things people are already relying on, why then would we need to do it? If we talk about warning traditional healers about toxicity of plants they are using, they probably know more about such properties than ministry personnel, who in any case, have little credibility in this area in the eyes of either healers or their clients using the traditional medicines. Moreover, experience has shown that it is difficult under the best circumstances to change traditional health practices.

Another problem is that the more-or-less established properties of medicinal plants relate primarily to the amelioration of common symptoms such as pain, cramps, fever, or chills; or to general conditions such as weakness, fatigue, or shortness of breath (high blood pressure).

For example, Oku Ampofo, in his practical guide for health workers, *First Aid in Plant Medicine* (1983: viii), lists remedies for the following conditions: cough, asthma, burns, skin rashes, snake bite, jaundice, cuts, wounds, diarrhea, and convulsions. (Even with these, Ampofo—a medical doctor—suggests that the health worker might want to use an allopathic medicine along with the traditional plant remedy!). Virtually none of these conditions except diarrhea are high-priority concerns among African health ministries.

Even if some of these plants were found to be effective in symptom reduction we again run up against the following problems (1) the plants could not be officially promoted without a great deal of "high-tech," expensive testing; (2) if a large pharmaceutical firm were to develop a drug from one of the promising plants, the Africans who were using the drug in its natural form could not afford it, nor would they receive royalties from sale of the new drug; and (3)—the ultimate nagging question—why has there apparently not been a single plant drug promoted officially elsewhere in Africa, for example in a country like Ghana where there has been years of ethnopharmocological research and where there is more money and better infrastructure than in Mozambique? On this point, even le Grand and Wondergem (1990:36) make this comment about the much-cited Traditional Medicine Institute in Ghana: ". . . after more than 10 years of research, no plants are presently recommended for use" (there has actually been more than fifteen years of research). More than ten years of research at the Department of Traditional Medicine, Muhimbili Medical Center in Dar es Salaam has likewise not resulted in official promotion of any herbal medicines in Tanzania (Mshiu 1993).

What if we used different, more relaxed standards for promotion of herbal medicines, arguably appropriate for the poor countries of Africa? Suppose we found a plant the medicinal use of which is well established in southern Mozambique, we establish that it seems to work quite well, we know from the literature that the same plant seems to work quite well elsewhere, and it does not appear toxic. Could this indigenous medicine be promoted? Again there are various problems: (1) the health ministry, as the promoter, could be accused of lowering public health standards for the poor and non-white, compared to the standards maintained in the rest of the world, and (2) the ministry would be reluctant to promote a medicine about which not enough has been established regarding toxicity, dosage, side effects, storage, etc. And a country like Mozambique cannot afford the requisite tests.

In sum, any possibility that involves the *medicinal* properties of plants seems to run up against a variety of insurmountable problems. On the other hand, possibilities involving the *nutritional* value of plants circumvent many of these problems, especially when considering known edible plants. If a plant is edible and its nutritional value is known—which is usually true even for tropical plants—then there is no need to investigate toxicity, optimal dosages, side effects, and so on.

One idea that seems viable is to look at high-priority, endemic diseases or conditions for which there are nutritional treatments. If it can be determined that there is an indigenous plant high in iron, for example, its use could be promoted in the treatment of child anemia, which is a major complicating factor in many infant and child deaths from infectious diseases such as malaria, according to a recent World Bank health sector report for Mozambique. True, it is very difficult to get tradition-bound people to adopt new foods, especially indigenous plants not locally regarded as edible. However, the approach could be to promote the plant through traditional healers as a *medicine* that can ameliorate the symptoms of anemia. Perhaps the healer could be encouraged to make a tea from the iron-rich plant. Traditional healers are open to adopting new medicines, they have a preference for indigenous plant medicines, and they have the influence and credibility to persuade their patients to adopt a new medicine. The plant with nutritional rather than medicinal value has several advantages starting with the fact that expensive, lengthy research to determine the active chemical compounds of plants as well as their toxicity would be unnecessary.

Another possible justification for ethnobotanical research might be in researching the toxicity of plant medicines in current use, then warning traditional healers and laymen about poisonous plants and toxic dosages of useful plants. This, in fact, is a responsibility of the Branch of Botany of the National Herbarium in Zimbabwe (under the Ministry of Agriculture). Although healers may already know a lot about plant toxicity, there nevertheless seem to be more poisonings and overdosings with traditional medicine than with allopathic medicine, even if most cases go unreported, according to a government botanist (Mavi 1991). It appears that urban healers nowadays buy herbs increasingly from retailers, and they often find themselves in areas with different vegetation from the area where they learned to practice, the result of both being that they may not be sure what they are mixing and prescribing. They may confuse unfamiliar with familiar plants. Therefore, there may be a need to provide healers and the public with certain information on medicinal plants.

Other than approaches such as these, I have been unable to find any real public health justification for allocating scarce funds of African governments to research the medicinal properties of indigenous plants. Moreover I am not certain WHO's role as a sponsor is justified. As a confidential memorandum circulated by a private, voluntary organization recently noted, even the WHO-supported ethnopharmacological database at the University of Illinois, Chicago (NAPRALERT, or Natural Products Alert), at least partially "serves the interest of the pharmaceutical companies who use WHO support to scour the world for plants which can be useful for pharmaceutical production." Ethnopharmacological and ethnobotanical research, of course, deserve support, but it probably should come from private industry and foundations rather than public funds. It can also come from private investors. Shaman Pharmaceuticals, a U.S. company established to develop new drugs based on traditional medicines in use, raised $42 million when it went public in early 1993 (WRI 1993:120).

Yet there are two ethnopharmacological research questions that should be answered because they could greatly help determine the nature of AIDS/STD collaborative programs involving healers: (1) Can at least some indigenous medicines be effective against any of the common STDs? (2) Can at least some indigenous medicines be effective against any of the opportunistic infections that characterize AIDS in Africa? A quick though preliminary answer to the first question could be provided by clinically testing clients under the care of a traditional healer before administration of any treatment. If the clients are clinically found to have an STD prior to treatment, and they are shown to be free of their STD after treatment, and it can be shown that they received no biomedical treatment from any source while under a traditional healer's care, the next research phase should be pharmacological analysis of indigenous medicines used in STD treatment. Such a study might violate codes of medical ethics if the STD sufferer were thought of as being denied treatment of known efficacy. However, if the patient prefers to use traditional medicine instead of an antibiotic anyway, the study ought to be ethical—especially if the patient were eventually treated with an antibiotic in case the indigenous treatment failed.

Regarding the second question, a WHO Expert Committee Meeting recently in Botswana concluded that it is appropriate for traditional healers to treat some of the opportunistic infections of AIDS, suggesting that the committee sees potential in their medicines (Staugaard 1991). Indeed, there are some tantalizing, preliminary findings from a small study in Pangani District, Tanga region, Tanzania, an area reputed to have powerful traditional practitioners and medicines (Mbura, Mgaya, and Heggenhougen 1985). Here, an experimental group was treated with a combintion of herbs administered by a traditional healer and "modern drugs." The latter consisted of antibiotics, antifungals and other commonly available medicines, but not AZT or other expensive antivirals. A control group was treated only with modern drugs. Of the twenty-one in the experimental group, four died within nine months and seventeen "improved." Among the twenty-seven in the control group, fourteen died within nine months. "Improvement" in the experimental group meant living longer, gaining weight, and scoring better in three clinical tests: hemoglobin, erythrolyte sedimentation rate, and white blood cell counts (although the last tests were not done with all patients.) The authors conclude, "Preliminary results indicate that taking the herbal regimen has a positive effect on people suffering from HIV disease" (Ulrich, Waziri, Nesje, and Scheinman 1991:8. Cf. also Mshana and Scheinman 1991; Scheinman, Nesje, Ulrich, and Malangalia 1992; Scheinman et al. 1992). The herbal medicines are currently being tested in Norway with AIDS patients, and in vitro at the National Cancer Institute in the United States, both with promising results (Scheinman 1993.) It should be noted that these herbs (*Steganotaenia araliacea, Harrisonia abyssinica Oliv., Aspilia mossambicensis, Steganotaenia araliacea,* and *Acalypha fruticosa*) came to the attention of scientists as a result of a collaborative workshop during which an elderly healer—who possessed little or no formal knowledge about AIDS—nevertheless recognized some of the opportunistic infections of the disease and offered to treat some AIDS patients provided by the European doctor who had initiated the workshop.

If the answer to either or both of our ethnopharmacological research questions is yes, then clearly the nature of collaborative programs in AIDS/STDs is different than if they were no. Instead of simply promoting Western-style contraceptives and looking for ways to reach healers' clients with antibiotics, we would also want to reinforce the use of certain indigenous medicines—even in the absence of millions of dollars of pharmacological research for each medicinal plant—in the context in which they are currently being used.

## Notes

1. A part of this chapter represents an update and expansion of material that appeared in Green, E. C., "Can Collaborative Programs Between Biomedical and Indigenous Health Practitioners Succeed?" *Social Science and Medicine* 1988, Vol. 27, No. 11, pp. 1125–1130.

2. Some anthropologists use "indigenous practitioners" or "traditional medical practitioners." "Traditional healers" seems to be preferred by Africans including healers themselves.

3. For example an international journal called Indigenous Knowledge and Development Monitor is published in the Netherlands, in English.

4. The number of U.S. and multinational companies had grown to at least 20 by 1993 (WRI 1993:8–13).

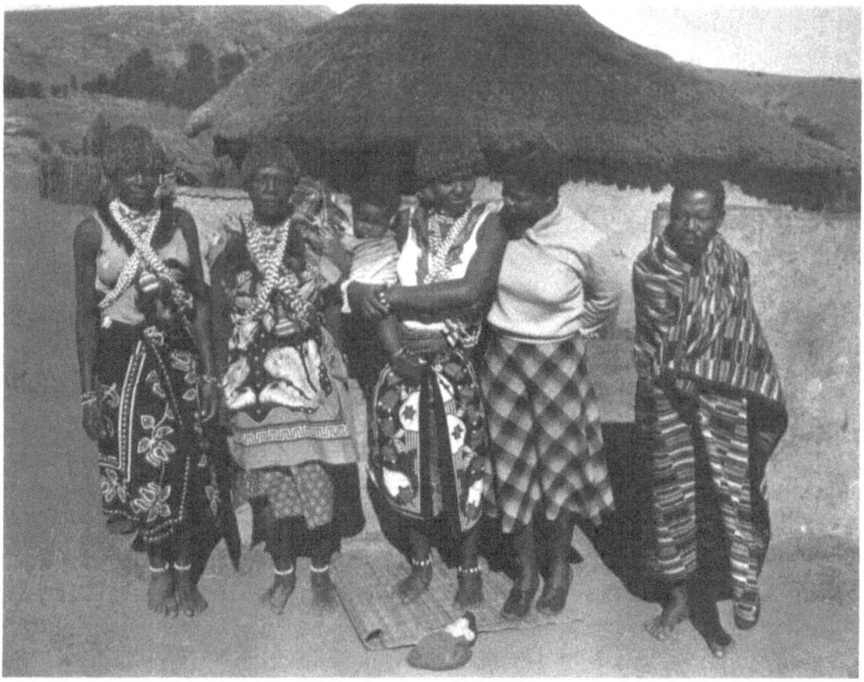

# 3

# Preliminary Research in Swaziland[1]

## Background

Let us turn to some of my first empirical findings related both to collaborative programs with indigenous healers and to sexually transmitted diseases. The findings emerged during fieldwork begun in Swaziland in 1981. I went to Swaziland that year to serve as an anthropologist on the AID-funded Rural Water-Borne Disease Control Project. I was a member of a multidisciplinary project team of U.S. technical advisers. The project called for a knowledge, attitudes, and practices (KAP) survey relating to water and sanitation in Swaziland. The survey was to be my primary responsibility, and the results were to be used to develop and implement a national health education program aimed at reducing the incidence of diseases related to water and sanitation.

The Kingdom of Swaziland had a population of approximately 600,000 people at the time of my arrival (it exceeded 800,000 in 1993). Some 80 percent of the population lived in rural areas, a percentage that was declining due to increasingly rapid urbanization, and 98 percent percent are ethnic Swazis. Economically, the country is relatively well off; GNP per capita is about $850, and the World Bank classifies Swaziland as a middle-income country. Income distribution, however, is highly skewed, with the rural majority having significantly lower incomes than urban, employed Swazis and whites. At the household level, most families have cash income from wage employment or income-generating activities in addition to the in-kind income they receive from agriculture. The high rate of population growth (3.4 percent), however, threatens to overwhelm Swaziland's reasonably healthy economy, and the health status of the population as measured by infant mortality and life expectancy is lower than that of countries with similar income levels.

Traditional Swazi culture and governance remain strong influences in the society. The king, assisted by the queen mother, is head of both traditional and modern government structures. In rural areas, the traditional government, led by chiefs, has considerable impact on peoples' daily lives. The influence of modern parliamentary-style government is primarily through the provision of education, health, and agricultural extension services and infrastructure.

In 1981 the Swaziland government had a rather ambiguous policy toward traditional healers. There had been an attempt in 1945–1946, during the colonial administration, to pass legislation that would provide for the registration and taxation of traditional healers and would attempt to control their activities. Prior to that time and dating back to 1894, all "witchdoctoring" was considered illegal in Swaziland (Green and Makhubu 1984; Booth 1992). Therefore, the 1945–1946 proposed legislation would have amounted to official recognition of healers on the part of the government. However, due to vigorous opposition by the incumbent director of medical services, the highest-ranking government physician, the legislation never went into effect.

King Sobhuza II (1899–1982) had always maintained that there was much that was valuable in traditional healing. He had recommended a scientific study of traditional healing should be undertaken before anyone attempted to restrict or alter practices and he believed that Swazis would ultimately benefit from a health service that combined the best aspects of both traditional and modern medicine. In 1954, the king issued an "order-in-council" by which much of the previously drafted legislation became law. Since that year, healers have been registered and taxed. However, the king's dream of a syncretistic health care system was no closer to realization in the early 1980s then it had been thirty years earlier.

In August, 1982 the Ministry of Health (MOH) requested through AID that I produce a report on indigenous healers in collaboration with Lydia Makhubu, a Swazi biochemist researching traditional medicines. The objectives of the report were to: (1) designate specific areas of possible cooperation between the "modern" and traditional health sectors; (2) evaluate the feasibility of a national association of traditional healers and make recommendations regarding the role of government in promoting, monitoring, and liaising with such an association; (3) assess the potential for paraprofessional training of healers; (4) summarize legislation, customary law and government policy regarding healers; and (5) assess the size and characteristics of manpower in the traditional health sector.

This was to be a "side job" for me apart from my regular duties on the Rural Water-Borne Disease Control Project. I was pleased to have a mandate to expand research with traditional healers, something I had begun in early 1981 in order to obtain sociocultural background and context prior to attempting a national sample survey relating to water and sanitation. By now (mid-1982) the water and sanitation survey had been completed and I was encouraged from the results to attempt a broader and more general study of traditional healers, since I was not sure how representative my findings to date were from the approximately twenty healers I had interviewed in-depth (some of whom allowed me to observe and even participate in their practices). For these reasons and because policymakers tend to require quantifiable data, I proposed conducting a national survey of traditional healers estimating the number and type of healers practicing in Swaziland.

## A National Survey and Census of Healers

Since no national lists of healers were available—at least complete, up-to-date lists—a strict probability sample was out of the question. It was also not certain what kind of cooperation we could expect from healers themselves, or whether permission to interview could be obtained from all local chiefs. It seemed best for two interviewers who had worked on the water and sanitation survey and were now working under me in the Health Education Unit, to begin by interviewing healers in their own home areas, where they were known and where permission to interview would not present a problem. We later expanded our interviews to include any areas where the interviewers had kinship or friendship connections, or where the Health Education Unit happened to be working on other surveys or evaluations. At the same time, we purposely sought a balance between the four topographic zones of Swaziland, between which meaningful social and economic differences are known to occur.

Between August 1982 and January 1983, my research assistants interviewed 144 traditional healers of all types (herbalists, diviner mediums, and faith healers). No adequate sampling frame of healers existed and thus a random or probability sample was not feasible. However, roughly equal numbers of healers were interviewed in the four major geographic regions of Swaziland. While the healer sample could have been more randomized by selecting only those healers who lived in randomly selected census enumeration areas, time and effort were saved by allowing interviewers to work primarily in areas where they had kinship ties or where they had interviewed during previous surveys. This also helped minimize suspicion and mistrust on the part of the healers. The usual procedure was for the interviewers to try to contact all types of healers (diviners, herbalists, and faith healers) in a chosen area by means of referrals based on the social networks of healers themselves. If any systematic bias entered our sample, it might have been in the type of community chosen for interviewing. Yet Swaziland is a small, culturally homogeneous country, and we found considerable similarity of knowledge, beliefs, and practices between healers in the four regions.

An open-ended questionnaire was used, which meant that considerable detail and serendipitous information was obtained. The interviewers collected data on things like the recruitment and training of healers, the types of diseases most commonly treated and methods of treatment, the problems commonly referred to clinics or hospitals, the degree of mutual cooperation between healers, the potential for cooperation with doctors or nurses, and healer attitudes toward receiving training in aspects of modern medicine. I checked information the interviewers were obtaining with my own sources among healers and I sought greater detail on things like traditional categories of illness, theories of disease causation, and attitudes toward cooperation with MOH personnel. I also tried to observe patient-healer interaction, curing ceremonies, preparation of medicines, and other behaviors.

In addition, we conducted a house-to-house census in four rural and four periurban communities in order to estimate the number and type of healers in Swaziland, along with certain of their characteristics. A total of 598 residential units in three geographic regions were covered in the census. We found healers in 48 residential units out of 598 surveyed, amounting to an 8 percent "coverage" of both rural homesteads or periurban households (we found rural/urban differences in "healer density" to be minimal). Assuming the surveyed areas to be representative of Swaziland, and having a fairly good idea of the mean number of residents in both rural and urban residential units, we were able to estimate a total of 1,292 healers in periurban areas and 4,150 healers in rural areas. This amounts to about one healer per 110 population, compared with a physician:population ratio of about 1:10,000 for Swaziland. It also meant there were some 5,400 healers in the tiny kingdom at the time (and closer to 8,000 at present). Some 50 percent of the total number of healers appeared to be herbalists, 40 percent were diviner-mediums, and 10 percent were Christian ("Zionist") faith healers. About half the healers were female, and the vast majority of these were diviner-mediums. Diviner-mediums tend to be more prestigious than herbalists because ancestor spirits are believed to work through them directly.

## Illness and Treatment in a Pluralistic Setting

The survey confirmed my earlier finding that most illness is believed to be ultimately caused by sorcery (human ill intention), or less frequently by loss of ancestral protection. However many healers were prepared to accept that there might be more immediate causes of illness about which doctors and nurses were quite knowledgeable. For example, a Swazi mother might accept the idea that her child will develop diarrhea if flies walk over the child's food; but she will also want to know how and why her enemies sent flies to harm her child.

We found that patients might seek treatment from both doctors and traditional healers for the same complaint. The doctor was thought capable of eliminating symptoms or treating the immediate cause of illness, and the healer was relied upon to explain the illness in culturally meaningful terms, and to treat or eliminate the ultimate source of the illness. Clearly, there already existed a basis for cooperation between the traditional and the modern health sector. In fact, some 90 percent of healers surveyed claimed to routinely refer some of their patients to clinics—in spite of the fact that very few cases of referrals from clinics to healers were encountered.

Swazis make a basic distinction between diseases or conditions regarded as "African," "Swazi," or indigenous, and those that are of foreign or recent origin. The former are regarded as best treated by traditional medicine and practitioners, while the latter may be conceded to be best treated by western orthodox medicine (Green and Makhubu 1984). Such a distinction has only arisen in the context of contact with Western medicine; a more traditional Swazi distinction is between diseases that are—or can be—spiritually caused, and those that are naturally caused. The latter are known collectively as *umkhuhlane,* and account for only a small percentage of locally recognized diseases.

Returning to the first distinction, *tilwane,* or madness caused by sorcery, is an example of a "Swazi" disease, while cholera, which seems to have first appeared in Swaziland only in 1980, is regarded as a foreign disease. Most diseases recognized by Swazis as being transmitted by sexual intercourse are thought to be Swazi diseases and therefore treated most effectively by traditional practitioners and medicines. Sorcery is believed to be the root cause of most such conditions, and Western medicine is considered ineffective in treating sorcery.

As shown earlier in Table 1.2, the survey revealed that doctors are much admired for their access to medical technology, however this is understood. Most commonly cited were various surgical practices, blood transfusions, and use of X-ray machines. On the other hand, diviners felt that their ability to diagnose the ultimate causes of illness (thereby answering the "why" or "why me" questions of misfortune) and to perform the *femba* ceremony through which agents of illness are removed—both of which involve cultivated relationships with spirits—are skills that are at least as important as those that doctors possess. Most of the healers interviewed either implied or made explicit their wish to be treated as equals by doctors.

The survey also sought to identify healing practices that seemed harmful. These included medicinal enemas that are used to prevent and treat several types of childhood diarrhea; induced vomiting to "clean out the chest" of TB patients; traditional vaccinations performed with an unclean razor; and use of powerful, mind-altering herbal medicines in treating madness. Since Makhubu and I were well aware of a strong negative bias toward traditional healers on the part of modern practitioners we were careful to point out traditional healing practices that were probably beneficial to the patient—and perhaps to the patient's family and community as well. These included use of herbal medicines that seemed to be effective in various ways; the reduction of stress through ritual and through explanations reassuring to the patient and his family; and the removal of a patient from a stressful situation at home to a therapeutic environment at the healer's homestead in which the patient can recover. We also pointed out that healers help ease pressure on overburdened clinics by treating minor, self-limiting, psychosomatic and certain other kinds of conditions for which traditional therapies are probably effective and appropriate.

### *Client Fees*

Although it was difficult to obtain information on client fees in the survey, I personally observed patients paying between $120 and $130 for treatment of a single condition such as *umtsebulo,* or soul loss. Healers in one area were earning about $140 for magical protection (*kubetsela*) of a homestead against mystical lightning strikes by enemies. A basic diagnostic fee of about $2 was standardized by a royal Order-in-Council in 1954, but healers earned an additional fee of between $10 and $20 to "open the bag" (*imvula sikhwama*) of medicines, which formalizes the beginning of any sort of treatment. In 1992, a small number of healers told me they were charging about $30 to $35 for tuberculosis (*lugola*) treatment over a period of eight weeks, and about $3 to $7 for treatment of the common STD *gcunsula* (considered by health workers to be syphilis) over a period of three to ten days.

Although Swaziland is a poor country, most people somehow find the money to pay the relatively high fees requested by traditional healers. This was all the more remarkable because modern sector clinic services at the time of the survey cost the equivalent of about $.20, whatever treatment was required. My findings on healing fees helped explain why a recent attempt by the MOH to train traditional healers as Rural Health Motivators (called village or community health workers in other countries) met with little success. Rural Health Motivators were being paid $20 a month. Several survey respondents were candid in remarking that healing is a lucrative and respectable profession, and perhaps the best one to which women and those lacking formal education can aspire.

However these were herbalists; diviner-mediums always emphasized that they had no choice in becoming healers—they were called by ancestral spirits and could not refuse.

### *Registration and Cooperation*

A system of registering healers began in Swaziland late in the British colonial period when it became recognized that doctors and nurses would not easily displace traditional healers and that the latter could not be completely ignored by the government. Registration represented a first step toward recognition of healers and exercising a modicum of control over their activities. It also provided tax revenues. Since independence, the Swaziland government has continued to register and collect taxes from healers.

In our survey, most healers (82 percent) reported being currently registered, and 8 percent said they had only recently qualified as healers and they intended to become registered. Even allowing for overreporting, the proportion of registered, tax-paying healers is higher than might be expected for a traditional African society. In addition, healers seemed in general to be favorably inclined toward registration. When healers were asked why they had registered, 30 percent commented that the police would support them in collecting overdue patient fees and protect them against complaints of patients only if they are registered healers. Other common remarks were that registration conferred legitimacy, respectability and authority on healers, and it also allowed them to travel and practice freely throughout Swaziland and neighboring countries.

Finally, the survey sought information on cooperation and paraprofessional training. An impressive (if slightly suspect) 98 percent of healers interviewed claimed they would like to achieve better cooperation between themselves and doctors and nurses. And 91 percent specifically expressed enthusiasm for the idea of undergoing some sort of training in modern medicine. The reason most gave was that they wanted to improve their healing skills and learn more about the treatments given in hospitals. However, several healers—most of them female—expressed concern that their lack of formal education would make "communicating with doctors" difficult.

## Swaziland's First Collaborative Program

In spite of the positive survey results, both Makhubu and I were aware of a certain amount of suspicion on the part of traditional healers regarding the motives of the MOH. And a great deal more suspicion and outright negative bias could be found in the modern health sector. Many local doctors preferred to pretend that the healers did not exist, and some took the view that healers should be arrested for practicing medicine without a license. This bias resulted from a failure to understand the traditional healer's role in Swazi society, from the nature of formal (Western) medical education and professional socialization, from a certain amount of professional jealousy, from the "bad press" healers tended to receive by local, sensation-seeking media, and from the fact that healers do engage in several practices deemed unacceptable by public health standards.

In view of the difficulties of developing a workable policy in an atmosphere of suspicion and mistrust, Makhubu and I recommended that the MOH proceed cautiously and not expect quick results. We suggested a policy of seeking cooperation rather than integration, a distinction described in Chapter 2. One of our primary recommendations was that the MOH conduct seminars (later called workshops) for traditional healers in order to upgrade healers' skills and to provide a forum for the exchange of information. The first such regional seminar occurred in June 1983. A major objective of the seminars was to train healers in the use of oral rehydration therapy and to develop an integrated, intersectoral approach to preventing and treating diarrheal diseases. Other areas of potential cooperation were discussed at the seminars such as appropriate patient referrals, the promotion of childhood immunizations, and the development of a national traditional healers association. Such an association did emerge independently from any recommendations in our report.

Since the first seminar in 1983, many others have been held in various parts of Swaziland. The numbers of healers attending grew from a handful to over a hundred per seminar, although it was found that groups of twenty to thirty seemed best for two-way learning and discussion. Responsibility for planning and conducting these seminars lay entirely in the hands of local staff of the Health Education Unit, cooperating closely with the Public Health Unit and coordinating through the new Traditional Healers Organization. The first seminars were popular with healers and many of those in the ministry who were directly involved. There was preliminary evidence of behavioral and attitudinal change on the part of healers and even of ministry personnel as a result of these efforts (Hoff and Maseko 1986), although this and subsequent collaborative efforts still await objective, outside impact evaluation.

By 1984–1985 various problems arose between the leadership of the Traditional Healers Organization and the Ministry of Health. There were also charges that the program had exceeded its mandate by branching into other areas of primary health care besides diarrheal disease, and that the program had become too American directed. These problems were exploited by those who had been skeptical about collaboration from the start, and formal collaboration between the Ministry of Health and THO came to a standstill in about 1985. By 1985–1986, however, THO had begun formal collaboration in public health programs with nongovernmental organizations (NGOs), beginning with Project Hope. Since 1990, UNICEF has spent about $100,000 in training workshops conducted through THO. UNICEF training has covered the full range of primary health care activities plus AIDS prevention. There is currently some official MOH involvement in the UNICEF/THO program, as nurses from Public Health and Health Education are assigned to work in the UNICEF collaborative effort.

The Swaziland government's latest seven-year plan (1993–2000) calls for training 200 traditional healers every year in control of diarrhea, during one–week workshops. Healers may also receive training in other areas of primary health care as well, according to the THO president. In late 1992, officers of Swaziland's National AIDS Program told me that program money had already been used to train traditional healers in the recent past, and their plan for the next few years calls for more of their training funds to be spent this way. The training focus is on general AIDS preventive education, condom promotion, and use of sterilized razor blades.

## Indigenous STDs in Swaziland

Illnesses and conditions related to sexual intercourse are important to healers and, it appears, to the general population of Swaziland. Therefore, whatever my research agenda in the early 1980s, it would have been difficult not to discover something about indigenous ideas about STDs. Most of these early findings derived from my own in-depth interviews and participant-observation research, although they are complemented by the findings of the traditional healer survey. Since these findings were peripheral to my primary research objectives, they must be regarded as preliminary and by no means a complete account of ethnomedical aspects of STDs in Swaziland. I returned to Swaziland in late 1992 for over two weeks of STD/AIDS-related interviewing. During this time I was able to confirm or update some of my earlier findings. My assistants and I also discovered some important new developments, to be described.

In Swaziland there are various emic categories or locally recognized conditions for which sexual intercourse is believed to be the vehicle—or *a* vehicle—of transmission and which might or might not correspond with sexually transmitted diseases recognized by orthodox medicine. The major group of these are believed to be caused essentially the same way: a possessive or jealous husband or lover who treats his wife or partner with special medicines intended to ensure her fidelity, especially while the man is working away from home. If another man has sexual relations with the woman, that man will develop symptoms of one of at least five distinct syndromes, depending on the medicinal spell to which the woman was exposed. Illness related to fidelity-protection medicines include (but may not be limited to):

1. *Idrop* (*dropu*): characterized by a pus discharge from the penis and pain in urination. A woman might have vaginal inflammation or sores. It "destroys the sperm" (causes sterility) if left untreated for a month. *Idrop* is considered a European disease. The root "drop" may come from the English word and refer to drops or discharge from the penis. It might also relate to the Dutch or Afrikaans word for gonorrhea (*"druiper"*). According to several healers interviewed in 1992, the medicine used to protect the woman is made from grinding up black and red dispensary-derived capsules that bear the inscription "500" (ampicillin) and mixing them with certain herbs and perhaps iron filings. Use of "modern" pills is offered as proof that *idrop* is of foreign origin. In another version, a woman takes birth control pills surreptitiously; these pills give her husband the disease. Other healers explained that *idrop* is caused by men taking traditional blood-purifying medicines, then having intercourse before the medicines have done their job (see below). Two healers said *idrop* is like bilharzia (*umthundungati*) because "You can get it from drinking bad water," and there may be blood in the urine of a victim. Another healer said the disease is caused by a husband wanting to protect his wife (see *likhubalo*, below.) Still others said they don't really know the cause of this disease; they can only cure it. *Treatment*: a patient drinks an herbal decoction (*imbita*) three times a day and is given an herbal enema three times a day except for the second day. Bits of coral from the sea might be mixed in the decoction. This is because of the similarity between the appearance of coral and the woman's vaginal sores. Treatment continues for four days. (See later chapters for descriptions of *drop* or *dropu* in Mozambique and South Africa.)
2. *Gcunsula* (*tilonza*): symptoms for both men and women include hot, burning, painful urination ("They may scream when they urinate"); sores or wounds on the penis or vagina; small pimples around the genitalia which eventually ooze pus; discharge from the penis; bad odors; and difficulty in walking due to clothes rubbing against the genital sores. *Gcunsula* can affect the fetus in the womb, although this can be avoided if the mother gets treatment before giving birth. If *gcunsula* is untreated, a baby will be born with sores all over his body. He will have yellow eyes and will eventually die. The disease is believed to be caused in the same

way as *likhubalo*, i.e., a man treats his wife with medicines believed to ensure her fidelity. Any subsequent lovers become victims of the man's revenge. Unlike *idrop*, it is considered an old disease.[2] Nevertheless, a number of healers interviewed in 1992 said *gcunsula* is caused by crushing "500" pills and mixing them with the same herbs used for the *likhubalo* spell. The husband takes this medicine thereby passing the spell to his wife or girlfriend. Potential lovers of the wife will then avoid her as she now carries this disease. One healer said that the sores of this illness can directly cause the disease in a sexual partner of one who has the sores. Another periurban healer believed that having many sexual partners spreads *gcunsula*, as does the taking of antibiotics as a preventive measure before sex with a risky partner. *Treatment*: the sores may be washed in a special medicine, and an herbal decoction (*imbita*) is drunk. Less often, herbal enemas are used. Treatment continues until symptoms subside.

3. *Likhubalo*: characterized by headaches, pain in the lower back or kidneys; swollen testicles; possibly a pus or blood discharge from the penis, mouth or other orifice. There are several types of *likhubalo* based apparently on different ways a man secretly exposes his wife to the medicine or spell. For example (1) a possessive husband puts the medicine on the ground where his wife will pass by (when this happens, a woman has symptoms of vaginal bleeding); (2) a man fortifies himself with the medicine through razor incisions (*kugata*), then passes it to his wife through sexual intercourse; (3) as with the second method, except that the medicine is prepared from the brains and/or boiled venom of a black mamba snake; (4) as with the second method, except that the medicine includes the sperm of two copulating dogs (this results in the illness variant *likhubalo lenja*, "dog *likhubalo*); (5) as with the second method, except that certain herbs are mixed with the head of a turkey and the head or heart of a tortoise.[3] Any future lover of the "protected" wife will find his penis turn greenish or bluish (like a turkey's head), then grow short and retract (like the head of a tortoise) to the point of disappearing into the body.

The first three forms of *likhubalo* are considered fatal. The male lover will die soon after sleeping with a woman who has absorbed this medicine/spell, and after his moment of death blood will dribble out of his nose, mouth, and/or ears. In *likhubalo lenja*, the illicit couple will remain stuck together. They can only become unstuck if someone summons the husband and he releases them from the disease/spell by obtaining medicines from the original healer to whom the husband turned to make the original medicine. These related illnesses or spells are so common in Swaziland that one healer said the basic mixture used to create the spell is referred to as *insiti yakangwane* (powder of Swaziland). *Treatment*: traditional vaccination (*kugata*).

4. *Imbune*: this involves a one-time "protection" for a woman that is said to last a lifetime. The medicine is prepared from the *imbune* plant (that wilts when touched), a ground-up turkey beak and a tortoise's head. A suspicious man will inoculate himself with this medicine through incisions in his groin; he then passes the spell to his wife without her knowledge through sexual intercourse. Any man attempting to have sex with a woman prepared with this medicine will be unable to achieve an erection. His penis will droop like a turkey's beak or wilt like the *imbune* plant. In a version of symptoms provided by some healers in 1992, an illicit male lover will develop incurable *idrop* or gonorrhea symptoms. A woman remains asymptomatic, although one healer explained that her vagina will feel "cold and windy" to her lover during intercourse, causing him to withdraw immediately.

   A woman can also secretly expose her husband to the *imbune* medicine in order to keep him faithful to her. If the exposed husband tries to have sex with another woman, he will lose his erection. There is also a nonfidelity protection form of this disease that seems closer to regular sorcery. If two men are very competitive, one man can sprinkle medicine made from this plant over a place where his rival will pass. Once the rival absorbs the medicine he will lose his erection forever. Another healer specified that a Tylenol pill is crushed up to make a destructive medicine/spell of this sort, causing kidney damage in the intended victim. In still another version or form of *imbune* from a periurban healer, the illness is caused by a woman taking birth control pills. *Treatment*: In order to cure *imbune*, the same plant and animal parts used in concocting the original medicine or spell must be involved. An herbal decoction is drunk over the course of a week, or until the symptom of impotence subsides.

5. *Timbilapho* (*timvilapho*): symptoms include lumps or oozing sores near the testicles, genital pain, fatigue, progressive thinness, wasting, walking awkwardly to avoid scraping sores against trousers, and a "stupid-looking" appearance." It is a fidelity-insurance medicine or spell like *likhubalo*. The medicine is made from herbs, perhaps mixed with avocado and potatoes and empowered with iron filings. In 1992, I encountered a form of this illness said to be caused by drinking *magazini* (potassium permanganate). When a man drinks *magazini* for medicinal purposes, it consolidates all the

accumulated impurities of his body and when he has intercourse, all these impurities are carried to his partner's womb by his sperm. A "foam" consisting of the man's "dirt" and his sperm stays in the womb, and the next man who sleeps with this woman will suffer from *timbilapho*. The woman has no symptoms. Another version was similar to this last except that pills or strong, purifying herbal decoctions are drunk instead of *magazini*. *Treatment*: traditional vaccination (*kugata*). Some healers said a smaller dose (or a less potent mixture) of the powder used to make *likhubalo* is used in the cure of *timbilapho*.

6. *Timbatane.*: this refers to lice on the genitals and inside the body, a condition affecting both men and women. Some say the disease destroys the sperm and ovaries. The plant used to create this illness or spell is similar to *imbune*. If one holds the leaf of the *Timbatane plant* up to the sun, one can see tiny, barely visible lice on the leaf. A suspicious husband mixes up this leaf, drinks it, and passes the medicine or spell to his wife through sexual intercourse. Any lover she has in the future will get this lice. If the husband manages to trick his wife into drinking some of this medicine, she will remain without any symptoms. The women who become infected with these lice include any partners of the male lover—such as his own wife. In a second version of *timbatane*, it is caused by people eating fruits with spikes on the skin, such as pineapple. These spikes combine with blood in the stomach and tiny, insectlike creatures develop there. They form little pimples or "bubbles" as they emerge from the body through the skin. They are spread through sexual intercourse or any other bodily contact with people who don't have the lice. In a third version, an enemy places the medicine causing this condition on the ground where an intended victim will pass by. *Treatment*: Certain herbs are mixed with vaseline, then rubbed on the genitals. However, the lice are really *inside* the body, "in the blood." Therefore, the patient must be given an herbal decoction to drink. This will cause the lice to exit the body through urine, while the externally applied medicine causes the lice infesting the pubic hair to fall off of the body. The vaseline is used to trap the lice so they "can't run away from the medicine," according to one healer.
7. *Shengele*: characterized by sores on the penis that begin on the crown and progress toward the body until they "eat up" the whole penis. It may tear the foreskin. One healer explained that the penis of a child (of an infected woman?) becomes reddish and he develops body sores, painful testicles, and swelling next to the anus. This is a fidelity-insurance medicine or spell like *likhubalo*. A

husband (or wife?) prepares the medicine and secretly puts it into something his partner will drink. *Treatment*: drinking herbal decoction (*timbita*), and washing sores with special medicine.

8. *Spanjolo*: characterized by genital sores, frequent urination, swelling in both male and female genital area. It "destroys the sperm," so that a man becomes sterile. There may be difficulty in walking due to genital sores rubbing against clothing. Hair becomes sparse and reddish.
9. *Horse disease*: symptoms include shaking or tremors of the thighbone or leg, as when a person has a stroke. Paralysis may occur on one side of the body. This is followed by wasting, thinness, and finally death. It's caused by a "pill" made by mixing horse sweat with "chemicals from the Portuguese." A man drinks it, apparently in order to pass the medicine/spell on to his wife in order to send the disease to her lover. *Treatment*: an herbal decoction is prepared from special herbs mixed with fish and other sea creatures such as seals. A one-liter dose is drunk three times a day for one week.
10. *Cauliflower* (*cornflower*, or *sifo semakhabishi*, "the cabbage disease" in siSwati). This disease takes the form of a genital growth that is said to resemble a cabbage or flower or cauliflower (see Chapter 7 for more). The growth may not be painful. On the vagina, the hairs first begin to disappear before the growth appears. The disease is considered difficult to get unless one has sex with a South African or Portuguese. It is caused by these foreigners taking antibiotic pills to prevent disease. To treat the disease, a patient must bring pills prescribed to him at the hospital in order for the healer to make the appropriate medicine to *really* cure the disease. *Treatment*: Ampicillin pills are mixed with a liter of herbal decoction and given to the patient to drink.
11. *Luhlanga*: characterized by the penis "drying up" and developing cracks or small cuts on the foreskin and under the foreskin on the crown. One healer said this is a hereditary STD: children inherit it from a mother or father who has the disease. Boys exhibit the same symptoms as the father. For mothers, they may have a vaginal itch during pregnancy which is rather pleasurable to scratch. The itch later becomes painful and a rash develops. *Treatment*: an herbal decoction is made up from a root which has cracks that resembles the cracks in the penis of a man with *luhlanga*. The whole family must drink the decoction together. Doctors cannot cure this new disease. Their "shots and ointments only take care of the outside symptoms. The disease is inside the body," requiring drinking the special decoction.

12. *sifo setifish* ("fish disease"): foreigners are said to be importing this disease; its English name signals its foreign status. In the outstanding symptom, tiny fish come out of the body during urination, then "turn to water" when they hit the ground. There's also pain during urination. The illness is caused by people taking pills as a preventive measure prior to having sex with a risky partner.

With illnesses 3–9, the spell seems usually to pass through women and only directly affect the intended victim, a woman's illicit lover. That is, the woman remains asymptomatic, while her male lovers fall victim to the illness. In some types of *likhubalo,* the woman may develop symptoms of vaginal bleeding and headaches.

*Shengele, spanjolo, cauliflower,* and the fish disease are not well known, and they seem to be regarded as foreign and/or new diseases. Some of these as well as older, indigenous illness were believed to be caused by people taking modern pills, including antibiotics (see section below), birth control pills, or analgesics such as Tylenol—but only during interviews in 1992, not in the early 1980s. I return to this point below.

In 1992, healers were also describing diseases that were so new that they had no name for them. In one of these, the penis swells up, then develops cracks or tears on the crown, under the foreskin. There is also pus around the crown indicating an infection under the foreskin. One healer called this disease *luhlanga.* In Chapter 7, *The Circumcision Factor,* South African healers offer observations and comments about such conditions under the foreskin. Another "new disease" is characterized by sores on the vagina in the woman and sores on the lower abdomen in the man. Both develop water blisters on the sex organs and there is pain in urination. If the disease is untreated, it leads to impotence. One healer said he might refer cases of this to the hospital.

Swazis recognize other indigenous illnesses believed to be transmitted or transmissible through sexual intercourse. Two of these are:

13. *Ligola* (*lugala*): characterized by symptoms similar to tuberculosis (some healers say this illness is exactly what the doctors call TB). Symptoms are said to include persistent coughing; progressive thinness; sunken eyes; body hair that sticks out and becomes sparse like that of a baby; very long fingernails; a personality that becomes harsh, aggressive, and quarrelsome; and cravings to eat roasted maize and meat. It is believed to result from a man having sex with: (1) a woman who has recently had a miscarriage, abortion, or stillbirth (some specified that these had to have occurred within six to seven months); (2) a woman within five months after a normal birth; (3) a woman while she is still menstruating. In

another type of *lugola*, an enemy puts harmful medicines into someone's food. In the case of violating the rule of postpartum abstinence, a man's blood will be affected and he may suffer low back pain. *Treatment*: special herbs are mixed with some menstrual blood. After burning this mixture, the resulting ashes are brought to the mouth with the fingertips, a process called *kucapha*.

14. *Sicitfo*: believed to result from a spell intended to ruin the victim's social life and romantic relationships. It is transmitted by contact with medicines deliberately placed at a doorway, by a bed, or directly on a woman's body. Either a possessive husband, an unprincipled healer, or a woman herself can place spell-casting medicines or poisons on her genitals. *Treatment*: induced vomiting, inhaling steam (*kufutsa*) from herbal decoction, traditional vaccination (*kugata*), burying the patient's blood in the ground with special medicines.

## The Ethics of "Fidelity Protection"

*Likhubalo* is considered the most common fidelity-protection illness, according to interviews in 1992 as well as our 1982 survey of healers. It is also considered the most powerful of fidelity-protection illnesses, since it results in death most often and since, as one healer put it, "A condom can't prevent *likhubalo*, yet a condom can defeat a disease like *timbilapho*." With *likhubalo*, the woman is not a voluntary or knowing participant. The husband ingests certain medicines himself through traditional vaccination (*kugata*) or drinking a decoction. Then, without his wife's or partner's knowledge, he passes the "protective" medicine/spell to her through sexual intercourse. He may also sprinkle some of the medicine along a place the woman is bound to pass, causing her to absorb the medicine. The severity of illnesses resulting from a male lover's exposure to the protective medicine is said to depend upon the degree of the husband's possessiveness and therefore the strength of the medicines he uses. Sometimes the intent is to kill, and indeed healers and other Swazi informants agree that men can and do die from *likhubalo*. Some tell-tale drops of blood may drip from the nose of the male lover, confirming *likhubalo* as the cause of death.

According to healer informants, insecure or suspicious men (or, less often, wives) must enlist the help of a traditional healer to prepare fidelity-protecting medicines or spells, since they themselves lack the knowledge to prepare these on their own. To the extent that such medicines have a negative effect on a victim—especially death—it would appear that healers are involved in a type of sorcery or quasi-sorcery to quite a considerable extent, given the high "prevalence" of especially *likhubalo.* Yet such practices would seem to contravene a code of ethics which Swazi and other African healers can readily describe. This code forbids healers to make medicines or spells that have the effect of harming people or even controlling their behavior or actions. In fact, healers normally refuse to name witches or other supposed perpetrators of harm or evil.[4]

Yet most healers seem to regard, or rationalize, fidelity-protection medicines as socially legitimate, and they are willing to speak openly about their involvement in their preparation. True, these practices involve the use of medicines for potentially harmful purposes, but it is in the cause of preserving marriage, family, and the proper rearing of children. With a few of these fidelity-insuring medicines, a couple is said to drink them together voluntarily and consensually.[5] In these cases, both partners in effect seal a pact that the woman (and perhaps the man) will remain faithful. However, most healers describe a *secret* administration of medicines associated with most of the fidelity-protection spells—almost always with the wife the unwitting carrier of the medicinal spell.

I was told that a generation or two ago, healers were not as willing as those of today to make fidelity medicines such as *likhubalo*; "It was seen as a type of witchcraft." Even nowadays, healers may not agree to make these medicines unless a patient beseeches them repeatedly, and even then they may ask for evidence that a wife is loitering about at shabeens (bars) or seeing another man before they are willing to make a potent fidelity protection medicine that could cause death.

One healer-informant reminded me that King Sobhuza II (who died in 1982) used to call together all traditional healers in the nation for meetings. In one such meeting before the king died, he urged the nation to give up *likhubalo.* This admonition was intended for traditional healers, self-styled "herbalists that play around with *likhubalo,*" and ordinary Swazis. This informant thought it unfortunate that King Mswati III (who has ruled since 1986) has not called Swazi healers together to admonish them in a way that preserves traditional ethics. Without royal guidance, some healers have begun to misuse traditional medicines. Yet this healer herself makes *likhubalo.* She said that people are demanding it and healers have to give people what they want. She attributed increased demand for *likhubalo* to promiscuity on the part of women, with a corresponding increase of worry and fear on the part of men.

However healers may justify their involvement in preparing *likhubalo* medicines, these are the sort of practices detractors of collaborative programs point to in arguing against government having anything to do with traditional healers. The argument goes that by dealing with healers in any way, governments officially recognize their existence, and by recognizing healers, governments implicitly condone sorcery practices. The counterargument is that governments must deal in some way with healers, for all the reasons discussed in Chapter 2, but this does not mean governments condone all traditional practices. Governments have no choice but to accept traditional healers as they are—but this does not mean attempts cannot be made to modify harmful practices while encouraging those that are health promoting.

The healer who makes the fidelity-protection medicine must also give the client the antidote formula to separate the couple if the wife takes a lover and becomes physically connected with him, in the case of *likhubalo lenja*. This is because healers will not publicly have anything to do with the dangerous medicine or spell they have concocted. If they are queried by the police, they will deny any knowledge of the whole business; the husband who commissioned the medicines must come forward with the antidote. A common treatment for *likhubalo* (as well as for *timbilapho* and *sicitfo*) appears to involve traditional vaccination (*kugata*) with powder derived from burning herbal medicines and perhaps animal parts. Cuts are made with razor blades on various parts of the body and the medicinal paste is rubbed into the bleeding cuts. The razor blades employed in *kugata* are usually unsterilized (although the Traditional Healers Organization is trying to change this), and they may be used on several people—usually family members—during a single treatment, allowing for "mixing of bodily fluids" or blood contamination since razors may be stained with drops of blood from others who have been vaccinated. We will return to this point later.

## Summary of Findings and Prospects for Referrals of STD Cases

I and my assistants found differences in perceived etiologies of indigenous illnesses related to sexual intercourse. These may reflect regional or rural/urban variations that need to be researched more systematically and thoroughly. As an example of individual differences, more than one healer interpreted at least illnesses 3–9 as all relating to fidelity-protection. However, one influential healer in western Hhohho interpreted the same conditions (except for *likhubalo*) in a different way. For her, illnesses such as *gcunsula, timbilapho,* and *cauliflower* are caused by a man taking herbal decoctions (*timbita*)—or nowadays, pills—to purify his blood, then neglecting to follow a healer's instructions to refrain from sex before his blood is purified. Because the man is impatient to resume sex, he passes the disease to a woman through intercourse. Both strong herbal purifiers and pills "collect the dirt" or the impurities that have accumulated in a man's body and then pass them through sperm to a sexual partner.

Although this interpretation differs from the fidelity-protection theory, they share some of the same important elements: (1) with both, a single, basic, causal explanation links several illnesses together into a group, with the result that these illnesses are understood and treated in the same way; (2) with both, men are usually the initial infectors, and women are the infectees. Certain other generalizations are possible about the beliefs and thinking behind virtually all of the foregoing conditions related to intercourse. First, for Swazis, most serious diseases do not simply happen. They are created and sent by a person of ill-will. This is as true for illnesses related to sexual intercourse as, for example, the more serious forms of childhood diarrhea (Green 1986). As discussed below, one healer demanded an explanation of how AIDS is *made*. Second, symptoms of the common STDs recognized by biomedicine (urethral discharge, pain in urination, genital sores and swelling) are all found among illnesses related to taking fidelity-protection or other medicines (including certain pills nowadays) and they all have essentially the same etiology. These are the illnesses whose symptoms correspond more or less to syphilis, gonorrhea, chlamydia, and chancroid, the diseases that facilitate the spread of AIDS, the diseases we are especially interested in curing and preventing. Third, virtually all of the illnesses described involve the violation of social rules, such as having sex with a married woman, sex with a woman who has been contaminated with death, sex with a menstruating woman, or failing to refrain from sex until one is well (or the medicines one has taken have done their job).

Finally, virtually all of the above illnesses save *drop* are considered Swazi or at least African illnesses. As such, they are considered conditions that Western-trained practitioners are unable to understand or treat. Even *drop* may be thought to involve causal factors thought to lie outside the domain of biomedicine, such as human intent (or spell) and traditional medicines.

The following case history is taken from my fieldnotes of May 1983. It illustrates the widespread tendency to consult only traditional practitioners in cases of conditions believed to be transmitted through sexual intercourse, as well as the common Swazi practice of consulting multiple healers for diagnosis and treatment of the same condition. It also touches upon the relationship between conditions regarded as sexually transmitted and the transgression of norms regulating sexual intercourse, a point developed further below.

## Case History of Gcunsula

Sipho has been away from his homestead for several weeks looking for work. He finally found a short-term job to help build a house at Lozitha.

However, he has been having pains he described as coming from his "kidneys" and soon after he began his job, the pain became overwhelming and he had to quit his job. Sipho told me that his condition was first diagnosed as *gcunsula* by a Christian faith healer (*umprofeti*). *Gcunsula* probably corresponds to syphilis.

One of the reasons Sipho consulted the faith healer is that this healer apparently doesn't believe that Christians should accept money for diagnoses or healing. (Note that Sipho's father is an herbalist of considerable renown; it may be that the somewhat shameful nature of Sipho's condition prevented him from consulting his father.) Sipho related that with no prior knowledge of Sipho's family situation, the faith healer informed Sipho that his father has three wives and that, as the eldest son of the father's senior wife, Sipho stands in line to inherit most of his father's property. Since all of this is true, Sipho was most impressed with the faith healer. The healer went on to divine that one of Sipho's "junior" mothers has sent *gcunsula*—by placing harmful agents on the ground where Sipho would be sure to pass and come into contact with the agents—in order to promote one of her own sons as principle heir. Although Sipho acknowledged that *gcunsula* usually results from sorcery on the part of a jealous husband, and that the outstanding symptom is external genital sores, Sipho at first accepted the faith healer's explanation.

A few days later I saw Sipho and told him that I might help him find treatment to relieve his "kidney inflammation." He said that would be fine, but only after his father takes care of him. It seems Sipho's herbalist father learned of the faith healer's diagnosis and divination but disagreed with it. He pointed out to his son that *gcunsula* is contracted only through sexual intercourse. He then asked Sipho if he had had any extramarital relations recently and when he was assured that his son had not, he concluded that the condition must be *umklwebho*, a commonly diagnosed type of sorcery. (Note that for the herbalist to accept the faith healer's divination he would have to have admitted that one of his wives was up to treachery.)

The herbalist has started his son on a regimen of medicinal enemas to counteract the *umklwebho* spell. The herbalist could not himself identify who sent the *umklwebho* since he is an herbalist and does not divine. However, Sipho consulted a Shangaan/Tsonga-speaking diviner (*sangoma*) and had the original faith healer's divination basically corroborated: Sipho was told his father has three wives and someone in Sipho's home is trying to harm him.

In his review of sexual behavior in Africa, Barton (1989:4) has observed that shame and "repressive public health measures" have led Africans with STDs to avoid doctors and to instead consult traditional healers, adding that "There are no statistics at all on traditional healer visits."

I have already cited the findings of our survey of Swazi healers showing that STDs—as locally recognized—are thought to be African diseases which are more amenable to treatment by African than biomedical healers. In another study (in which I was not involved) specifically focused on STDs in Swaziland, a small random sample of periurban Swazis was surveyed. There were also systematic interviews with clinic personnel. These findings seem to support my healer-derived information. Clinic personnel acknowledged that "a large proportion" of Swazi STD patients consult traditional healers for treatment, that others use antibiotics "to protect or prevent transmission of disease," and that some STD patients exhibit antibiotic resistance (Masango and Rakolojane 1987:1, 5).

A more recent, still-unpublished study in Swaziland showed a continuation of all these trends including significant growth of antibiotic resistance (Guinness 1990). Fully 31 percent of respondents from the 1987 survey cited traditional healers as the therapists of choice for most people with an STD, which is high considering respondents were selected only in urban areas where modern biomedical health care is available. The figure is also high considering that Swazis, like other Africans, have shown a marked reluctance to admit in the context of formal interviews that they consult traditional healers for any reason. Moreover emic disease terms such as *likhubalo* and *gcunsula* were apparently not used in interviewing. Sixty percent of survey respondents also expressed beliefs that having an STD is shameful or damaging to one's reputation and gave these as reasons for not seeking medical treatment.

## A Framework for Analysis

A reading of the anthropological literature, as well as my own experience in Africa, suggests the presence of certain basic conceptual themes, or dominant cultural metaphors of health, that underlie traditional African thinking about health. Drawing on the work of Janzen (1986, 1989: 232–235), I find it useful to distinguish four basic themes that relate to health in its broadest sense among (especially) Bantu speakers: *purity, coolness, balance,* and *social harmony.*

1. *Purity* refers to the absence of contamination or pollution. Contamination may be conceived in natural terms ("dirt") or mystical terms (the pollution of sin, evil spell) or something in between (menstrual blood, which may be regarded as an agent of mystical potency). (Negative expression: contamination or pollution);
2. *Coolness* refers to lack of "heat." Resembling (and perhaps influenced directly by) traditional health beliefs from the circum-Mediterranean and Islamic regions, Africans healers may attribute intrinsic hot and cool qualities to both illnesses and their cures. (Negative expression: heat, although any imbalance of hot/cold attributes can explain illness);

3. *Balance* refers to the maintenance of harmonious relations with nature and the spirit world; (Negative expression: may be disfavor of spirits; withdrawal of ancestral protection);
4. *Social harmony* refers specifically to maintenance of harmonious relations with kinfolk, neighbors, and others with whom people come into regular social contact. Social *dis*harmony leads to resentment, anger, envy, jealousy, etc., and often to sorcery and witchcraft. (Negative expression: sorcery, witchcraft).

Janzen refers to the first three of these as elements of wellness. I saw value in adding a fourth concept, social harmony, even though it could be considered a subcategory of "balance," if social balance is added to balance with nature and the spirit world. Social harmony is offered as a separate category to account more directly for the centrality in at least Bantu thought of what Janzen himself calls "... the invisible cause of misfortune and injury arising from the specifically human social dimension of evil-wishing, envy, gossiping, cursing, and mystical hurt projected within social relations" (1989:233).

Of course, these are not necessarily discrete conceptual categories. As Janzen (1989:234–235) notes, coolness is a quality that may be invoked to counteract pollution and balance may relate to the hot/cold dichotomy in treatment. Hammond-Tooke (1981:112–130) also relates pollution concepts with the Sotho ethnomedical concept of heat. Nevertheless, he notes the distinctiveness of pollution (*fisa*) beliefs among the Sotho-speaking Kgaga:

> This complex of beliefs is clearly analytically separate from that concerning ancestors or witches. Firstly, it does not involve the actions of intelligences, whether human or "spiritual".... Secondly, there seems to be little, if any, association with morality (Hammond-Tooke 1981:112).

Hammond-Tooke suggests that the Kgaga concept of pollution is better understood as "impersonal causation." He describes a Kgaga "pollution complex" wherein contamination occurs through "no fault of one's own," an idea supported by Mary Douglas' work among the Lele of Zaire. She notes that Lele rules of pollution depend not upon intention but only "whether a forbidden contact has taken place or not." (Douglas 1966:155 quoted in Hammond-Tooke 1981).

Aided by this framework, several patterns emerge from an analysis of indigenous Swazi illnesses believed related to sexual intercourse. First, the major apparent grouping of such illnesses is believed to originate in the mind (or heart) of an angry (suspicious, jealous) person. One becomes exposed to the illness—or becomes a victim to the spell—by violating a fundamental social rule, that of sexual fidelity within marriage or at least a socially recognized, stable relationship. The basic conceptual theme in this interpretation of illness is social harmony—or the lack of it.

The violation of other rules or norms governing sexual behavior (avoidance of widows or other women who have been associated with death or menstrual blood) is believed to result in *ligola*. The theme here is purity—or the lack of it. Both death and menstrual blood are regarded as highly polluting or contaminating in many parts of Africa (Douglas 1966; Ngubane 1977; Hammond-Tooke 1981; Janzen 1989). One Swazi healer explained that *ligola* can be caught by eating from plates or kitchen utensils that have been handled by a widow; she, in effect, passes the contamination of her husband's death on to the one who eats from a plate she has touched.

The high prevalence and perceived upsurge of illnesses of the fidelity-insurance type probably reflects the insecurity of men—even women—in their attempts to maintain stable sexual relationships in time of enforced separation of spouses due to labor patterns, erosion or abandonment of traditional norms, rapid urbanization, and general social upheaval.

A third pattern that emerges from my 1992 Swazi fieldwork is an apparent recent introduction of Western medicine, in the form of pills, into the interpretation and treatment of several STDs. The evidence of this will now be presented.

## Use of Antibiotics and Other Recent Trends

During two weeks of key-informant interviews in 1992, when I was assisted by two interviewers who had worked with me in the early 1980s, some significant new findings emerged. There was evidence that traditional healers, at least those practicing close to Swaziland's towns, were beginning to use antibiotics in the treatment of certain STDs. Neither I nor my assistants had seen any evidence of this in the early 1980s, nor had we heard of any government officials or doctors alleging such use. Therefore, we assumed antibiotics began to enter traditional practice in the mid- or late 1980s.

By the time of our interviews in 1992, healers were describing an increase in diseases related to sexual intercourse, especially *gcunsula, idrop,* and *emakabishi* (probably syphilis, gonorrhea, and chlamydia respectively.) They also described the appearance of new diseases imported by foreigners from neighboring countries. Some of these diseases were believed to be *caused* by antibiotic pills, specifically by men taking such pills prior to intercourse with women suspected of having a communicable disease. It may be that healers noticed that such self-medication prior to intercourse in fact did not prevent communicable diseases, therefore in healers' thinking, it was the pill that actually caused these diseases.

One of the patterns evident in Swazi ethnomedical thought is the notion of an intrinsic connection between natural materials involved in the cause or creation of a disease, the symptoms of the disease, and its treatment. For example, a man or woman connives to ensure the sexual fidelity of his or her partner by preparing a medicine from *imbune,* the name of a plant said to wilt when it is touched. The illness or condition passed on to a wayward husband, or to a male lover of a wayward wife, is also called *imbune.* The penis of the illicit lover or the unfaithful husband wilts like the *imbune* plant. And finally, the *imbune* plant is used in the cure or neutralization of the illness.

With the introduction of antibiotics into traditional treatment, we again encounter belief in an intrinsic connection between materials involved in the cause or creation of a disease, and at least the treatment deemed necessary. The "500" pills (ampicillin) seem to have caused the illness, therefore the same pills must be used in treatment—too sparingly to be effective, it seems. In treatment for the "foreign" disease cauliflower, one healer uses either one "500" pill or two "250" pills per liter of herbal decoction. The pill(s) are added *after* the decoction is cooled, in order not to "destroy the power of the pill." Note that one liter (and one or two pills) are considered sufficient to cure this disease, which was equated with chlamydia during my South African research (Chapter 7). This would seem to be an example of a healer using antibiotics in such a way as to promote antimicrobial resistance among patients.

It is interesting—and perhaps important—to speculate as to how and why antibiotic pills have apparently entered Swazi indigenous practice in the first place. First, beginning in the late 1980s, warnings about a new, fatal sexually transmitted disease have been assaulting Swazis from all sides, which understandably has raised everyone's anxiety level about such diseases. Second, the Swazi government's greater efforts to control standard STDs have probably had the effect of introducing more antibiotic pills into Swaziland. In any case, there has been a recent proliferation of antibiotics among the public, evidenced in part by the rise of a cadre of pill hawkers at the bus "ranks" and markets. Perhaps healers are beginning to resent what they perceive as encroachment on their treatment domain by pill hawkers and indeed doctors. These new developments in the age of AIDS may be seen by healers as a threat to their prestige and practice. If so, they may feel they are "evening the odds" a bit by using the newly proliferating pills in their own practice.

Another reason simply may be that healers are having difficulty curing STDs nowadays, and they think they would be aided in their efforts by borrowing some of the *materia medica* of doctors. Of course, healers would not—and did not—give this sort of explanation.

Supporting the threat-to-prestige hypothesis, we found healers warning against people treating themselves with pills. There were healers who told me "500" pills are a kind of poison (*sidliso*), and they assured me they could drive them out of a patient's body with traditional herbs. We also found evidence of healers' disapproval of clients' use of birth control and analgesic pills. Indeed, pills were not seen by healers as the only danger, or threat. Some warned that mixing a "hospital injection" with the traditional medicine required to cure (locally recognized) STDs would result in the patient's death. And potassium permanganate was said to cause the disease *timbilapho*. It seems the only way people can use pills safely, in healers' thinking, is for them to bring the pills to healers who can then mix the pills with traditional herbs.

At the same time, and in this atmosphere, healers also began to hear about and see what they regard as new STDs. They may have connected the proliferation of pills and the introduction of new diseases in their minds in a way that they became causally connected. And as with traditionally recognized STDs, the "hair of the dog that bit you" principle applied: the same medicine (in this case, pills) that caused the disease must also be used in its cure.

According to some of the healers we interviewed in 1992, they ask their clients to bring them the pills they are given at the hospital so that the healers can empower them, or use them in the proper way in the treatment of their clients' illnesses. That this happens even sometimes is further testimony to the faith many Swazis have in healers and their corresponding lack of faith in biomedical practitioners. There may be other ways healers obtain antibiotics. According to a pharmacist acquaintance of mine in Mbabane, traditional healers have asked him for "500" pills at the rate of about once a month since he opened his pharmacy in the mid-1980s. When he has refused on the ground that antibiotics can be sold only on prescription, the healers have sometimes become indignant and pointed out that they can buy these pills at bus stations and at the Mbabane market. (I have also heard that pharmacists will in fact sell antibiotics without a prescription.)

My pharmacist informant, a physician at a government hospital, and a member of the National AIDS Program all confirmed in conversation with me that ampicillin seems to be freely available without a prescription, that Swazis often take one or two of these before intercourse to avoid diseases, and that there is a great deal of resistance to both ampicillin and tetracycline. The physician told me that virtually 100 percent of her STD patients have already consulted traditional healers before consulting her. They often have multiple venereal infections,[6] and these often do not respond to either ampicillin or tetracycline.

In sum, some Swazi healers seem to be using at least ampicillin to treat certain illnesses in such a way as to increase resistance to commonly available and less-expensive antibiotics. This practice seems to have developed since the mid- or late 1980s. Further research is needed to demonstrate how widespread such use is and to supply details of the practice. It may be confined to healers practicing in periurban areas. Most of my 1992 interviews were conducted with healers practicing near towns or major roads in Hhohho and Manzini provinces. More than half were using antibiotics and the others reported knowing other healers who use such pills. Reasons for *not* using pills included: (1) not wanting to depend on something for treatment that may not always be available; (2) mixing pills with *timbita* (decoctions) "makes the *timbita* too strong;" and (3) using pills is not traditional, not the way healers were trained.

My purpose in reporting practices that are not in the interest of public health in Swaziland—practices that in fact indirectly facilitate the spread of HIV—is not to suggest that the full force of the law should be brought to bear on errant or unscrupulous healers. Repressive measures would simply drive healers further underground. Some more realistic ideas about what might be done regarding healers and antibiotics are presented in Chapter 5 in reference to Mozambique.

## Note on AIDS and Condoms

In 1992, I was not interviewing specifically about perceptions of AIDS, which was still a relatively new disease in Swaziland. However a master healer (*gobela*) I had known for twelve years made some unsolicited and revealing comments about both AIDS and condoms. She said that Swazis including traditional healers believe that AIDS is fictitious. It is a European plot to trick Swazis into using family-planning devices in order to reduce the size of their families. In reaction to this, "people are being defiant and they are being more promiscuous—they are having *more* sex." This healer, who always has between three and six healer-trainees (*ematfwasa*) studying under her, said she herself accepts that AIDS is a form of *gcunsula*. She noted that both diseases eat away at the genitals slowly. She also likened AIDS to the sorcery-induced condition *umklwepho*: both are slow acting and fatal. She went on to say that Swazi healers resent the fact that doctors have withheld the explanation of how AIDS is *made*. They would like to know "What did the first person who got AIDS *take*?" She said that until doctors are forthcoming about the *cause* of AIDS, healers will not disclose the cause of *likhubalo*, a disease which doctors cannot understand let alone treat.

She complained that white South Africans have come to the Ezulweni Valley (an area of hotels, casinos, and prostitutes). They sleep with local girls, then disappear, leaving a note revealing that they have AIDS. They may leave money for the girl, "to pay for her coffin, because she might die at any moment." Moreover, with the arrival of AIDS, people are experimenting with all kinds of new things, such as taking pills. At this point I asked whether a condom can prevent the diseases we had been discussing. She said yes, *idrop, cauliflower,* and even *likhubalo* can be prevented because diseases are passed by sperm. If it is the woman who has—or is carrying—the disease, the man absorbs her fluids from *her* ejaculation and thus gets the disease.

## Swazi Attitudes Toward Contraceptives

A recent study of male and female attitudes toward modern contraception revealed the following constraints in the course of male and female focus group discussions (McLean 1990). Many of these are typical throughout Africa (cf. Lamptey and Goodridge 1991):

- family planning will emasculate Swazi culture; white culture will predominate;
- contraceptives actually cause STDs;
- both oral contraceptives and condoms weaken or kill babies in the womb;
- condoms burst and can threaten woman's life;
- it is immoral to discharge semen in a "container" or "over oneself";
- condoms leads to sterility, impotence;
- condoms are associated with prostitution and promiscuity—in any case, they are used only for extramarital sex;
- condoms diminish sexual pleasure;
- condoms are a psychological barrier to intercourse, partly due to the interruption of foreplay when putting a condom on;
- even if a man wants to use a condom, his partner might be insulted by doing so;
- men said they were not ready to pay for condoms. Some said if men had to pay for them, they'd use them more than once.

If men in these focus groups are to be believed, they worry a lot about the effect of contraception on the health of women. If any advantages to condoms were noted (and usually none were), it was that they prevent disease rather than prevent pregnancy. There was also a lot of ignorance and misinformation about proper use of condoms, their side effects, and related topics. Many men got first-hand information about condoms only when they were treated for STDs at clinics. Radio broadcasts from the national Family Life Association of Swaziland (FLAS) was another accurate source mentioned.

Among female attitudes and general constraints to contraceptive use were:

- women were generally afraid of the health side effects of contraceptives;
- there is often opposition to contraceptives by the woman's partner;
- family and lineage expectations are such that Swazi women must prove their fertility before considering contraception;
- oral contraceptives destroy the uterus, causing sterility. They also cause side effects such as vaginal wetness as well as gain or loss of weight, birth defects, etc. (An experienced Swazi nurse told me that Swazi men feel threatened to the point of impotence when they find their partners overlubricated during intercourse. The fear is that the woman has been unfaithful. "Orals" can cause women to oversecrete, and both spermicides and lubricated condoms can also have the effect of excessive vaginal lubrication);
- condoms can burst and stay lodged in the vagina. IUDs circulate around the body in the bloodstream and can kill an unborn child.

Many expressed religious opposition, sometimes observing that contraception is associated with promiscuity. Swaziland seems to currently be undergoing a wave of Christian fundamentalist revivalism, evidence of which can be found in prayer services that are held in government offices around the country. It was not clear in 1992 which sects or denominations were ascendant, but it appeared that evangelical churches such as Jehovah's Witnesses and Church of Jesus Christ of Latter Day Saints had recently intensified proselytization and evangelical efforts through importation of foreign missionaries. Some indigenous evangelical churches such as the Zionist Christian Church drink a sacramental "tea" believed to neutralize birth control pills if they are taken, so adherents are advised to avoid them. I do not know what position, if any, the far larger Apostolic Zionist and Jerico sects take on contraception. However, two Jerico "prophets" who treat indigenous STDs expressed negative attitudes toward oral contraceptives when I interviewed them.

## The Traditional Healers Organization and Condoms

Although not all Swazi healers belong to the Traditional Healers Organization (THO), it is the only such national-level organization. The Ministry of Health as well as nongovernmental organizations such as the Family Life Association of Swaziland and Project Hope have worked collaboratively with the THO since the early 1980s in areas such as diarrheal disease, breastfeeding, referrals for child immunizations, and AIDS/STDs. THO has a network of 8 "field officers" and 200 "senior promoters" who have been trained in AIDS and related topics under Project Hope. One controversial aspect of this organization is that field officers are not themselves traditional healers.

In interviews with the THO president in 1991—in connection with a proposed family-planning project that in the end was not approved by the government—I learned that THO had been opposed to the use of condoms for any reason prior to the workshops on AIDS organized by Project Hope. Since these workshops, THO has come to endorse the use of condoms for disease prevention. Some of the rank-and-file of the organization have even begun to distribute condoms, as have a few healers outside THO. However, at the time of project design in 1991, Swazi healers remained at least formally opposed to use of condoms for family planning. However, the THO president believed that if healers were "properly trained in family planning," they could be expected to endorse the use of condoms for contraception.

Although THO as an organization was interested in receiving training in family planning, its president cautioned that healers did not want simply to become "condom sellers." He had publicly criticized what he referred to as the "dumping" of condoms in toilet vending machines, hotels and shops, commenting that this amounts to license for teenagers to engage in sex. (Many Christian leaders in Swaziland support this view.) He also criticized MAN TALK's seemingly haphazard manner of simply supplying condoms to people[7] before they have had what he called proper education in their use. He claimed that the "nation's elders" were offended that they had not been consulted. In fact, some men in Swazi regiments (*emabutfo*) were said to be singing anticondom songs. Satiric songs of current topical interest are often sung by regiments during the discharge of royal duties; these may reflect or influence popular sentiment.

After several meetings with me and others on the project design team, the THO president concluded that traditional healers were prepared to provide their clients with a comprehensive consultation on either child spacing or AIDS/STD prevention. As part—but only part—of such a consultation, the healer could sell or give the client a strip of condoms. The president felt that a healer would also be willing to refer a client to a hospital to obtain hormonal contraceptives for his partner if the client shows resistance to using condoms himself. To provide such a consultation, healers would need additional training in family planning, one that teaches about the full range of available contraceptive methods.

As noted, the proposed family-planning project was not approved by the Swazi government, or at least not in time for USAID funding. As of this writing THO continues to promote condoms for AIDS and STD prevention, but is not formally involved in "modern" family-planning efforts.

I have made no formal recommendations to the Swaziland government or to USAID in Swaziland concerning STDs or AIDS. My research in the early 1980s was incidental to my work in primary health care and that in 1992 took place because I was in the region and I wished to update and expand my earlier findings. However, my general conclusions are that: (1) STDs must be controlled in order to limit the spread of HIV infection; and (2) this is not possible without developing—or expanding—collaborative programs and involving traditional healers who already see and treat most STD cases. Indeed, to ignore healers is to turn a blind eye to their role in spreading antimicrobial resistance through apparent misuse of oral antibiotics.

Yet many biomedical practitioners would prefer to ignore traditional healers. Before leaving Swaziland in December 1992, I discussed my findings and recommendations with an expatriate doctor at a government hospital. She agreed with all my premises and in fact was the same doctor who told me that virtually 100 percent of her STD patients have already consulted traditional healers before consulting doctors. Yet she disagreed with the notion of training healers—even in condom promotion. Her preferred solution was health education for the general public. Later in this conversation she lamented how superstitious and unscientific people still are in her European country of origin, because they still consult alternative healers and believe in astrology. I asked the obvious question: how much impact has many generations of scientific and health education had there? How many generations and how many AIDS deaths will it take for Swazis to reach even this level of public sophistication about science?

## Notes

1. A part of this chapter represents an update and expansion of material that appeared in Green, E. C., and Lydia Makhubu, "Traditional Healers in Swaziland: Toward Improved Cooperation Between the Traditional and Modern Health Sectors," *Social Science and Medicine*, Vol. 18:12, p. 1071–74, 1984.

2. Bryant (1909) describes this disease among the Zulu and equates it with syphilis.

3. With ingredients like these, I thought it wouldn't surprise Swazi healers to learn that medical science's most effective drug for AIDS, namely AZT, comes from herring sperm. When I told one healer this, her only questions were where does one find this fish, and how does one tell a male from a female?

4. Healers themselves sometimes describe this code as a way to protect themselves from retribution from those who believe themselves victimized by healers.

5. In this regard, one healer explained that except for the long-lasting *imbune* medicine, a couple must drink decoctions together more than once to ensure each other's fidelity.

6. Several healers mentioned that if a person has one (indigenous) STD, he may develop symptoms of another STD.

7. This refers to a contraceptive social marketing program in Swaziland started by an indigenous Health Maintenance Organization.

# 4

# STDs and AIDS in Liberia[1]

**Background to Study**

I had the opportunity to design and supervise a study of STDs and AIDS in Liberia in 1988 when I was working on an AID "centrally funded" or global family-planning social-marketing project known as SOMARC (Social Marketing for Change). The SOMARC project had been successful in using existing private-sector channels to promote contraceptives in developing countries, and with the exponential growth in HIV seropositivity in Africa we were interested in learning how to promote condoms to limit this growth. At the time, I had recently completed an evaluation of an effective and innovative AIDS prevention/condom promotion campaign in the Dominican Republic (Green and Conde 1988), where I had been managing a social-marketing program for family planning. The evaluation had stimulated my interest in finding new ways to intervene in the spread of AIDS.

HIV seropositivity in Liberia had not been accurately estimated at the time of this study, but preliminary serological surveys indicated that HIV-2 was already prevalent. Only two confirmed cases of AIDS (HIV-I) had been reported, although another sero-survey was in progress. The hope of Liberian health officials was that timely intervention could prevent the spread of the more life-threatening HIV-I. In our study, we tried to establish a preliminary information base for interventions to prevent HIV-I dissemination. In light of the importance of standard STDs in HIV transmission, there was considerable focus on ethnomedical beliefs and practices related to well-established STDs such as gonorrhea and chancroid.

Although an AIDS-related KAP survey had already been attempted in Liberia just prior to fieldwork for the present study (Spielberg 1987), it seemed to us that too little was known about patterns of knowledge, attitudes, and behavior related to AIDS and STDs to attempt to *measure* such patterns through survey methods. Instead we employed a mix of qualitative research methods, described in the next section. It should be noted that some six to seven months prior to the study (September 15–November 8, 1987) there had been an intensive AIDS education campaign broadcast by the Liberian Rural Communication Network. Five radio stations broadcast a total of 2,004 minutes of AIDS education during this period. Prior and subsequent to this effort, there had been a fairly regular supply of interviews and news-type programs related to AIDS on television and radio (Huntington 1988).

## Research Methods

Two qualitative data-gathering methods were used: focus group discussions (FGDs) with 53 participants, and key-informant interviews with 103 informants. "Discussants" and "informants" are referred to below to distinguish findings from FGDs and key-informant interviews respectively.

In the first procedure, there were eight focus groups divided on the basis of gender, rural/urban residence, and ethnic group (Kpelle or Kpelle-related versus Bassa or Bassa-related language groups). Urban discussants were selected from Monrovia; rural Kpelle were recruited from Bong county; and rural Bassa were recruited in the area of Buchanan's hinterland. I developed a topic guide, and my assistants pretested it in a practice FGD. All FGD moderators were Liberians with previous experience as moderators in focus groups, and all received further training from both myself and Dale Huntington, a FGD expert from Johns Hopkins University.

I also trained four experienced survey interviewers in key informant interviewing techniques. The key-informant interview schedule, which was open ended and fairly flexible, was pretested and modified prior to use. Basic frequency distributions were calculated for responses to open-ended questions, although since the sample was nonrandom, statistical findings could not be projected to geographically based or other naturally aggregated populations.

Key informants were chosen on the basis of their knowledge—and therefore their ability to shed light upon—both wider Liberian society and the particular subgroups they represented. The subgroups themselves were selected both because of their representative's special ability to provide insights into AIDS/STDs-related knowledge, attitudes, and practices, and because they may be potential conveyers of AIDS education information themselves and perhaps even distributors of condoms. There was selection emphasis on informants in the private and traditional sectors because they are socially and culturally "close" to the majority of Liberians and because their mobilization in anti-AIDS efforts (or their sanction of such efforts) cannot be taken for granted as might be the case with salaried government workers or members of modern-sector private voluntary organizations.

Key informants were selected among peripheral-level health workers (HWs) such as village health workers or MCH nurses; local political leaders (LLs) such as paramount chiefs, clan chiefs, or "town chiefs"; traditional healers (THs) including subtypes such as herbalists, "sandcutters," or diviner-mediums, and *zoes* or cult priests; religious and spiritual leaders (RLs) including Christian and Muslim faith healers; and urban prostitutes (the term sex workers is a less value-loaded term, but was not in general use at the time).[2] The characteristics of our key informants are summarized in Table 4.1. The mean age was 42.

A descriptive note about traditional healers is warranted. Liberia appears to offer the variety of indigenous health practitioners found in most parts of sub-Saharan Africa, such as herbalists, diviner-mediums ("sandcutters" in Liberia), cult priests (*zoes*), Christian and Muslim faith healers, as well as various specialists such as bonesetters. There are also untrained allopathic medicinal hucksters or injectionists, locally known as "black baggers," who give injections for STDs.

Both FGD discussants and key informants were located in a "snowball" technique that relied on the social networks of individuals in various informant categories. Care was taken not to bias the nonrandom sample by selecting in a way that skewed variables such as age, sex, or level of education. There was no overlap between the two groups of informants and discussants.

The findings derived from both methods are now presented. When

TABLE 4.1 Characteristics of Key Informants

| *Age Group* | *Health Worker* | | *Local Leader* | | *Traditional Healers* | | *Religious Leaders* | | *Prostitutes* | | *Total* |
|---|---|---|---|---|---|---|---|---|---|---|---|
| | *M* | *F* | *M* | *F* | *M* | *F* | *M* | *F* | *M* | *F* | |
| 15–19 | 0 | 0 | 0 | 0 | 0 | 0 | 0 | 0 | 0 | 4 | 4 |
| 20–24 | 1 | 1 | 0 | 0 | 0 | 0 | 0 | 0 | 0 | 8 | 10 |
| 25–29 | 1 | 3 | 0 | 0 | 1 | 0 | 4 | 0 | 0 | 4 | 13 |
| 30–34 | 3 | 1 | 1 | 0 | 2 | 0 | 4 | 1 | 0 | 2 | 14 |
| 35–39 | 3 | 2 | 0 | 0 | 2 | 0 | 3 | 1 | 0 | 2 | 13 |
| 40–44 | 1 | 1 | 2 | 0 | 1 | 0 | 2 | 1 | 0 | 0 | 7 |
| 45–49 | 0 | 1 | 3 | 0 | 3 | 0 | 2 | 1 | 0 | 0 | 10 |
| 50–54 | 0 | 1 | 5 | 0 | 4 | 0 | 0 | 0 | 0 | 0 | 10 |
| 55–59 | 0 | 0 | 4 | 0 | 3 | 1 | 1 | 0 | 0 | 0 | 9 |
| 60–64 | 1 | 0 | 1 | 0 | 2 | 0 | 0 | 0 | 0 | 0 | 4 |
| 65–69 | 1 | 0 | 4 | 0 | 0 | 0 | 0 | 2 | 0 | 0 | 7 |
| 70–74 | 0 | 0 | 0 | 0 | 0 | 0 | 0 | 0 | 0 | 0 | 0 |
| 75–79 | 0 | 0 | 2 | 0 | 0 | 0 | 1 | 0 | 0 | 0 | 3 |
| Total | 11 | 9 | 22 | 0 | 19 | 1 | 19 | 3 | 0 | 20 | 103 |

appropriate, note is made regarding agreement—or lack of such—between the two sources of information.

### Sexually Transmitted Diseases

Many diseases are thought to be sexually transmitted or transmissible, according to informants and FGD participants. Traditional healers alone offered some twenty-two names of diseases of this sort, and some of these had two or three subtypes. Both Western/scientific and indigenous names in English and African languages were given (English is the first and sometimes only language for a small percentage of Liberians). Gonorrhea was mentioned most frequently by key informants, followed by AIDS, syphilis, chancre, trichomonas, crab lice, and herpes. The following also received at least one mention by informants: hookworm, "displaced womb," "high malaria," jaundice, "weak spell," tuberculosis (*tobeh* in Kpelle), hernia, leprosy, piles (*kpogboi* in Mende), seizures, and stomach ache.

We encountered the belief common in Africa that diseases or other misfortune can be "sent" through sorcery or witchcraft—or "African science" as some informants describe it—and that sexual intercourse provides one common point of contact for the medicine or spell causing such diseases. As one traditional healer informant elaborated:

> A country doctor (traditional healer) cuts sands (i.e., performs divination) before he tells someone whether a disease is transmitted through sex only. Gonorrhea can be transmitted mostly through sex, but also through the air, through food we eat, through clothes, and in many other ways. For example, a headache can be contracted through sex. Why? Simply through African science. A man can go to a country doctor and say, "I want you to make any man who sleeps with my wife sick." After intercourse with the man's wife, the boyfriend will then start to complain about a headache, stomach ache or some other pain in his body and he will eventually die. Sometimes if such a person seeks treatment from a country doctor, the doctor will tell him to leave this man's wife alone, and that is the only way the boyfriend will get better. So you see, from having sex one can have different sicknesses, small as well as big sickness (paren. mine).

This healer went on to describe his own method of mystically divining whether a man contracts a sexually transmitted disease from his own wife or from another person's wife. It is in the latter case that witchcraft or sorcery is suspected. Women involved in non-sanctioned sex such as adultery might remain symptomless, but the male seducer is believed to become sick from the medicine or spell from the husband, and the symptoms might take the form of gonorrhea or another common STD. Variants of this theory of STDs can be found in other parts of Africa such as Ghana (Warren 1979:39), Zimbabwe (Gelfand et al. 1985), Botswana (Ingstad 1990:34), Swaziland (Chapter 3), Mozambique (Chapter 5), and South Africa (Chapter 7). Common to these societies is the belief that transgression of social norms, as in adultery, provokes mystical punishment either by means of sorcery or retribution from ancestor spirits.

### *Gonorrhea*

A disease with gonorrhea-like symptoms is locally recognized. In Bassa or Kpelle it is known as *kanyan, kianyan* or *porkay*; in Mende as *kainyen*; in Kissi as *korseena* or possibly *esiagwen*; in Vai as *gwanma jede* or *khanyan*; in English slang as "gon" or "gun." (No standard orthography is used in renderings of Liberian disease names; spellings are given as interviewers wrote them.) It is not possible at this stage of research to know the extent to which indigenous and scientific nosological categories actually correspond. For example, it is quite possible that nongonococcal urinary tract infections and perhaps other scientifically recognized diseases are lumped together with gonorrhea under an indigenous African disease name.

Informants and participants believed gonorrhea-like illness to be the most common sexually transmitted disease. It is known primarily by the symptoms of painful, burning or difficult urination, and a yellowish or milky pus discharge. Symptoms mentioned less frequently by informants include "itch inside the penis," "red urine" or blood in the urine, swollen penis or pain in the genital region, stomach pain in the woman, and eye problems in babies of an infected person.

As might be expected, traditional healers tended to have more to say about these diseases than lay informants or discussants. Some healers described two or three major subtypes of *kanyan,* which may represent different stages of gonorrhea if it is left untreated. The subtypes are regular or ordinary *kanyan,* which is not very painful and is characterized by a whitish discharge; yellow *kanyan* which is far more painful and is characterized by yellowish discharge and genital rash; and "bloody *kanyan,*" the most serious type, characterized by blood in the man's or woman's urine as well as swollen genitals and/or genital sores. The last type was said to sometimes result in death. (Blood in urine is not a clinical manifestation of gonorrhea.)

Gonorrhea was believed to result from having sex with a person who has the disease, or an "unclean" person, a "stranger," or a prostitute. It may also result from "strenuous sex." Some healers observed that men or women who "sleep around" with many sexual partners are more likely to have the disease. Gonorrhea was also said to result from contact (usually through feet) with urine or "itchy urine" from an infected person or dog (fully 25 percent of key informants mentioned this); from "bad breezes" (reflecting a fairly widespread African view that disease may be spread by vapors or by winds carrying destructive medicines or spells); from dirty toilets, underclothing or towels; from "not minding one's own business"; and from masturbation. Gonorrhea was also attributed to sorcery; for example, a jealous woman might "throw" the disease against a co-wife to make the husband avoid the co-wife. Many of these causal theories were found to apply to other STDs as well as to gonorrhea. Table 4.2 summarizes the more common theories mentioned by key informants.

"Promiscuity" or having numerous sex partners was thought to cause or at least contribute to the spread of a number of locally recognized STDs. Some informants and FGD participants referred to sex with "infected" people as well as "protected" women. Although these terms were used in the government-sponsored AIDS education radio campaign (IIR 1987), they usually had different connotations when used by informants. For example, protection usually referred to medicines and amulets believed to ensure fidelity, not to condoms or abstinence. And in elaborations by traditional healer informants, a woman's fallopian tubes were said to become blocked by "infected sperm," or a "worm" was said to get into a man's urethra after sex with an infected woman. A cure for gonorrhea relating to the worm etiology is for an "infected" man to have sex with a virgin, because the worm is thought to be killed when it comes up forcibly against an intact hymen. This finding has obvious public health implications.

Some traditional healers used separate disease names such as *esiagwen* or *alornu* to distinguish a gonorrhea-related condition that only women suffer from. One healer said this of *esiagwen*:

> It prevents pregnancy (and) causes the tubes to be blocked due to infected sperm which accumulates in the tubes over a period of time. This may not

TABLE 4.2 Causes of STDs According to Key Informants

| | *Health Personnel*[1] | *Local Leader* | *Tradit. Healers* | *Relig. Leaders* | *Prostitutes* | *Total* |
|---|---|---|---|---|---|---|
| Promiscuity | 9 | 10 | 7 | 13 | 7 | 46 |
| Stepping in infected urine | 2 | 4 | 7 | 6 | – | 25 |
| Sex with infected persons | 3 | 7 | 6 | 3 | 4 | 23 |
| Witchcraft, sorcery | 1 | 5 | 4 | 1 | 3 | 13 |
| Dirty towels, underclothing, etc. | 2 | 4 | – | 1 | 3 | 10 |

[1]includes village health workers

> be discovered early. The time of discovery varies from woman to woman. It can last undiscovered for up to five years. At this stage, it becomes difficult to cure. (Other symptoms are) chills and continuous abdominal pain.

Another healer, referring to *alornu,* also noted that sufferers are unable to conceive and that the disease is caused by having many sexual partners. Although difficult to cure, *alornu* was said to be treatable by traditional healers.

### *Other STDs*

In response to an open-ended question about diseases that can be transmitted by sexual intercourse, 35 out of 100 informants mentioned syphilis (*gbo* in Bassa; *mahun* in Fanti). Both informants and discussants provided information about the disease. Syphilis was said to be characterized by genital sores, patches on the skin, pus discharge, bumps on the body, "holes in the penis," and/or pain and swelling in the genital region. One healer said that only men suffer from this disease, that sufferers become sterile after two years, and that symptoms are not easily noticed. In fact "this disease causes no pain until after . . . five to six years. . . ." He went on to say that men with *mahun* pass the disease to a woman as *esiagwen* (i.e., gonorrhea symptoms).

Another locally recognized STD that may correspond to chancroid is *bubos* or blue ball(s) in English slang; as *kpo* in Bassa; or as *gbele* in Mende. It is described as a single, prominent, painful boil in the genital region that becomes very hard and solid a few days after appearing. Men were said to catch it from women, and vice-versa. It may be caused by "a mixture of different sperms," from sex with older men, or from stepping on infected urine.

A disease mentioned by several traditional healers ("tear-tear" in English; *meleemate* in Kissi) was said to "eat away" the genitals, or make them "disappear." One healer called this disease *porkay* (see above), but rather than characterizing it with symptoms usually identified with gonorrhea, he claimed that with this disease, "All of the penis and vagina are eaten up by maggots. One has to keep the (genital) area covered because when a breeze blows on the affected area, it becomes worse. People die instantly from this."

Those thought to be at most risk of contracting an STD include sexually active men and women, especially in urban areas, and those with multiple partners such as prostitutes. Some informants thought that everyone is at risk for STDs, noting that innocent babies can be born with eye infections if the mother has gonorrhea. Rural Liberians tended to think of STDs as primarily urban diseases, with rural people being at less risk than urban dwellers. Some FGD participants regarded pregnant women as being at special risk, which may be related to the fact that such women are more likely to visit clinics and therefore to be examined and diagnosed.

## AIDS

AIDS was mentioned spontaneously as a sexually transmitted disease by 40 out of 103 key informants, and it was discussed in all FGDs, either because it arose spontaneously in connection with discussion of STDs or because the topic was prompted. Almost all informants had heard of AIDS, which was identified as a new disease and one that was not thought to be common in Liberia. Some referred to AIDS as "the killer disease." Kpelle speakers referred to it as *fair-ank'bah*, meaning "until I kill it"; it was known as *ah-munehun* in Kru; and some Fantis were calling it African Kimping.

Information about AIDS was reported to derive primarily from radio. Allowing multiple responses, 78 out of 100 informants cited radio as a primary source of information; 51 cited television; and 30 cited friends or other individuals conveying information personally. Findings among FGD participants were similar, although some urban participants also mentioned schools, books, and magazines as sources of information. The three main messages about AIDS that seem to have been retained by both informants and discussants are that "it kills easily," "there is no cure for it," and "it is transmitted through sex." These three messages were, in fact, emphasized in the recent AIDs education radio campaign in Liberia (IIR 1987). A fourth message stressed by the campaign, namely that AIDS can be prevented, seems not to have been understood or retained as easily as the others.

Other characteristics of AIDS mentioned less often were that it is transmitted by blood contact or by homosexuals, that it has to do with a weak immune system, that it originated in Africa or America, or that it is contracted from animals.

Symptoms associated with AIDS were weight loss ("becoming thinner every day"), diarrhea, and fever. Most traditional healers reported they knew little or nothing about AIDS, including those who had a lot to say about other STDs that are well established in Liberia. However, a few healers, prostitutes, and others expressed the belief that Liberians can and do cast spells in the form of AIDS sickness on their enemies. Thus, it appears that some Liberians are beginning to view the new disease in frameworks of interpretation compatible with traditional ethnomedical beliefs. It is possible that such views are more widespread than research findings indicate because throughout Africa, people in formal discussion contexts are often reluctant to express views that they feel may be ridiculed by interviewers.

TABLE 4.3 Messages Key Informants Heard About AIDS

| | *Health Personnel*[1] | *Local Leader* | *Tradit. Healers* | *Relig. Leaders* | *Prostitutes* | *Total* |
|---|---|---|---|---|---|---|
| Kills easily | 6 | 14 | 5 | 8 | 9 | 42 |
| Has no cure | 8 | 9 | 3 | 9 | – | 29 |
| Transmitted through sex | 4 | 1 | 5 | – | 4 | 14 |
| Transmitted by blood contact | 4 | 1 | – | 3 | 1 | 9 |
| Transmitted by homosexuals | 3 | – | 4 | 1 | – | 8 |
| Weakens immune system | 2 | 1 | – | 2 | – | 5 |
| Originated in Africa | 1 | – | – | 2 | 1 | 4 |
| Contacted from animals | – | – | 1 | – | – | 1 |

[1]includes village health workers

AIDS was said to result primarily from promiscuity or having many sexual partners, from punishment by God, from prostitution, from homosexual practices, and from sexual or other contact with animals that have the disease. Less frequently mentioned by informants as causal agents were sinners, Europeans or whites, baboons or other monkeys, witchcraft/sorcery, nuclear or atomic waste, or mulattoes or albinos. (The notion of sex with monkeys may reflect scientific discussion at the time that linked HIV with SIV, the latter found in Central African green monkeys.) When asked specifically about modes of transmission, informants mentioned sexual intercourse (seventy-seven mentions), followed by contaminated or dirty needles, blood transfusion, kissing or hugging, sharing cups or eating utensils, and having sex with animals.

It is interesting to note, especially among FGD participants, that quite different reasons were given for the presence of the disease and for specific modes of transmission. Its presence related to God's will, to sexual contact with animals (i.e., with a notion of sinful or abhorrent behavior, whether or not such behavior has ever occurred), and with sorcery or witchcraft; while transmission modes resembled the scientific explanations promoted by health educators. It is common in Africa to make a distinction between the ultimate and the more immediate cause of an illness; in fact this can help reconcile traditional belief systems with scientific explanations taught in school and broadcast through mass media, as in the case of the recent AIDS education radio campaign in Liberia.

As Gluckman (1956) has observed about African traditional thought, every misfortune involves two questions: *how* it happened, and *why* it occurred at all. The "how" question is answered by common-sense empirical observation. In the case of a new disease like AIDS, Liberians seem prepared to accept the radio campaign proposition that person A can catch the disease from person B through sexual intercourse. But even scientific explanation cannot fully—certainly not simply—explain why this disease transmission does not always occur, that is, does not occur in every case of intercourse between an infected and an uninfected person. Thus, the "why" or "why a particular person" question arises.

Religion, witchcraft, and sorcery provide theories of ultimate causation that can explain the "whys" of even a new disease like AIDS; the idea that AIDS is God's punishment is such an explanation, as is the notion that enemies cast a spell ("throw AIDS") on a victim. Such dualistic thinking about causation must be kept in mind by AIDS educators and researchers who might encounter survey evidence showing that samples of Africans and others, for example, Americans "score" much the same on a survey question about the causes of AIDS. This should not be taken as evidence that Africans and Americans understand the disease in the same way.

Informants and FGD participants believed prostitutes to be at greatest risk of getting AIDS, since they have sexual contact with "strangers" and foreigners. Homosexuals, heterosexual adults with many sexual partners, and "grow-now" girls and boys (slang for sexually active teenagers) were also thought to be at risk.

Regarding treatment for AIDS, most believed that the disease has no cure. It is noteworthy that traditional healers shared this view, and that no healer claimed to have medicine for AIDS. Most informants and participants spoke of consulting a doctor for diagnosis and perhaps advice about the disease, but few believed that doctors could provide effective treatment. Several informants said they would simply pray and wait for death if they had AIDS. Some thought people would change their behavior if they knew they had AIDS, mostly by stopping or reducing sexual activity. Only four informants volunteered the belief that some AIDS victims would begin to use condoms. Most participants and informants thought that a majority of people with AIDS would tell no one about the disease and would continue to spread it, either because of carelessness, hopelessness, or—in the view of some—revenge or some other motive that would make someone spread AIDS intentionally. Although such statements were almost always about what *other* people would do, one prostitute key informant said she herself would "get revenge" by giving the disease to her clients.

In focus group discussions about possible behavior change resulting from awareness about, or fear of, AIDS, some male participants thought that Liberians might now be more likely to confine intercourse to a single partner and that some will be more careful in the selection of new part-

TABLE 4.4 Informant-Designated Methods of AIDS Prevention

| | *Health Personnel*[1] | *Local Leader* | *Tradit. Healers* | *Relig. Leaders* | *Prostitutes* | *Total* |
|---|---|---|---|---|---|---|
| Sticking to one partner | 13 | 17 | – | – | 10 | 30 |
| Sex only with known partners | 2 | 6 | 7 | 10 | 1 | 26 |
| Use condoms | 6 | – | 1 | 2 | – | 12 |
| Don't eat monkey meat | – | – | 1 | 2 | 4 | 7 |
| Regular medical check-up | 2 | – | – | 3 | 1 | 6 |
| Avoid unclean toilets | 5 | – | – | – | – | 5 |
| Pray | – | – | 2 | – | – | 2 |
| Traditional mark | – | – | 1 | – | – | 1 |

[1]includes village health workers

ners. But the predominant perception was that most Liberians have not changed their behavior because the disease was not thought to actually exist in the country, or because of fatalistic notions. Regarding the latter, one discussant commented, "Man dies but once."

When asked about prevention of AIDS, a slight majority of informants mentioned confining relations to a single or a known partner, as illustrated in Table 4.4. Among the principal messages of the recent AIDS education radio campaign in Liberia were that AIDS is preventable and that sticking to one partner, along with regular condom use, are ways to prevent AIDS. In spite of this, we see once again that condom use was rarely mentioned, except by health workers.

## Prevention of STDs and AIDS

Ideas about preventing STDs were found to relate directly to theories of disease causation, not surprisingly. For example most of the 25 percent of key informants who attributed gonorrhea to stepping in infected urine recommended wearing footwear to protect against contact with urine. An informant who attributed STDs to sorcery believed there was no way to prevent such diseases "because no one knows who hates him" and therefore might attempt sorcery. Yet others who shared this theory of causation believed a "tribal mark on the back," magical amulets or protective medicines could prevent STDs.

When asked about possible ways to prevent AIDS, 41 percent of key informants mentioned restricting sexual activity to single partner, followed by limiting intercourse to only known and trusted partners, using condoms (twelve citations by key informants, six of them health workers), avoiding monkey meat, having a regular medical check-up, and avoiding unclean toilets. With the exception of health workers, there was little spontaneous mention of condoms in connection with AIDS prevention. Or, if condoms were mentioned, they were generally not ranked first or as one of the more effective preventive means.

When prompted to think about condoms in association with AIDS prevention, 47 percent of informants (or only 35 percent if health workers are excluded) said they thought condoms could be effective in protecting a partner from either receiving or giving AIDS during sexual intercourse. Thirty-five informants deemed condoms ineffective. However, fifty-nine informants thought condom use would increase in the future, largely because of concern about AIDS and other STDs but also because of family planning. Findings from FGDs were similar: once the AIDS/condom association was prompted, many participants guessed that more people will use condoms in the future in order to avoid AIDS, in accordance with advice broadcast by radio. Although women were far less informed about condoms than men, many female FGD participants seemed supportive of condom use to protect against STDs and AIDS.

The topic of whether or not there should be mass media education or advertisement about condoms arose in the FGDs. Women generally supported condom education and advertising, while men were generally opposed—rural men strongly so. Those opposed thought that sexual self-control was preferable to condom use, and made comments to the effect that condoms are unnatural and unaffordable to some. Supporters tended to think that the disease prevention function of condoms should be stressed more than their contraceptive function. Some urban male participants thought that discussing both condom functions would be confusing.

## Sexual Behavior

As Barton (1988a:1) has noted, "Current events in Africa surrounding the occurrence and spread of AIDS have brought into the foreground many issues of sexuality and sexually related behaviors that have previously received insufficient attention by the scholarly community." Although there is a fairly substantial body of medical literature related to STDs in Africa, there is surprisingly little reliable information relating to social and behavioral aspects of STDs, perhaps especially to sexual behavior (O'Reilly 1986; Brokensha 1988; Mann et al. 1988:85–86). In the nineteenth century there were a number of highly ethnocentric, sensational, moralizing accounts of "native" sexual behavior written by explorers, adventurers, missionaries, and amateur anthropologists whose intent was to shock and perhaps titillate the reader, or to show that Africans were "oversexed" or lacking in moral restraint. Typical is this account of the Masai in the 1880s:

> Life in the warriors' kraal, as may easily be conceived, was promiscuous in a remarkable degree. They may, indeed, be described as a colony of free lovers ... no one confined his or her attentions to one only. Each girl, in fact, had several sweethearts, and, what is still stranger, this seemed to give rise to no jealousies ... in their savage circumstances it was really pleasant to see how common it was for a young girl to wander about the camp with her arm round the waist of a stalwart warrior (Thomson 1887).

In later years, trained anthropologists sometimes seemed equally intent on countering the effect of such accounts. In the 1950s Gluckman observed of the Zulu:

> ... old records on the Zulu ... indeed affirm that they were a 'moral' people among whom divorce, adultery, and illegitimacy were rare. Chastity was highly valued, and was part of the ethical code enforced by the age-set regimental organization which was directly under the king. Regiments could only begin to marry when the king gave them permission as a set to marry a younger age-set of girls, who by this time would be well in their twenties (Gluckman 1958:181).

Of course, differences by ethnolinguistic group are found in sexual and other behavior. In his same report, Gluckman says this of the Lozi of (former) Rhodesia, who are related to the Zulu as southern Bantu speakers:

> ... early travellers to Loziland, and every missionary and administrative record, describe men and women as promiscuous and marriage as unstable.... Texts, life-histories of old men, and genealogies, confirm this.... Seduction, adultery, and abduction of wives were undoubtedly rife.... Adulteries, divorces, and abductions did not come to court at the capital until 1918–20, when the paramount chief issued an edict saying that his court would hear these cases. To-day it does little else.

By and large, anthropologists have been reluctant to formally report details of sexual behavior of the African peoples they study in part because they fear accusations of prurient interest (Barton 1988a:2–3) or violation of the trust that typically is established over the course of long-term ethnographic research. Pellow (1990:71) notes, "For a Western (white) social scientist to write on the topic opens the door to charges of voyeurism and prurience, even racism." A perusal of professional anthropological writings regarding sexual behavior shows that most of it focuses on marriage rules including polygamy, the stability of marriage, adultery, beliefs regarding sexual intercourse with spirits, the teaching and learning of norms regarding sexual intercourse, sexual discovery among adolescents, courtship behavior, beliefs associated with the magic potency of sex, control of female sexual behavior through infibulation, popular and ritual expressions of obscenity in song, dance, etc. There is evidence of multiple sexual partners and high frequency of extramarital relations in some societies (see below), but little reliable evidence on non-standard practices relevant to AIDS etiology such as homosexuality or anal intercourse.

Since the outbreak of AIDS and subsequent intense speculation over the African origin of the disease, Africans have understandably become very sensitive to what they perceive as treatment by foreigners amounting to "blaming the victim," unfair discrimination against overseas Africans proven or assumed to be HIV-positive, and unwarranted Western interest in, and hypercritical condemnation of, African sexual behavior. Further exacerbating the situation is the widespread belief among Africans—including some Liberians, as found in the present study—that AIDS originated in the West, and then spread to Africa, not the other way around as most Westerners seem to believe (Waite 1988:154). The association of AIDS with sexual deviance and promiscuity, as well as intravenous drug abuse, further heightens African sensitivities. Thus we face a situation in which there is an unprecedented need for accurate, reliable, and objective information on sexual behavior in Africa—and elsewhere where AIDS is prevalent—in order to find ways to break the cycle of AIDS transmission, yet sensitivities have perhaps never been higher about research in this area, particularly if conducted by Westerners.

It should be noted at the outset that based on admittedly limited information, the current consensus is that homosexual activity, anal intercourse of any kind, and intravenous drug use seem to account for only a small amount of AIDS transmission in Africa, especially when compared to the United States and Europe (Biggar 1986; Imperato 1986; Quinn 1987:288; Brokensha 1988; Piot and Harris 1990:10–15). In an anthropological review, Hrdy (1987: 1113), citing Murdock 1959 and Textor 1967 who have drawn conclusions from reviewing the Human Relations Area Files[3] summarizes the question of homosexuality:

> Homosexuality is not part of traditional societies in sub-Saharan Africa. The few instances of homosexuality noted are related to societal institu-

> tions where an older man has authority over younger males.... Homosexuality probably also exists to some extent in migrant labor camps, where few women are present. These anecdotal accounts do not indicate widespread homosexuality like that which seems to occur in some societies. Nowhere in traditional African society is there the kind of sequential homosexual activity between men that is found in urban Western societies.... It is likely that, as elsewhere in the world, there are pockets of homosexuality in Africa, but homosexuality does not seem to be practiced as overtly and commonly as in other parts of the world.

Pellow (1990), reviewing the research of Moodie and Beinart (1988), describes male homosexual behavior in the South African gold mines where men live in close quarters and isolation from women. Stable relationships develop between senior men and teenage boys that exhibit aspects of marriage, with the "wives" carrying out domestic chores and being supported financially by "husbands." Sexual intercourse tended to consist of nonpenetrative "thigh sex." However, there are also accounts of anal rape and seduction of boys in the mines, described poignantly in the autobiography *Kaffir Boy* (and see Beinart 1987). My own findings from South African healers tend to confirm the foregoing conclusions.

In a review of evidence of heterosexual anal sex in Africa, Hrdy (1987:1113–1114) concluded that the practice seems to occur predominantly in certain Muslim areas where infibulation is found, but in any case is relatively rare. However, some recent studies suggest that male/female anal intercourse may be quite common among certain groups in certain areas, such as commercial sex workers along a major truck route in Tanzania. Some sex workers were found to offer anal intercourse as an alternative during their menstrual periods. Others were offered more money by truck drivers who preferred anal sex, or perhaps they were simply forced (O'Connor, Leshabari, and Lwihula 1992).

Nevertheless, if African sexual behavior is broadly compared with that of Western Europeans and Americans, it appears to be more conventional in the sense that practices other than heterosexual vaginal intercourse are almost certainly less common in Africa. And although there are allegations of "promiscuity" among certain categories of African males, such as middle- and upper-class urban dwellers or geographically mobile truck drivers, the actual number of sexual contacts may be no greater—and may actually be fewer—than the number of contacts and partners of certain categories of Westerners, for example those belonging to mate-swapping associations.

Still, the Western image of the hyper-sexed African male persists. In a recent review of the epidemiology of AIDS in "Third World countries," Meheus and De Schryver (1991:202), citing references to Africa but no evidence regarding sexual behavior, observe that the pattern of HIV transmission is different from "Western countries" due to "level of sexual activity, not sexual orientation. . . ." They cite the association between STDs and HIV transmission as a secondary risk factor.

In Barton's essay summarizing findings in an annotated bibliography on Sexuality and Health in Sub-Saharan Africa, evidence of sexual mobility or "poly partnerism" is acknowledged, but not without explanation. He notes that Western, colonial impact on Africa led to labor migration, disruption of sex education for adolescents, changed bridewealth patterns, increased age of marriage for men, and decline in polygamy among peoples who practiced periods of pre- and postnatal sexual abstinence. "The various delaying and destabilizing influences on marriage and the numbers of women abstaining at any given time have all contributed to forms of rural poly partnerism, including 'prostitution' conducted either for barter or cash" (Barton 1989:9). The destabilizing effect of labor migration on marriage and its contribution to the spread of STDs appears to have been recognized at least a half-century ago (Furnivall 1948:356).

In his review of sexual behavior in sub-Saharan Africa, O'Reilly (1986:47) notes that although there is great intercultural variation, "Age at first intercourse is earlier in Africa than America, with over a third of African women reporting sexual activity by age 14, and 90 percent by age 17 . . . (moreover) premarital sexual activity is high." Rapid population growth has combined with labor migration patterns to result in certain demographic and health patterns characteristic of Africa:

> Current population growth in Africa has skewed the population towards the young, there has been rural to urban migration, and there are skewed sex ratios with many more men in cities: all of these factors predispose to STD. The high prevalence of untreated STD, resulting in increased infertility acts paradoxically to increase rather than decrease the fertility in Africa. Infertility is devastating for an African woman, resulting in divorce and diminished social status that often leads to prostitution (O'Reilly 1986:47).

Biggar (1991) also makes the point that the services of prostitutes are in great demand in African cities where young men greatly outnumber young women. As Caldwell et al. (1993:4) point out, most of these cities are in East and Southern Africa. They find it not coincidental that the two West African cities with high male-to-female sex ratios, Abidjan and Dakar, happen to also have HIV levels that are unusually high for West Africa (they do not discuss the possible role of male circumcision).

Caldwell, Caldwell, and Quiggen (1989, 1991), in their review of anthropological and related literature, suggest a pattern of sexual permissiveness in sub-Saharan Africa due to a relative lack of moral and institutional constraints on sexual practices, particularly in women. However Le Blanc, Meintel, and Piche (1991:501) take issue with this conclusion:

> They (Caldwell et al.) imply that sexual promiscuity, particularly among women, is the norm in Africa, and that "lack of control" of women's sexuality is the key to the AIDS epidemic in that region. It is our view that, in fact, the sexual behavior of women is subject to a great deal of social regulation and that norms are highly variable from one African society to another.

I too have found evidence of a great deal of social regulation of (especially) female sexual behavior, both in my own research and in the literature. However, economic, population, migration, and other factors seem to have led to a weakening of such regulation. As Le Blanc, Meintel and Piche (1991:502) themselves note, "Many ethnographic studies point to stricter norms about sexuality, particularly female sexuality, in the past than at present." Most traditional healers interviewed for this book who commented on the issue—spontaneously or in response to a question—agree that there has been an erosion of what they describe as morality in the past few generations, and that this has led to increased sexual permissiveness. To account for the new permissiveness, some healers, such as those in South Africa, pointed to factors such as "Western lifestyle" and its promotion of womens' freedom; neglect of traditional culture; poverty or "lack of financial security"; overcrowding in housing; alcoholism and erosion of traditional healers' moral authority due to church influence, apartheid, and exclusion from government health programs (Green, Zokwe, and Dupree 1992:64–65).

### *Prostitution*

Being a prostitute or engaging in intercourse with a prostitute are both known risk factors in the spread of AIDS in Africa (Quinn 1987:287), however there is disagreement over the magnitude of this risk (Ward and Day 1991). Prostitution in Africa has not been well researched scientifically and therefore it is not well understood. Since AIDS became a recognized health problem in Africa, there has been considerable focus on African commercial sex, much of it ethnocentric and based on the assumption that patterns in Africa are variants of European or American prostitution. David Brokensha has noted that the term prostitution is often used loosely and inaccurately by Westerners in reference to Africa and that "Western cultural stereotypes and moral judgments can also present a problem in analysis" (Brokensha 1988:169). He further observes:

> Unquestionably, each large city, and many small towns (even some villages) has a group of "professional" prostitutes who earn their income in this way. But many other women "exchange sexual services" to augment their income, or to meet special needs. Sometimes women are steady

> partners of one man, referred to as "spares" (Zimbabwe), "meanwhilers" (Ghana) or "town wives" (West Africa). Variations of such relationships include forms of courtesanship in northern Nigeria among Hausa women who are generally uneducated, with few marketable skills, and hence few employment opportunities.

It is important to note that while women may be rewarded in cash or gifts for sexual favors, they are not necessarily prostitutes any more than would be the case with unemployed or lower-income single women in the West who are economically dependent on a succession of lovers (Brokensha 1988:169). However, in some areas women may engage in open, short-term, high-client-turnover exchange of sex for a standardized price, known as *wazi wazi* (open, nonhidden) prostitution in Kiswahili. For a variety of social, economic, and historical factors women of a certain ethnolinguistic group may develop partial monopolies of such business, for example the Haya in urban Tanzania (Kaijage 1989). In a recent ethnographic study of East African truck drivers and their sexual partners, the authors identified seven categories of women who may engage in some form of commercial sex, ranging from "brothel girls" to bar maids and lodge attendants, free-lance sex workers, traditional beer sellers, "intermediaries," adolescent girls and regular partners (O'Connor, Leshabari, and Lwihula 1992:15).

A good deal of female sexual behavior in Africa can best be understood as strategies for economic survival and adaptation to patterns of male dominance in low-income countries (Green 1988a:180). As Barnett and Blakie have summarized it, African women gain access to economic resources through a range of sexual relationships with men, including monogamous and polygamous marriage, long-term relationships lacking de jure recognition, stable nonresident relationships involving visits on a regular basis, casual liaisons, and the type of commercial prostitution familiar in industrialized countries. "The economic transaction may not be the main or express aspect of the relationship for the participants, but given women's underlying unequal access to economic resources, sexual favours and reproductive potential are powerful resources—sometimes the only resources—on their side of the transaction (Barnett and Blakie (1992:77–78)."

It has been recognized by demographers that the economic and jural empowerment of women leads to lower fertility rates, which in Africa are currently the highest the world has ever known. Such empowerment would also do much to reduce poly partnerism, including various forms of commercial sex. A woman with direct access to economic resources would have less need to enter into many types of sexual relationships; a woman with more legal rights and protection is in a better position to "just say no" to coerced sex.

### *The Cultural Context of AIDS-Related Behavior*

Sexual behavior and indigenous health practices exist in a cultural context that—along with the behavior itself—must be adequately understood before attempting to direct behavior change. For example, in patriarchal societies where men control economic and other resources, those who control more resources are able to maintain sexual relations with a greater number of women. This includes more permanent relations with wives and mistresses, as well as less permanent ones with prostitutes, bargirls, and casual girlfriends. In any case, men achieve status in part by the number of women with whom they maintain sexual relations. Women may be rewarded in cash or gifts for sexual favors, which does not necessarily make them prostitutes.

Patterns of male dominance also make it possible for men to coerce women, including teenage girls, into sexual intercourse—without much fear of having to account for their behavior so long as the woman is currently unmarried. Unmarried and younger women have little power to resist sexual advances from older men in particular and they may have little recourse, even in cases of outright rape. Cases of rape are traditionally settled (and most still are settled traditionally, rather than in civil courts) by requiring the offending man to pay a fine to the woman's family. While some may regard this as "paying for services," the victim is certainly not a prostitute. In any case, sexual practices must be understood in their cultural context in order to understand the transmission of AIDS, the necessary intervention points to interrupt transmission, and realistic strategies for intervention.

Understanding cultural context can also help to explain certain epidemiological findings in Africa, such as differences in seroprevalence by age and sex. Ryder et al. 1987 found "The overall female:male infection ratio in our study (1.1:1) is similar to the figure widely used in describing the epidemiology of HIV infection in Africa. However, we found that cases of infection clustered in two risk groups, young women (ages 13–25) and middle to older aged men." In a study of AIDS patients in Kinshasa, Zaire, Piot et al. (1984:65) likewise found that "Female AIDS cases were younger than male patients with AIDS (mean ages 28.4 versus 41.1 years, respectively), and were more often single. . . ." In light of the earlier discussion of how younger, unmarried women are forced or coerced into sexual relations with older men, it is possible to offer some explanation for the age-specific prevalence differences found between men and women. Still, a fuller explanation should be explored through behavioral research in Africa.

Although it has been fashionable for decades to blame many of Africa's ills on colonialism, European influence has, in fact, impacted on sexual behavior and women's status in the areas of high HIV prevalence in Africa. A recent analysis in Zimbabwe concludes:

> ... land expropriation, rural impoverishment, and the forcible introduction of male migrant labor fostered new patterns of sexual relations, characterized by multiple partners. Traditional patriarchal values reinterpreted in European law resulted in further subjugation of women as even limited rights to ownership were withdrawn. For many women, sexual relations with men, either within marriage (for the majority) or outside, become inextricably linked to economic and social survival. In this setting, all sexually transmitted diseases became rampant, including genital ulcer, which facilitates transmission of the human immunodeficiency virus (HIV) (Bassett and Mhloyi [1991]. Krieger and Margo (1991) make a similar argument).

### *Commercial Sex in Liberia*

The term prostitute is reserved to denote women (and theoretically at least, men) who more or less actively market their sexual services and who accept cash for such services. Liberian informants and FGD participants tended to distinguish two types of prostitutes: a higher-class and usually older prostitute who receives clients at home, and a lower-class, usually younger, woman who solicits clients in the streets (who may be called a lane girl) or in hotels (who may be called a rally girl). Some informants made a distinction between those who practice prostitution more or less full-time versus those who practice it temporarily or intermittently. Others distinguished between those who are experienced and "highly trained" and therefore expensive versus those who are less experienced and inexpensive.

When asked why women become prostitutes, many answers related to economic reasons: women need money; they may have no education or skills or other means of support; there are few alternative job opportunities; or they must support children or other dependents. Other reasons were that certain women have been frustrated or mistreated by men; or they are not satisfied with home life; or some women love engaging in sexual activity; or prostitution is a relatively easy way to earn money and a way "to avoid responsibility."

A distinction is usually made between prostitutes and "grow-now" (also "gronna" or "go around") girls. The name refers to the tendency of some immature, irresponsible women to regard themselves as mature or "grown now" (whence the name) before they really are. "Grow-now" mocks this self-assessment. Grow-now girls or boys were described as young people who loiter around the streets and in bars, do not listen to their parents, do not attend school, and have sex with many partners.

One informant explained that prostitutes may be forced by financial circumstances to engage in commercial sex, but that they may still treat people with respect just as if they were market women dealing with customers. By contrast, grow-now girls and boys treat people disrespectfully, are rude and headstrong, and may be involved in crime. They tend to engage in sex with many partners, although they do it for pleasure or excitement rather than for money.

### *Rape and Coerced Sex*

With the exception of some rural Bassa in the focus groups, informants and participants believed that rape or coerced sex is common in Liberia. Men with special authority over younger women or girls might use their authority to persuade or coerce them into sexual relations. Patterns of this sort identified by FGD discussants include male teachers seducing/raping pupils under their charge (a pattern noted by Brokensha [1988:170] for Africa as a whole); foster fathers seducing/raping their wards; and older boys seducing/raping younger—including very young preteen—girls. Some participants attributed a measure of blame or responsibility to women or girls who are "materialistic" or "after money" or act sexually provocative, a defensive charge one also hears in discussions of the sexual abuse of minor girls in the United States. Some participants observed that if girls get into sexual trouble because they are "after money," their parents are partly to blame for lack of economic support and lack of closer supervision. Girls staying away from their parents while visiting friends or relatives were another special risk group identified by FGD participants. It was acknowledged that it is not uncommon for schoolgirls to become impregnated by teachers, older men, or schoolmates, which may result in the early termination of girls' schooling. Such girls were said to often keep their pregnancy secret from their parents for as long as possible.

Rape and coerced sex is found in varying degrees in most parts of the world, and it is not my intention to offer or discuss general or universal theories that purport to explain such behavior. However, it can be noted that there may be some region-specific cultural patterns that shed some light on the subject and may suggest preventive interventions, for example the traditional beliefs discussed earlier that appear to impel men to seek intercourse with a virgin in order to cure gonorrhea. Furthermore, in the context of coerced sex, some informants observed that some Liberians believe it brings luck to sleep with a virgin.

Legal constraints to rape seem relatively weak in Liberia. Some urban Kpelle men even thought rape was acceptable behavior. Many cases are settled privately, out of court, in order to preserve the victim's reputation and that of her family. In rural areas, village elders or the local chief may help settle the case. When cases are publicly tried, prison sentences tend to be short, however, they may, to some extent, serve as constraints to rape. Other constraints, which may operate more at the village level, include beliefs about supernatural protection of a woman through medicines intended to make a man sick—even mortally so—who has nonsanctioned relations with a woman. Loss of reputation and public ostracism of the offender may also serve as constraints.

*Multiple Sex Partners*

A number of AIDS investigators who focus on Africa believe that since available evidence suggests that "... vaginal intercourse is the dominant behavior in sub-Saharan Africa... (then) frequency of sexual contact is the primary factor governing the transmission of HIV there" (Mann et al. 1988:86). In fact, there was general agreement among informants and FGD participants that there is a great deal of casual sex these days in Liberia. Although adultery contradicts normative statements about the rules and expectations of marriage, it was thought to be common for married partners of both sexes to have liaisons outside marriage, although some believed that such liaisons are less common among women. Men were said to have outside relationships because they want variety, because they lose sexual interest in their own wives or become alienated from them for some other reason, because their wives may have a lover, because their wives refuse them sexual relations, or because of peer expectations. Women may have outside relationships because of want or need of money or gifts, because their husbands do not satisfy them—possibly because they have an outside woman—or because of the husband's attitude or a desire to "get even" with the husband. A need for variety is thought to be more inherent in men than women. A polygamist man might be as likely as a monogamist to have one or more outside relationships, although there was divided opinion on this.

Generalizing about Africa as a whole, van de Walle (1990:10) observes that practices such as differences in age between men and women at marriage and a long period of postpartum abstinence, have contributed to the frequency of extramarital relations and to the spread of sexually transmitted diseases. It is noteworthy that many traditional healers I and my colleagues interviewed in all five countries believed that extramarital relations are common nowadays. All respondents in a small sample of South African healers said they thought it "very common" for married partners—both male and female—to have outside lovers nowadays (Chapter 7).

Liberian informants and discussants also believed it was common for single men and women to have multiple sex partners, although less common for women. Such behavior in men was explained as looking around for the right partner, as proving a man's sexual power, as yielding to peer influence, as reflecting a man's desire for sexual variety, and as relating to a single man's belief that he has no obligation to any particular woman. Such behavior in women was more likely to be explained in terms of seeking economic support or "love of material things."

Extramarital sex was generally thought to be morally wrong and in violation of Christian and Muslim commands; it was also considered a bad practice because it leads to domestic disunity and divorce, to illegitimate children, and to the spread of disease. As might be expected, religious leaders were likelier to cite scriptural reasons for condemning adultery, while health workers and traditional healers tended to cite the spread of disease and domestic disharmony.

Although having multiple sex partners was more likely to be disapproved or condemned in the case of married as distinct from single men and women, most participants and informants also viewed such behavior as unacceptable even for unmarried Liberians. Reasons for disapproving multiple sex contacts among single Liberians were that it spoils a woman's chances of getting married, it becomes more difficult to settle down with a spouse later, a woman will lose self-respect and the respect of others, it wastes money, a man will be "overstrained," it conflicts with an ideal of "one woman for one man," it discourages the development of responsibility, and it can spread diseases.

There appears to have been no specific mention of AIDS in this context. Considering the high prevalence of STDs in Liberia, the fear of AIDS found in most of Africa including Liberia, and the intensive AIDS education campaign broadcast by the Liberian Rural Communication Network some six to seven months prior to the present study, it is surprising that there was not more mention of AIDS and other STDs as reasons to discourage the practice of having multiple sexual partners.

On the other hand, it may be noted that traditional healers, prostitutes, and others readily identified a number of dangers, including AIDS, that result from indiscriminate sex, sex with prostitutes or "grow-now" girls or boys, or simply sex with multiple partners. Hence, there is a clear basis for building upon what people already believe in an AIDS campaign that advises people to stick with one sex partner.

### *Nonstandard Sexual Practices*

Since certain male homosexual practices, as well as anal intercourse whether homosexual or heterosexual, are known risk factors in the spread of AIDS, information was sought on nonstandard sexual practices. Because the topic is sensitive—especially if information were sought about the informant's own behavior—and because the interviewing method employed cannot yield projectable, quantifiable data, only indirect questions were asked and the questions assumed that the practices *exist* in Liberia. For example, informants were asked what kind of people might engage in oral or anal sexual practices, how common and acceptable the practices are in Liberia, and why such practices might be engaged in at all. In the study design phase, the topic was deemed unsuitable for group discussion in the FGDs or for private, one-on-one interviews with informants expected to be unknowledgeable about, or offended by, the topic. On the other hand, preliminary discussions and the key-informant interview pretest suggested that health workers and prostitutes were both knowledgeable (and/or opinionated) and willing to discuss nonstandard sexual practices, and so these informants were interviewed on the subject. It should be noted that information in this section derives from only forty informants, therefore findings must be regarded as very tentative and preliminary.

Few if any informants disagreed with the presumption that oral, anal, and general male homosexual practices occur in Liberia, at least in urban areas. There was some consensus that all such practices tend to be associated with wealthier, better educated, urban Liberians and those exposed to or influenced by foreigners. A few informants concluded that some men are "feminine" or simply are not sexually interested in women. Others suggested that older men initiate younger males into homosexual activity, enticing the latter with money or gifts.

Some informants expressed negative attitudes toward homosexuality and viewed it as deviant or pathological behavior, referring to people with "bad minds" or "bad habits." However, others expressed no ideas suggesting pathology, noting that homosexuals tend to be "intelligent higher-ups" who read books and have "good and strong family ties" and are "normal."

There was diversity of opinion about the types of people who are likely to engage in anal and oral sex. Informants mentioned prostitutes or "highly trained prostitutes," homosexuals, "grow-now boys/girls," people of either sex who are looking for new experiences or sensations, students, poor or abandoned teenagers, older people, and people wanting to prolong intercourse. There was somewhat more consensus that oral sex is practiced mostly by women, either because they are prostitutes or want to satisfy their male partners, or because they are homosexual or bisexual and they practice this with female partners. One health worker observed, "(Oral sex is practiced) mostly by professional people and people who have travelled extensively. They are the ones who introduce these sexual practices in our society."

Most health workers and prostitutes felt that male homosexuality, as well as anal and oral sex practices, are not very common in Liberia, although some practices were believed to be fairly common within certain subgroups. For example, a few informants felt male homosexuality was somewhat common among wealthy, urban-residing men from prestigious families, or that oral sex is common among prostitutes or female homosexuals.

However, our overall Liberian findings seem to support the conclusion of a group of international AIDS experts who observed, "... available studies strongly suggest that vaginal intercourse is the dominant (sexual) behavior in sub-Saharan, reinforcing the supposition that frequency of sexual contact (rather than, e.g., homosexual intercourse) is the primary factor governing the transmission of HIV there" (Mann et al. 1988:86, paren. mine). The experts further note that "... homosexuality ... has not been documented to any appreciable extent among AIDS cases in sub-Saharan Africa" (Mann et al. 1988:85). There is further discussion about homosexuality and other sexual practices in Chapter 7, based on South African findings.

## Discussion of Liberian Findings

AIDS appears to have not yet become widespread in Liberia, nor has seropositivity to the HIV-I virus, however conditions are present in Liberia for AIDs to become a major public health problem. It is hoped that timely interventions can prevent this from happening. Gonorrhea and other STDs that probably serve to facilitate the sexual transmission of AIDS in Africa are present in Liberia, and some are probably of high incidence. The study found clear evidence that, as elsewhere in Africa, STD treatment is often inappropriate: sufferers treat themselves with antibiotics (not necessarily in medically appropriate ways) or traditional medicines, or they consult traditional healers who administer therapies that healer and patient seem to have faith in, but that are probably ineffective. The role of the "black bagger" (an untrained, itinerant injectionist) was inadequately explored in the study; but he is known to treat STDs, therefore further research in this area seems warranted. Furthermore, it has been suggested that "parenteral contact with unsterile needles used for STD treatments" may partly account for the high incidence of HIV seropositivity in parts of Africa (Van de Perre et al. 1987), and if this is so, black baggers and their counterparts in other countries may rank high among those responsible.

It was beyond the scope of our limited study in Liberia to estimate what proportion of STD cases are treated by medically trained practitioners as compared with traditional healers and self-treatment. Even large sample survey results providing such estimates would be confounded by the not uncommon practice of Liberians trying two or more STD therapies simultaneously, and by a disinclination to give candid responses about reliance on traditional healers. However, the apparent high incidence of gonorrhea and several other STDs in Liberia suggests that many STD cases are treated ineffectively.

Thus, to limit the establishment and spread of AIDS in Liberia, it will be necessary to intervene in several ways, including mass education about diagnosis and treatment of STDs in order to reduce the incidence of several already established, common STDs. This will not be easy. In some countries reduction of STDs can be accomplished in large measure by providing more standard antibiotics and in-service training for medical personnel. In Liberia we face not only the problems of: (1) insufficient trained personnel capable of treating STDs; (2) unbalanced distribution of trained personnel, resulting in segments of the population having little access to treatment; and (3) inadequate funds for STD medicines and the related perennial problems of medicine storage and resupply. We face the additional problems of: (4) persistent ethnomedical beliefs that discourage people from even presenting STD cases at clinics and hospitals, and (5) resistance to standard antibiotics due to uninformed self-treatment with antibiotics. Any interventions aimed at reducing the incidence of common STDs must take these factors into account and must be anthropologically informed about relevant aspects of Liberian culture.

## Condom Promotion and Its Problems

Condom provision and promotion is another logical and potentially effective AIDS intervention, one that the sponsors of the study—a contraceptive social-marketing program—were and are especially well equipped and positioned to plan and implement. As mentioned in this book's introduction, the prevailing view among donors such as WHO and USAID has at least until very recently been that apart from sexual abstinence or partner restriction, condoms are the only effective means for preventing the sexual transmission of HIV (e.g., Goldberg et al. 1989)—assuming they are of good quality and are correctly used. There has even been support of this view among anthropologists (USAID and NIAID 1988). Condoms also have the advantage of protecting the user against most of the curable STDs as well.

However, due to innumerable factors—well documented in qualitative and quantitative studies throughout Africa—there is great resistance to using condoms. As one recent summary puts it:

> The failure of vending machines in Botswana . . . rumours that the USA is providing sub-standard condoms to Zimbabwe, beliefs that condoms are part of the South African government's efforts to reduce the rate of black population growth, or that condom use is all part of some other kind of

> conspiracy against Africans, or simply men's unwillingness to recognize the risk and the issue of trust between partners in a steady relationship . . .—all these factors make condom programmes difficult to introduce (Barnett and Blaikie 1992:162–163).

To this we might add the problems of transportation, storage, hygienic disposal, distribution, and affordability of condoms. Condoms also have a relatively high failure rate in Africa, due to incorrect use but also to the poor quality of condoms often found in poor, tropical countries. Furthermore, condom use depends upon male cooperation; African women are in no position, or at least a weak position, to insist that their partners use a condom.

The present study showed that condoms were not well known or well thought of by most Liberians—even if they were easily accessible. With the exception of health workers, there was little spontaneous mention from either research group of condoms in connection with AIDS or other STD prevention. For example, only 28 out of 100 key informants (excluding those who were health workers) said they thought condoms could be effective in protecting against AIDS transmission, and that was after prompting to think about condoms in the first place. It was also in spite of a recent AIDS education radio campaign that promoted condoms as a major AIDS preventive. A larger number (35) offered the view that condoms would not be effective in AIDS prevention.

A far more detailed study of condom perceptions and attitudes undertaken just prior to the present study similarly found major obstacles to condom acceptance among Liberians (Subah-Bellah Associates 1988). Indeed, "aversion to, and high cost of, condoms" have been recognized as obstacles to limiting HIV infection for sub-Saharan Africa as a whole (Prual, Chacko, and Koch-Weser 1991). Prospects therefore seem unpromising for a significant rise in condom prevalence levels in Liberia within the next five years or so, even without the present civil war conditions. In any case, promotion of condoms and "safer sex" practices are probably insufficient in themselves to significantly impact on rising HIV seropositive incidence without parallel efforts to lower the incidence of standard STDs. This is not to say that promotion of condoms and safer sex practices should not be undertaken simultaneously as complementary elements of an AIDS prevention strategy.

A condom education campaign would have to convey a number of messages of varying degrees of complexity and detail. First, Liberians would have to come to understand and accept the role of condoms in preventing AIDS and other STDs. Second, the prevailing aversion to condoms would have to be overcome by somehow improving the condom image. Third, since Liberians are not currently very familiar with condoms and since user failure has been found more important than product failure in cases where condoms do not protect against STDs (CDC 1988:1925), there would need to be clearly presented information about correct use, handling, and storage of condoms. With regard to the last, perceptions about the tendency of condoms to break or tear are often grounded in actual experience in countries like Liberia. An AIDS education program in Liberia will have to direct some of its efforts at ensuring that those who store and sell condoms know how to store and handle condoms in ways that minimize product deterioration.

The promotion of condoms for disease—especially AIDS—protection can be more complex and pitfall prone than promotion of condoms for contraception. A man about to use a condom may not want to appear to either have AIDS or to suspect that his partner has AIDS, perceptions that can be avoided if one or both partners think of the condom as protection against unwanted pregnancy. An appropriate promotional strategy for condoms might be what could be termed "purposeful ambiguity": to remain nonspecific and not make too strong an AIDS-condom connection, especially in a country like Liberia where the condom already has a negative image, one that associates condoms with prostitutes and disease. A simple, ambiguous message such as "protection when you need it" might work well in Liberia. Protection against pregnancy can be either the overt or the unspoken, understood function of the condom between partners, while protection against possible exposure to disease could actually be motivating one or both of the partners to use the condom. Alternatively, a promotional strategy could take advantage of the association that already exists between condoms, STDs and nonsanctioned sexual behavior including sex with multiple partners.

Liberian healers claimed little experience with, or knowledge about, condoms. As influential health opinion leaders, perhaps especially in matters related to STDs, their support—or lack of opposition at a minimum—could be crucial to the success of a campaign designed to promote the adoption and continued, correct use of condoms on the part of sexually active Liberians. The study showed that healers were more ignorant of, than specifically opposed to, condoms. Special education or training efforts aimed at traditional healers should be considered. These could be designed as TOT (training of trainers) programs since trained healers could be expected to pass information on to other healers as well as to their many clients, as experience elsewhere in Africa has shown occurs (Hoff 1986; Warren and Green 1989). A collaborative TOT program in South Africa with emphasis on condom promotion is described in Chapter 7.

**Spermicides**

Condoms are not the only contraceptive that could or perhaps should be promoted for disease prevention. There is in vitro and limited in vivo evidence that spermicides such as nonoxynol-9 kills bacteria, viruses, and parasites that cause many STDs including AIDS, gonorrhea, chlamydia, herpes, and trichomonas (Cates 1988; Tice et al. 1990; Rosenberg 1991; Rosenberg et al. 1992). Other widely used spermicides are octoxynol-9, menfegol, and benzalkonium chloride—like nonoxynol-9 all "surfactants" that can inactivate STD-causing bacteria and viruses by damaging bacterial cell membranes and viral envelopes (Benson 1988:8). Therefore, AIDS/STD programs in Liberia and elsewhere in Africa may want to consider promoting contraceptive sponges and diaphragms used with spermicides (which most already are), vaginal foam (which contains spermicide), and condoms lubricated with nonoxynol-9 to limit the spread of STDs (a public health goal in itself), to limit possible cofactors in the spread of AIDS, and to directly limit the spread of AIDS itself.

True, more research is needed to clarify the STD- and AIDS-prevention role of spermicides, but there is enough suggestive evidence to at least begin the planning of how spermicides and female barrier methods could best be promoted in Africa for STD prevention (there is considerable experience already in their promotion for family planning). These methods have the significant advantage over condoms in that women can initiate and have some control over them. In male-dominated societies (and all societies are probably such to varying extents), women may not be in a position to insist or even suggest that men use a condom. A woman, however, can use vaginal foam, thereby exercising a measure of control over her health and fertility. She may be able to use spermicides secretly in cases of uncooperative or recalcitrant partners.

There is even evidence that female-controlled barrier methods used in conjunction with spermicides may be superior to condoms in preventing common STDs. A recent retrospective study of 5,681 women at a Denver STD clinic looked at the relationship between recent use of three popular forms of barrier contraceptives and prevalence of common STDs. Women using the contraceptive sponge, diaphragm, and condom all had significantly lower rates of infection of three common STDs: gonorrhea, trichomonas, and chlamydia. However, those using the sponge or diaphragm had significantly lower rates than those using condoms (Rosenberg et al. 1992:670–671). Part of the reason for these findings is poor or inconsistent use of condoms. While condoms are highly effective in the lab (about 99 percent) in preventing STDs, they are far less so in actual practice. And condom failure rates tend to be higher in Africa where products may be of poor quality, where inadequate storage and transportation under tropical conditions may lead to further product deterioration, and where male resistance to their use in the first place is strong.

I agree with the conclusion of Rosenberg et al. that STD control efforts should be oriented more toward women, toward female-dependent or female-controlled methods. This argument is bolstered by the finding that STDs including HIV infection can be transmitted more easily from men to women than vice versa (Platt, Rice, and McCormack 1983; Rosenberg 1992:673). However, two problems might emerge with promotion of spermicides. One is that some women seem to develop allergic reactions, including inflammations that might conceivably facilitate HIV transmission (O'Farrell and Barlow 1992). However, Bird (1991:791) notes that "most literature reviews on nonoxynol 9 concluded that any reports of local toxicity were only minimally significant." And as Voeller (1992:341) suggests, "... products PH buffered into tissue-tolerable acidic ranges ..." could be developed thereby reducing the possibility of allergic reaction, plus there are a number of spermicides besides nonoxynol 9.

Another problem is that in parts of central and southern Africa where men prefer "dry sex," it might be difficult to promote any agent that lubricates the vaginal canal (Runganga, Pitts, and McMaster 1992).

## Addressing Risky Behavior

Another appropriate intervention or element of an AIDS education campaign in Liberia should be to advise about the risks associated with visiting prostitutes or having sexual intercourse with a number of partners and partners of unknown or at-risk sexual background. The simple message probably ought to be to stick with one sex partner. There seems to be a clear basis for building upon what people already believe about the hazards of having sex with strangers or with a multitude of partners. Traditional healers, among others interviewed, were unequivocal and even moralistic on this subject. Here again, healers could be enlisted along with religious and political leaders and health workers to convey and reinforce the message of staying with a single partner—or in the cases of polygamous marriage, confining relations to the marriage. Seventeen out of twenty local leaders suggested sticking to one partner as the best way to avoid AIDS, and interestingly, fully half of prostitutes interviewed offered the same opinion (Table 4.4).

As Ward and Day have observed (1991:189) commercial sex cannot be eradicated by legal acts or police crackdowns; this simply drives prostitutes underground and beyond the reach of the health care worker. Prostitutes are in special need of treatment and prevention services, and when these are available, the health payoffs are evident. There are some areas of the world where STD infection rates among prostitutes are virtu-

TABLE 4.5 Presumed First Action upon Learning of STD Infection

| *1st Action* | *Health Personnel*[1] | *Local Leader* | *Tradit. Healers* | *Relig. Leaders* | *Prostitutes* | *Total* |
|---|---|---|---|---|---|---|
| Visit hospital/ clinic | 15 | 18 | 10 | 14 | 9 | 56 |
| Visit traditional healer | 1 | 8 | 14 | 2 | – | 27 |
| Consult friend | 3 | 3 | 4 | 3 | 4 | 17 |
| Visit pharmacy, self-treatment | 4 | 1 | – | 1 | 4 | 10 |
| Traditional self-treatment | 1 | – | 1 | – | – | 2 |

[1]includes village health workers

ally zero, especially in Western Europe but also in parts of Africa and East Asia.

## STD Therapies and Therapy-Seeking Behavior

Summarizing our earlier discussion, the following seems to characterize STD therapy-seeking behavior in many parts of Africa: (1) a disinclination to seek modern-sector therapy because of cost, shame or embarrassment over having an STD, lack of access to a medical facility, and beliefs that traditional healers have effective cures for STDs; (2) self-treatment with antibiotics (often without asking pharmacists for guidance or advice), much of which is inappropriate and may lead to resistance to standard antibiotics; and (3) reliance on traditional healers for treatment. With regard to the last, there is evidence in a number of African countries of the belief that traditional healers have effective medicines for treating STDs—or for diseases with indigenous names and etiologies that are characterized by symptoms that modern biomedicine would associate with STDs. In fact, many healers and their clients believe traditional therapies to be superior to modern medical therapies.

Liberia seems to conform to this pattern. Although nearly twice as many informants and participants mentioned consulting clinics, hospitals, or doctors than those consulting traditional healers, as illustrated in Table 4.5, the latter is typically underreported and the former overreported in formal interview or group discussion situations in Africa. Even in such a context, about 26 percent of informants mentioned consulting a traditional healer and 27 percent mentioned visiting a pharmacy for treatment, or consulting "a friend." The latter suggests self-treatment with antibiotics or perhaps traditional therapies. Some self-treatment with herbal medicines was also mentioned. About 75 percent of formal-sector health workers thought STD sufferers would first visit a clinic or hospital for treatment, while the same proportion of traditional healers thought people would first consult traditional healers (or try traditional medicines on their own or with advice from a friend) and would visit clinics/hospitals only if traditional therapies failed.

Before describing traditional Liberian STD therapies, some general observations are in order to help explain the existence and persistence of faith in traditional STD medicines in Africa. Since biomedical treatment of common STDs usually entails use of antibiotics that show rapid and marked results, it might be expected that faith in traditional medicines would quickly give way to faith in antibiotics. Yet if this is happening in Africa, it is happening surprisingly slowly, and this demands explanation. It has been well-documented that African traditional therapies provide culturally meaningful explanations, lend psychological comfort to the patient, restore some measure of social and family harmony, and reduce fear and stress, thereby positively impacting the psychosomatic component of disease.

But what about the actual medicines used in STD treatment? It seems unlikely that traditional medicines are pharmacologically effective for STDs requiring antibiotics. It appears more likely that most healers use medicines for STDs that lack antibiotic properties but nevertheless seem effective because many STD symptoms clear up spontaneously as the disease enters a latent phase. When symptoms return, treatment is again administered and symptoms may again disappear, although not because of treatment. In short, there may be apparent cause and effect relationship between administration of traditional STD treatments and the disappearance of symptoms such that both healers and patients believe in the efficacy of the treatments. There may be other reasons accounting for the faith of healer and client in traditional STD medicines (Spielberg 1987:56–57. See Chapter 9.)

In the present study, Liberian healers seemed sincere in the confidence they expressed in their STD medicines (excluding AIDS) and several were quite candid about revealing details. One healer noted that a number of STD sufferers he sees try self-treatment with tetracycline and lime, but he believed this has "zero" effect. After identifying four traditional disease categories believed to be sexually transmitted—at least one of which probably corresponds to gonorrhea—he went on to say:

> There are different kinds of roots and herbs in the bush for (each of) them. There are also different pots to cook these medicines in. Each of these pots have different prices. After treatment, if the person is cured, he or she is to break the pot and throw it away. . . . If you keep the pot, you will contract the disease again. (After) the medicine is cooked, women take the treatment for 2 to 3 days, and men take it for 4–5 days.

Another healer even revealed the name of the source for his herbal medicine for gonorrhea:

> There is a tree in the bush called *gbulie* that the Bassa people use. I usually boil the leaves of this tree and have the patient drink it three times a day for about three days. During this period, my patients are not to have any sexual intercourse. I also stop them from drinking anything other than water. No alcohol, because it counteracts the strength of the leaves.

He went on to say he would be thankful if someone would teach him how to treat the new disease AIDS.

Most healers described making decoctions from the leaves and roots of various medicinal plants and administering these as teas to be taken over a two- to four-day period. Chalk or kaolin marks on the body may also be part of treatment. One healer mentioned adding lime to an orally administered herbal decoction that cures *khanyan*; he claimed that *khanyan* is a very easy disease to cure. Another healer described the therapeutic action of his herb tea as "cleaning the system," a necessary measure because gonorrhea "is an inside disease." Some healers prescribe herbal decoctions that are taken by enemas or vaginal implants in addition to, or instead of, teas. The herbal enema was said to "help clean the spinal cord" or "the system." As one healer elaborated:

> I have two methods. I use the tube and pump this person and help to clean his system. I boil some herbs and tea for him to drink for about two days. This also helps to clean out the system. Syphilis is treated the same way but the difference here is that chalk is given to the victim to help clean the sores from all over the body. Blue Balls can be treated by cutting the swelling when it is ripe and squeezing out the pus.

Evidence from the study suggests that an STD sufferer may try two or more therapies in quick succession, or even simultaneously, either because of impatience to experience results or because he is not sure where to place his trust. A patient who receives simultaneous treatment from a clinic and a traditional healer may put himself at risk of overdose, or the two types of medicine might tend to counteract or neutralize one another (Asuni 1979:37). Even if a traditional medicine is ineffective for STDs, it may still have toxic, potentiating or other pharmacological effects.

Of course, the simultaneous use of multiple therapies is common throughout Africa and elsewhere where traditional or other nonallopathic therapies are available and popular. Liberia is certainly not unusual in this regard. What is striking is that alternative therapies for AIDS appear not yet to have emerged in Liberia. This may be attributable to the newness and fatal nature of the disease. Healers may not want to set themselves up for failure in the form of dying patients—at least until it is well recognized that AIDS patients die in spite of modern medical therapy, by which time traditional, alternative, or religious faith healers may feel they have nothing to lose by trying some sort of therapy on dying patients.

Liberia, like other nations of Africa, is undergoing culture change that is so rapid that even "traditional medicine" is experiencing significant transformation and upheaval. Some healers may share their patients' ambivalence about choice of therapies. In the words of one:

> Before the white man came to Liberia, people used to go to the *zoes* (cult priests or diviners) for treatment. The *zoes* at that time had power to cure any kind of disease. At that time, people had faith in the *zoes* too; but now things are changing. People including myself prefer going to the hospital to seek medical attention rather than seek traditional treatment. Also some country (traditional) medicines are not working good today because people are not taking time to learn them. They are also not taking time to cure people the right way, the *zoes* just want to make fast money. In the past, people stayed in the bush for about seven to eight years before getting cured. But now people don't have the patience to stay in the bush too long. Now the primary role of a *zoe* is to be a teacher and not a doctor.
>
> Also we prefer going to the hospital because the doctor takes the disease away forever, but the country doctor will only cool the disease down for some two to three years. Later, it (the STD) will develop and eventually kill you. This is why people are learning to forget about the country medicines and are moving towards the hospital if they are sick.

It is of interest that at least one traditional healer regarded some of his colleagues as out to make "fast money" and recognized that traditional medicines for STDs might provide only a temporary cure—and that the STD may return after two or three years in a worse form that may eventually kill the patient. This probably reflects what is often the actual situation when ineffective treatments are given by healers—even though the healers may be sincere and well meaning—for syphilis or gonorrhea. Another traditional healer accused sandcutters (diviner-mediums) of attributing virtually every malady to witchcraft, thereby "creating all kinds of enemies" for the afflicted person. This healer believes diseases such as leprosy and TB are witchcraft caused, but not gonorrhea. His comment about witchcraft accusation suggests not only candor and reflection, but perhaps changing cultural patterns and the impact of modern and scientific education on traditional modes of thinking as well. Of course, it may also reflect rivalry between classes of healers if not between individuals, but in this case the healer further commented that he admires "hospital treatment."

### Liberia in the Future

Neither AIDS nor HIV-I seropositivity had become widespread in Liberia at the time of fieldwork (MHSW 1987; Nimpson 1988), however conditions were present for AIDs to become a major public health problem. The outbreak of civil war since fieldwork has doubtless increased opportunities for HIV transmission, if for no other reason than the breakdown of government preventive and curative health services. Assuming the restoration of political stability—at least central government—and resumption of national health programs, it is hoped that timely interventions can prevent or delay major spread of HIV.

Gonorrhea, syphilis, and other STDs that probably serve to facilitate the sexual transmission of AIDS in Africa are present in Liberia, and several appear to be highly prevalent. Some two dozen locally recognized STDs were described (and named in local languages) by informants and participants. Sorcery, taboo violation, and contamination were believed to be causally involved with most STDs; and more "naturalistic" explanations were often based on simplified notions of human anatomy and biochemistry. Three basic messages about AIDS that were broadcast in a recent campaign were retained, namely "AIDS kills," "there is no cure for it," and "it is transmitted through sex." There was also evidence that some Liberians were beginning to interpret AIDS in ways compatible with what Janzen (1989) calls "the broad orienting hypotheses of African medicine," including sorcery.

The study found clear evidence that, as elsewhere in Africa, STD treatment is often inappropriate: sufferers treat themselves with antibiotics (not necessarily in medically appropriate ways) or traditional medicines, or they consult traditional healers who administer therapies that healer and patient seem to have faith in, but that are probably ineffective.

The study's qualitative methods were ill suited to estimate what proportion of STD cases are treated by medically trained practitioners, traditional healers, or self-treatment. Had a large sample survey been undertaken, resulting estimates would be confounded by the common practice of Liberians trying two or more STD therapies simultaneously, and by respondent disinclination to give candid responses about reliance on traditional healers. However, the apparent high incidence of gonorrhea and several other STDs in Liberia suggests that many STD cases are treated ineffectively—as elsewhere in Africa.

I feel the Liberian study demonstrates the value of both the standard anthropological research method of key informant interviewing as well as focus group discussions in illuminating indigenous knowledge systems relating to AIDS and STDs, shedding light on sexual and therapy-seeking behavior, and generally discovering new information. The combined methodologies were mutually complementary, relatively inexpensive to administer, and quick to provide results, therefore I believe they should be considered by those planning AIDS education or intervention programs elsewhere in Africa. In any case, qualitative research of some kind should probably precede behavioral/attitudinal surveys in countries lacking a good knowledge base for AIDS planning. In the case of Liberia, a survey deigned by outsiders would probably contain no questions about "grow-now girls" or indigenous categories of STDs such as "bubos," therefore it would miss much useful and pertinent information. And a survey response that made reference to intercourse with a virgin as treatment for gonorrhea would make little sense without an understanding of the indigenous worm-in-the-urethra theory of gonorrhea.

## Notes

1. This chapter is an expansion of material that appeared in Green, E. C., "The Anthropology of Sexually Transmitted Diseases in Liberia," *Social Science and Medicine* Vol. 35, No. 4, 1992, pp. 1457–1468.

2. On the other hand, politically aware prostitutes may reject such euphemisms as reinforcing the view that prostitution is an immoral occupation. For an account of the First and Second World Whores' Congresses, see Pheterson (1989).

3. The Human Relations Area Files (HRAF) consist of descriptive ethnographic data from over 300 cultures—with an emphasis on those which are non-Western and nonliterate—drawn from a wide variety of published sources. Created at Yale University in the 1930's, they are now computerized for easy retrieval of topics and subtopics.

# 5

# STDs and AIDS in Mozambique[1]

## Background on Mozambique

The physical and social infrastructures of Mozambique at the time of independence (1975) were as weak as any African nation that had gained independence in the 1960s or even in the 1950s. The new Frelimo government, in its attempt to create a modern, nontribal, nonracial, equitable nation, embarked on a radical program to transform the country's economy and society as quickly as possible. The "traditionalism" of the various ethnolinguistic groups seemed to stand in the way of "scientific socialism," and so there was an attempt to abolish traditional practices such as bride-price (*lobola*), polygamy, initiation rites, land tenure, and traditional healing practices. The rural masses were obliged to regroup into communal villages in order to engage in new forms of collective agriculture. Frelimo attempted to achieve full equality of women—in societies for the most part strongly patriarchal—through legislation. In 1978 "Peoples' Tribunals" were set up to be headed by judges chosen on the basis of having "good sense." This was an assault on traditional adjudicative systems, including the traditional authorities who convened and presided over adjudicative councils.

Chiefs, formerly known as *regulos* or *chefes de zonas*, were recognized and often appointed by the Portuguese during the long colonial period, although their positions no doubt pre-dated that period. Soon after independence, Frelimo embarked on a program to break the power of traditional chiefs. Part of the rationale for this is that chiefs were often used as instruments of control of the masses by the Portuguese colonial administration. Another reason may be that chiefs appeared to Frelimo reformers as guardians and purveyors of the old, traditional order targeted for radical transformation. Still another is that Frelimo quickly established a highly centralized government characterized by urban-based, top-down decision making. Chiefs—particularly those who questioned the wisdom of government decisions—constituted a challenge to a government of this sort. And no doubt many chiefs questioned the wisdom of abolishing bride-price, polygamy, initiation rites, traditional land tenure, etc.

With Frelimo's "marginalization" or suppression of traditional political authorities, many went underground or simply continued to exercise power informally and behind the backs of Frelimo officials. Still, chiefs have not existed officially since the early postindependence period. The abolition of chiefs meant that many of them did not oppose Renamo, which they might well have otherwise done if their authority had been left intact. In a parallel development, traditional healers, spirit mediums, and cult figures were discouraged—sometimes oppressed—as purveyors of "obscurantism" and superstition. The alienation of traditional and ritual leaders and healers was a major factor in Frelimo's loss of political control of most of the geographic area of Mozambique.

The overthrow of chiefs and other traditional political and spiritual authorities was supported by fanciful and monolithic historical notions of the existence of "theocracies" that enjoyed absolute power in Mozambique. Such anthropologically uninformed thinking provided a rationale and justification for Frelimo's attempts to overthrow indigenous power structures in the name of scientific socialism or even democracy. It is an irony of Mozambique's history that the founding father of Frelimo, Eduardo Mondlane, was a U.S.-trained anthropologist. According to K. B. Wilson, citing Steven Thomas, the image of Eduardo Mondlane tends to be spared during occasions of Renamo's ritualized destruction of Frelimo symbols and icons (Wilson 1992:11).

Beginning in the mid-1980s, there was growing awareness within the ranks of the Mozambique government that it had made a number of serious mistakes. It did not go unnoticed that much of Renamo's early success could be attributed to its ability to manipulate traditional beliefs that it had the approval of ancestor spirits as well as magical protection from local spirit-mediums. By the mid- to late 1980s, Frelimo began to successfully manipulate the same cultural symbolism against Renamo. Wilson (1992:17–23) notes that in some areas such as Northern Tete, ". . . it appears that Frelimo worked quite closely with local chiefs who in such areas generally have some ritual authority and access to ancestral spirits." During roughly the same time (1989–1990), a third force arose in Northern Mozambique in the form of the Naprama "cult of counter-violence" (Wilson's term), which exhibits many of the features of what anthropologists call cultural revitalization movements (Wallace 1956). The Naprama movement consists of citizens led by a charismatic traditional healer who protects his followers with magical medicines and amulets. These citizens fight against Renamo and other bandits using only "traditional weapons" rather than firearms, which are easily available in Mozambique.

By the 5th Frelimo Party Congress (1989), the government formally recognized the mistakes it made in its zeal to create a new, equitable, unified, national society. In an April 1992 national workshop held in Mozambique, a presenter noted that Frelimo's attempt at radically transforming society:

> ... was extremely altruistic, but the way it was implemented entered into direct confrontation with the cultural system hitherto existing in the countryside, which was ignored or set aside to make way for the new, modern progressive and urban culture. A phenomenon which in Europe had taken centuries to evolve was attempted here from one day to the next, and in general the results were not good. There was resistance, difficulties, and failures which might not have occurred if there had been an attempt to conciliate the culture of the peasants and the new forms being proposed, in order to achieve a more gradual and less confrontational transition. A situation of contradictory norms emanating from the traditional authorities and the central government generated disrespect for norms of any kind" (CDC et al. 1992:39).

## The Genesis of a Policy and a Program

Late in 1990, I was asked by the Department of Traditional Medicine (DTM), a small unit within the Mozambique Ministry of Health, to help develop a policy regarding that country's traditional healers, and to advise on any necessary legislative modification. The initial consultancy was supported by the European Community between November 1990 and March 1991. At the end of 1991, AID funded a later two-month consultancy through its HEALTHCOM project. In 1990 there was no formal/legal recognition of healers by the Frelimo government, nor was there any program of cooperation or collaboration with the exception of some informal, uncoordinated local-level efforts on the part of a few health workers. On the contrary, intersectoral relations were among the worst in Africa due to the Frelimo government's attempt to suppress traditional healing.

It has already been mentioned that Frelimo reversed its policy in 1989. A quick, small survey by the DTM in 1990 found that 76 percent of doctors and 82 percent of other health workers were in favor of "collaboration"—a high proportion by African standards. However, it was not known whether traditional healers wanted to have dealings with the government. The DMT survey of ministry health workers found a "medicocentric" attitude on the part of doctors and others; many were found to hold negative attitudes toward traditional healers, attitudes based on hearsay rather than on direct or scientific observation (de Jong 1990). However, it should be noted that support within the Ministry of

Health—including its highest ranks—was unusually strong by African or any standards. Perhaps Mozambique's desperate economic, political, and health situation discouraged the luxury of looking down on traditional healers. A senior ministry official told me, "People here need to be more self-reliant in health than people elsewhere. We just don't have trained health personnel in many rural areas."

After my initial briefings and immersion in reports, I proposed and reached agreement with my colleagues on a rationale for developing a collaborative program between the National Health Service and traditional healers. We presented it in a simple outline form which we hoped would be convincing. Our argument was couched in public health rather than political terms:

1. Government health services are inadequate in manpower, distribution of manpower, and rural outreach. The physician:population ratio is less than 1:50,000, and there are less than 1,500 health workers of any kind;
2. Mozambicans are dying from preventable and treatable diseases;
3. Traditional healers have the numbers and distribution needed to serve the population, as well as other advantages over allopathic health workers such as cultural acceptability (there is a traditional healers:population ratio of roughly 1:200, suggesting there are approximately 85,000 healers in Mozambique;
4. For a variety of reasons traditional healers want to improve their healing skills, to learn more about allopathic medicine, and to collaborate better with modern health practitioners—which is not to say they wish to stop being traditional healers;
5. The government of Mozambique, since the 5th Congress (July 1989), is seeking ways to collaborate with healers in order to improve the public health;
6. WHO and UNICEF, OAU, the Non-Aligned Countries, and other international bodies have recommended to member states that strategies to develop traditional health humanpower be developed;
7. Therefore, it is not a question of whether, but rather *how* best to, collaborate with traditional healers.

We took the position that traditional healers constitute a separate, parallel, and largely self-regulating health service that with the right approach can formally collaborate with the government in the realization of specific public health goals, such as lowering morbidity and mortality of major life-threatening diseases through prevention and treatment. We pointed out that in a pluralistic health system such as Mozambique's, traditional healers are not and should not be part of the National Health Service. Traditional healers serve a useful, complex function in Mozambican society and the ministry should not attempt to transform them into ill-prepared, unpaid nurses or village health workers.

### The Issue of Village Health Workers

Another question that arose—as it often does in discussions about traditional healers—is why not simply develop a new cadre of minimally trained health workers, situate them in villages, and have the villages provide some sort of salary or compensation? The short answer is that cadres of village health workers have been trained in a number of African countries and have been found to have serious drawbacks, not the least of which is that village health workers compete with the established person who already enjoys credibility and prestige as a health expert, the traditional healer. The WHO *Global Medium-term Programme* (Programme 12.4 Traditional Medicine, March 1984) seemed aware of this when it noted, "Some countries tend to create new community health workers rather than incorporate practitioners of traditional medicine into their health delivery systems, especially at the primary health care level." Whatever we think of "incoporation," the implication is that upgrading traditional healers is more reasonable than creating new cadres.

Mozambique, in fact, had trained a cadre of village health workers known as *Agentes Polivalentes Elementares* (APEs). The program was designed along the lines of similar programs in Africa: an APE is volunteered by his/her village, then receives a six-month training course after which he or she is returned to the village. The village is supposed to pay a small salary or provide in-kind subsistence allowance. The APE carries out preventive and some curative health care. For the latter, there is a basic kit with antimalarials, analgesics, ORS packets, and the like. The program was developing as well as can be expected until Renamo banditry and resulting economic conditions meant that communities could no longer pay APEs, whereupon the program began to deteriorate. Training stopped in Maputo in 1985 and elsewhere in the country by 1989.

My colleagues and I argued that traditional healers enjoy certain advantages over village health workers—to return to their generic designation—inherent in their roles. These can be summarized in Table 5.1, which is based on the actual situation of the APE. It should be kept in mind that the main strengths of VHWs are that they are considered trained, albeit minimally, and to some degree supervised by the government.

TABLE 5.1 Comparison Between the Traditional Healer and Village Health Worker in Mozambique

| *Comparison* | *Traditional Healer* | *Village Health Worker* |
|---|---|---|
| Qualifications | Years of training as well as a spiritual basis rooted in traditional religion | 6 months of training. No previous health background or credibility |
| Age (a factor related to respect, prestige and credibility) | Tends to be older | Tends to be younger |
| Financial sustainability of service | Has own established income base | Has no source of income, even as a VHW. A proposed new plan would pay the VHW less than 60% of the minimum wage. |
| Cultural "fit" | Culturally acceptable | Seen as an agent of an alien system |
| Approach to health care | Holistic | Of necessity, fragmented and narrowly focused |
| Materia medica, agents of therapy | Well-supplied, easily replenished | Health kits usually unreplenished |
| Practical experience in health matters | Has much experience | Has little or no previous experience |
| Career stability | Stable. Practitioners are content and take pride in their respected role | Unstable. VHWs want to be trained to become salaried health workers like nurses |
| "Coverage" of country | 100% | Less than 30% |
| Caseload | About 1 practitioner per 250 population estimated | Has risen from 1 VHW per 250 *families* to 1 per 1–3 *villages*. |

## National Policy and Pilot Project in Manica Province

As part of my initial consultancy, my colleagues and I were asked to make recommendations for the modification or repeal of existing legislation so that MOH policy would be compatible with the nation's laws. Accordingly, we recommended a policy of official recognition of traditional healers and proposed draft legislation that specifies details of the relationship between government and healers. We further recommended the immediate creation of an interministerial task force (Health and Justice) to recommend and implement new legislation relating to the legal status and practice of traditional medicine. We kept our legislative recommendations simple, advising that the government adopt the widely accepted definition of traditional medical practitioners provided by the World Health Organization; that properly constituted professional associations of healers be legally recognized, which implies legal recognition of all formally registered members of such associations; and that registration of healers be the responsibility of the associations themselves, based on their own criteria of membership (Green, Jurg, and Tomas 1991).

We also designed a pilot program after consultation on key elements with not only government health officials but one national and one provincial-level association of traditional healers. It should be noted that the previous year, 1989, the Maternal/Child Health section of the health ministry had initiated formal training intended to upgrade the midwifery skills of traditional birth attendants—another example of an African nation willing to collaborate with TBAs before traditional healers.

We recommended that the department begin two pilot projects for traditional healers early in the first year of the new program, one in Manica and one in Gaza provinces. These were to serve as models for planning and implementing a local program of collaboration between government and traditional healers. The pilot projects would concentrate, at least initially, on child diarrhea and on AIDS/STDs, but the model would serve to guide the establishment of programs in any area of health.

Diarrhea and STDS/AIDS were initial focus areas because both were and are high-priority health concerns for government and donors (we had little data indicating community-identified health priorities). Other selection criteria were the potential to have substantial health impact in the short to medium term and to able to begin a collaborative without undue delay. We noted there had been fruitful collaboration with traditional healers in child diarrhea elsewhere in Africa (Hoff and Maseko 1986; Warren and Green 1989; Hogle and Prins 1991), therefore there was a fund of practical experience to draw upon. In the case of AIDS and STDS, Mozambique's National Program to Combat AIDS (1988–1990) had already recognized the important potential role of healers in reducing the spread of HIV and the prevalence of other STD infections. The AIDS/STDS program had also set aside funds for efforts involving healers, some of which could be available to our program in order to begin without delay. Finally, my colleagues had already conducted preliminary ethnomedical research related to AIDS and STDs in the Maputo area, and they were excited by the idea that we might be able to limit the spread of HIV infection in Mozambique before it became as widespread as in many neighboring countries.

In the DTM/MOH pilot project in Manica Province, Mozambique, we first conducted research to establish an adequate knowledge base to develop a training strategy specifically for traditional healers. Our aim was to improve intersectoral cooperation in the prevention and treatment of STDs (and child diarrheas). A more general goal was to demonstrate the value of quick, low-cost anthropological or ethnomedical research for the development of culturally sensitive health education strategies and related public health interventions—whether or not there is interest in collaborating with traditional healers.

Intermittently between February and October 1991, fifty-one traditional healers claiming specialty in sexually transmitted diseases were interviewed in depth as key informants. An additional fifty-three healers were interviewed on related health topics. Interviews were conducted in the homes of these healers in the five districts of Manica province accessible by road. Follow-up interviews were occasionally conducted with a particularly helpful informant to pursue a topic in greater depth. A random sampling technique was not attempted since we lacked an adequate sampling frame. However, selection was assisted by the Manica branch of AMETRAMO, the national healers association, which sought to provide balance by gender, age, and district. As with the membership of AMETRAMO itself, there may have been a selection bias in favor of more urbanized, Portuguese-speaking healers.

Interviewers were drawn from the Manica Provincial Health Department, Radio Mozambique, and the Department of Traditional Medicine, with me assisting and supervising. A semistructured, open-ended interview schedule was used, and interviews lasted an hour or more. The instrument was refined and modified as incoming information was assessed and new lines of inquiry—or new ways to ask questions—were suggested.

In addition, we conducted five focus group discussions (FGDs), two of which focused specifically on STDs. One group consisted of male traditional healers, the other of female healers. There was an average of seven healers per focus group. Discussions lasted about two hours and were conducted in the chiShona-related dialect of the particular district. FGDs were held in villages and/or in the compounds of traditional healers to help participants feel relaxed and unintimidated by any of the trappings or symbols of Western biomedicine. Segregation by sex was more to remove any barriers of decorum than because we expected male and female healers differed significantly in knowledge, attitudes, and practices. In-depth interviews conducted earlier in fact suggested otherwise.

In sum, data gathering was qualitative and derived solely from traditional healers. Survey findings, especially among clients with STDs who consult local healers would obviously have provided a more complete picture. However, time and financial constraints limited us to interviews and group discussions with traditional healers. Still, in my experience, healers usually represent the beliefs of clients who consult them and they are often better able than their clients to explain such beliefs, both because of their specialized knowledge and because their status in the community makes them less likely to be intimidated by an interviewer.

As noted in Chapter 1, indigenous classification of "STDs" may not correspond with scientific categories, and, in fact, are often broader. Illnesses and conditions not classified as sexually transmitted in biomedical nosology may be regarded as such by indigenous healers, and presumably their clients who share a common belief system. For example, earlier surveys of traditional healers and their clients in Maputo and in Inhambane province, suggest that tuberculosis is believed related to sexual intercourse in various ways (Pateguane 1983; Jurg, de Jong, and Tomas 1991), something we saw in both Swaziland and Liberia. In the Pateguane study, TB symptoms were ascribed to the violation of sexual taboos such as intercourse with widows or with women who have recently had an abortion. Most patients were found to seek traditional therapy for TB.

In our studies of STDs in Liberia and Swaziland, we found that symptoms relating to (urinary) schistosomiasis, hernia, leprosy, tuberculosis, piles, seizures, or hookworm might also be seen as related to sexual intercourse, ideas also found in Malawi (Helitzer-Allen and Allen 1992). This does not mean that these other conditions are necessarily sexually transmitted (i.e., always), but rather that they and others are sexually transmiss*ible*—that is, they *can* be transmitted by at least certain types of sexual intercourse. To understand this, we need to recognize the prevailing belief in traditional African thought that many diseases or conditions can result from contamination or spiritual punishment, or from sorcery or witchcraft, and that sexual intercourse provides one common point of contact for the contamination, medicine, or spell causing or transmitting such diseases.

## Profiles of Locally Recognized STDs

A number of diseases believed to be transmitted through sexual intercourse are recognized by Manica healers. An even larger number of diseases are thought to be "caused" by sexual intercourse in the sense that their underlying cause is believed to be intercourse with a prohibited person. As elaborated in the Analysis section below, Manica healers classify several common sexually transmitted diseases together under the rubric *siki*.

The following are composite profiles of the more important locally recognized diseases believed to be transmitted through sexual intercourse. There may be conceptional differences between language group, area, and individual practitioner in details of diagnosis, treatment, etc. Sometimes this is noted in the sketches that follow.

Less clinically oriented readers may wish to skip to the Analysis section that follows. For them, Table 5.2 summarizes the most important diseases discovered.

TABLE 5.2 Summary of Important Locally Recognized STDs in Manica Province, Mozambique

| *STD* | *Men* | *Women* | *Newborn*[1] | *Outstanding Symptoms* | *District or Area* |
|---|---|---|---|---|---|
| Chikazamento[2] (Dropu) | X | X | X | Pus discharge, painful urination, infertility | All districts |
| Chimanga[2] | X | X | X | Sores, blisters around genitals, symptoms in newborns | All districts |
| Mula[2] | X | X | – | Painful lump like furuncle in groin | All districts |
| Songeia[2] | X | X | – | Pain in urination, saffron-colored urine and eyes, and pus discharge | All districts |
| Chikeke[2] | X | X | – | Sores, blisters, discharge, painful urination | Gondola Amatongas Vanduzi |
| Gobela[2] (Keni) | X | X | – | Little holes or tears in the penis or vagina | Chimoio Vanduzi |
| Nyoka Kundu | X | – | – | Painful, swollen testicles | All districts |
| Nyoka Dzoni | – | X | X | Menstrual problems, miscarriage | All districts |
| Sida | X | X | – | Diarrhea, thinness, death | All districts |
| Rikaho | X | (X) | – | Oozing sore on the head, black vomit, partners stuck together. | More common in north |

[1]NB=disease causes problems or symptoms in newborn children.
[2]All categorized as "SIKI" diseases by healers.

1. *Chimanga*. Symptoms: sores in the genital area. In men, these may be located on the head or "point" of the penis. There may be a white discharge from the penis. Some healers claimed that women can also have genital sores or boils, and that these are of similar size and appearance. Some healers claimed the sores or boils do not run, others said they ooze a watery liquid. The sores might begin inside the genitals and then spread to the outside. The sores were characterized as red, sometimes white. Some described little holes or punctures on the penis. There is also pain in urination and men walk stooped over due to "pain in the lower backbone." Some describe the manner of walking as wiggly, "like a duck." Several healers said that the disease, or its symptoms, can remain hidden, perhaps especially in women.

   One healer described "Type 1 and Type 2 *chimanga*," and provided considerable detail about the appearance of symptoms, e.g., a man's urine turns from very yellow to colorless by the third day in Type 1.

   There was disagreement over whether a man becomes sterile or impotent if *chimanga* is not treated. Most healers seemed to believe a woman becomes infertile if the illness remains untreated for, variously, one to six months. Some thought a cured woman can still have children in the future—we know this because "she can still menstruate." The newborn child of a woman with *chimanga* can have sores on the skin, mouth, or nose. The newborn can die from the illness, either in the womb or some time not long after birth.

   A woman with *chimanga* might have no visible sores, therefore the disease might be overlooked unless she is pregnant and miscarries. In this case, "The baby dies inside her and then for about four days little bits of the foetus come out of her." The miscarriage is due to contamination. In the words of one healer, "There is something dirty inside her uterus and the baby eats this dirt and then dies."

   *Cause*: This and most other common, locally recognized STDs are usually described as resulting from intercourse with a person who has the disease, specifically from transmission of an agent of transmission known as *khoma*. *Chimanga* is considered a disease of adults, not children: one must be sexually active to get it. Many healers designated or implicated having many sexual partners as a contributing factor, noting the disease is found in men who "go around" with many women. The presence of Zimbabwean troops in the province has led to an increase in this disease in recent times.

   *Chimanga* can be transmitted in ways other than intercourse, namely by stepping in urine or feces, wearing clothes or touching cloth contaminated with the agent *khoma*.

*Prevalence*: *Chimanga* was described as very common and dangerous. Some claimed this disease is transmitted in both directions (male-female, female-male) with equal ease, which explains why it is found in both men and women in equal numbers. Others thought men more susceptible than women.

*Treatment*: an herbal decoction for drinking as well as a poultice applied directly to the sores. The latter medicine may also be put inside the vagina. One healer commented that the genital sores or boils may disappear quickly but they "go inside," so treatment must be continued for at least a week. The patient must drink the decoction three times a day and there are certain taboos such as avoiding alcohol, smoking, Coca-Cola, and *peri-peri*, or hot pepper (note this seems compatible with what doctors would advise in cases of prostatitis). Eating *peri-peri* is said to interfere with treatment because it "stimulates *khoma* in the abdomen." Healers stressed the importance of following the correct treatment regimen and beginning treatment within the first week.

Chimanga is described as a uniquely traditional disease, therefore "hospital medicine" is considered unable to cure it. Specifically, hospital medicine "cannot kill the *khoma*," and in fact can make the *khoma* "hide in the body" and thus become impossible to "finish" with traditional medicine. Some healers said—perhaps diplomatically—that both modern and traditional medicines were effective. One older healer commented that in earlier times, hospital treatment worked quickly. Nowadays, it does not work this way (evidence of antibiotic resistance?) so patients come to her instead of going to the hospital.

*Prevention*: *Chimanga* can be prevented by boiling some roots in clean water and then keeping a bottle of this available with the roots still in solution. The decoction is taken "as needed." Healers noted that preventive medicine is different from *chimanga* curative medicine. The factor that determines susceptibility to *chimanga* is said to be in the blood. If one's blood is fortified with the preventive medicine, one should not get this disease.

At the same time, healers advised against having many sexual partners and sex with prostitutes and others who might carry the disease as a way of preventing *chimanga*. Healers were emphatic in their advice that sexual relations must be suspended during treatment lest the patient continue to spread the disease.

A female healer commented about foetal contamination with *chimanga*, noting that it can be avoided if the mother with this disease takes the traditional preventive medicine once a week until she delivers the baby, in which case the child will be normal. Without such treatment the baby can die in the womb or might be born with the same sores as the mother.

*Etiology*: *Chimanga* was believed by some to be fatal unless treated by either traditional or modern medicine. People may try to hide the disease for some time due to shame or fear, thereby delaying treatment. However the pain and discomfort of *chimanga* is such that people eventually seek treatment. *Cost*: Chimanga patients usually make repeat visits to the healer or they may actually stay in the healer's compound for about a week. There are certain advantages to a patient in residence, e.g., the healer can make sure the medicine is taken at the right times and in the right dosage, and he can also enforce the dietary proscriptions. However, "in-patient" fees are higher because the patient must be fed and housed. The cost of a week's treatment would be about three chickens or its cash equivalent (about Mt15,000). Cost of treatment was a sensitive topic, therefore it was not part of the interview schedule. Although some cost information was revealed during discussions, it must be regarded as very preliminary and not necessarily reliable.

2. *Chikazamentu* (*dropu, gobela*). Symptoms: a white, milky discharge from both penis and the vagina, characterized by some as "dirt" or impurity. There is also painful, burning or difficult urination for both men and women. There may be abdominal pain, slight fever, itching, weight loss, and/or—according to some—sores or boils on or around the genitals that secrete a milky fluid. However, several healers specifically mentioned that there are no sores with *chikazamentu*. At least one healer saw *chikazamentu* as equivalent to what the hospital calls gonorrhea. The alternate term "*(i)dropu*" is also used by Swazis and Zulus to designate or approximate gonorrhea.

   Another symptom may be "heat" in the waist or groin. Another, in both men and women, is a wet groin from the discharge which they're always trying to hide. A female healer characterized female symptoms as stomach pain, "heat," stools that change from normal to yellowish/milky, and boils on both sides of the vagina.

   *Cause*: Sexual intercourse with someone having the disease. Single women who have had many partners are likely to transmit *chikazamentu*, according to some. As with *chimanga*, it is also believed possible to become contaminated with the disease from contact with bodily waste or clothing of a person with the disease. A few mentioned toilets and "lack of hygiene" as ways to catch it. Those who mentioned stepping in infected urine referred to little creatures (*bichinhos* in Portuguese) in the urine as agents of transmission.

*Treatment*: Similar to *chimanga* and other "*siki*" diseases (see below), all of which seem to be treated in much the same way. Special roots are placed in water and the solution drunk over a period of a week. Some said *chimanga* may lead to infertility (or impotence) within six months if not treated. Others disagreed. A few healers emphasized that one has to "treat all partners of the patient to avoid new transmissions" of the disease.

*Incidence*: Most said *chikazamentu* was very common, although there was disagreement whether it was more or less common than *chimanga*. A number of healers believe that men are more likely than women to get the disease.

3. *Mula*. Symptoms: painful lump, furuncle, abcesses or sores around the genitals. Some described "dirty discharge," painful urination, little creatures in the genitals, sores inside the bladder, difficulty in walking, and/or sores that disappear then return. A few healers volunteered that the disease is fatal if not treated. Specifically, the untreated sore "opens up inside" allowing the impurity to go inside the stomach and cause death. There was disagreement over whether an infected pregnant woman can pass the disease to her unborn child. Some in any case said the condition causes miscarriage and still-birth.

   *Cause*: Intercourse with an infected person. *Khoma*, the same causative agent that transmits the first two STDs (above) was sometimes specified as the thing that transmits *mula*. Others, using Portuguese, called the agent a little creature (*bichinho*.) *Mula* is also transmitted by contact with contaminated feces, urine, dirty toilets, etc. Prostitutes or Zimbabwean soldiers are likely carriers.

   *Treatment*: There are several curative plants. The roots of these may be combined with each other or used as alternatives. These are left in cold water until the solution looks bubbly or frothy like beer. Treatment lasts for five days. As with the first two diseases described as sexually transmitted, *mula* patients should avoid sexual relations and hot pepper until they are completely cured.

   The invisible "little creature" that transmits *mula* is impervious to "injection" (e.g., penicillin.) A few healers said that hospital treatment can be effective in the early stage of the disease, but if the secretions become heavy, traditional medicine is needed.

4. *Songeiga*. Symptoms: characterized by a yellowish, malodorous pus discharge from the penis or vagina. It is also characterized by pain in urination—those afflicted are said to "scream" when they urinate. Other symptoms may include swollen groin, abscesses in

groin, yellow feces and/or urine, pain in the waist and legs, and blood in the urine. As with the first three conditions described, untreated *songeiga* can lead to infertility and the "impurity goes inside the stomach and causes internal abscesses." A few healers said that *songeiga* and *mula* are the same. In men, there are little boils inside the penis. In women there are external sores and menstrual problems. A few referred to stillbirths. A syndrome with the same name and symptoms is found in Malawi (Helitzer-Allen and Allen 1992). The name may suggest belief that the illness first came from Songea, a town in southern Tanzania.

*Cause*: *Songeiga* is caused by either men or women sleeping with a contaminated person. As with other STDs, it is also transmitted by contact with contaminated feces, dirty toilets, little creatures of an infected person, etc. Also like other *siki* diseases, the Portuguese are thought to have brought the disease to Mozambique. Zimbabwean soldiers are likely to spread it nowadays.

*Prevention*: People can prevent this disease, perhaps especially men. If a special medicine is taken, a man or woman can have intercourse with a sick partner and probably not get *songeiga*. There seem to be a number of different medicines that can be used in this way.

*Cost* of treating *songeiga:* one healer revealed that it costs MT3,000 for treatment and it costs Mt4,000 for prevention. Clients apparently come to traditional healers for prevention as well as treatment of this and other STDs.

5. *Chikeke*. Symptoms: include blisters or sores like little tears in the male or female genitals, milky discharge, painful urination, genital boils and swellings (causing stooped walking), yellow or bloody urine, sores spreading to the rest of the body, and genital discharge. The sores can spread to the rest of the body including the mouth. Some describe *chikeke* as in many ways similar to *chimanga* and *chicasamento*, in any case it is regarded as a disease in the *siki* category (see below) and, indeed, shares many features of symptoms, prevention and treatment with other STDs. It is believed to have come from Malawi.
6. *Nyoka Kundu* and *Nyoka Dzoni* (*Nzoni*). There are two *nyoka*-related diseases (discussed later) believed to be sexually transmitted, *nyoka kundu* which affects men and *nyoka dzoni* which affects women. They will be discussed together.

   *Symptoms*: In men at least, the disease is in the upper groin. The testicles are swollen and painful. The stomach is upset and "noisy." The lower back may ache and both men and women may have trouble walking upright. There may also be hernia (*phuzi*) symptoms or even paralysis in the lower waist and back. In women we find miscarriage, menstrual irregularities, infertility, and premenstrual problems.

*Cause*: The male variant is believed caused by a man having intercourse with a menstruating woman. The man is thought to become contaminated with the impurities the menstruating woman's *nyoka* is expelling. A man who has many sexual partners may become contaminated in this way, then pass the contamination to his wife.

Likewise, the female variant, *nyoka dzoni,* is believed transmitted when a woman has intercourse with a man with *nyoka kundu.* A woman gets the disease by contact with bodily fluids believed contaminated by *nyoka kundu.* It can also be contracted from a mother who, if she doesn't treat her *nyoka dzoni* with traditional medicines, can pass her disease on to her unborn daughter. Women appear to also be able to get the disease from contact with the menstrual blood of another woman with the disease, for example by stepping in the place where such a woman has bathed. Thus, in a general sense, the *nyoka* diseases with genito-urinary and related symptoms are caused by contamination and subsequent provocation of a person's *nyoka.* They can also be caused by violation of behavioral norms, such as a menstruating woman jumping over a man or a child.

*Treatment*: A topical medicine rubbed in the upper groin. Also a decoction is drunk. Treatment for *nyoka dzoni* is aimed at regularizing menstruation and preventing infertility.

7. *Gobela, Keni, Madjuru.* Symptoms: "holes in the penis." This condition obstructs the flow of urine and therefore urine is said to leak out of little holes at the end of the penis. Another symptom is pain in urination. Men also have a wet crotch which they may try to hide, but this symptom can not be hidden for long. Females also get this STD; it may appear as sores or also as wetness from discharge.

   *Treatment*: Drinking an oral decoction. There is also an herbal medicine that treats the external sores.

8. *Rikaho, Rukawe.* We saw in Swaziland (Chapter 3) that there are several illnesses with STD-like symptoms that are believed caused by medicines used deliberately to ensure a wife's sexual fidelity. Some Manica healers recognized a syndrome believed to result from a special medicine that a man secretly rubs on his wife to "protect" her from sex with another man. If such sex occurs, the woman's partner will exhibit symptoms which include pain in urination and pus discharge. The illness is called *rukawe* or *rikaho* in Manica, and *rukawe* among the Shona of Zimbabwe. In one form of

this, a man surreptitiously puts a special medicine in the food that he and his wife will eat together. If the wife sleeps with another man after ingesting the medicine, the latter will fall ill with genital and urinary symptoms. The man might also vomit a dark substance and develop an oozing sore on the top of his head as well as headaches and stomach pain. The condition was described as incurable and fatal.

As we saw in Swaziland, in one form of *rukawe* or *rikaho,* a woman committing adultery becomes stuck to her partner in such a way that they cannot separate. The same syndrome has been described in Tanzania (Swantz 1990:125). Some Manica healers described this condition as well known locally and quite common, although it was better known during the colonial period, especially in Tete province to the north. One healer commented that many old men would protect their young wives this way; he made the analogy of laying an explosive mine to protect one's property. Many whites were said to die this way when they slept with local women.

10. *Chitheta* (or *chiterera*), *iumanga, mugarapadima.* (See below, *Nyoka-Related Conditions.*)

## Discussion and Analysis of Findings

It is only for the purposes of translating our findings into a biomedical framework and developing an educational strategy that I will now attempt to simplify the ethnomedicine of STDs and related conditions in Manica. Manica traditional healers recognize two broad categories of illnesses believed to be sexually transmitted: *siki* and *nyoka* related. Both will be described, as will AIDS which falls into neither category.

### *Siki Diseases*

A generic term, *siki,* exists in several Manica languages and dialects to designate the more serious diseases that are considered sexually transmitted, namely *chimanga, chicazamentu, mula, songeia, chikeke,* and *gobela.* These seem to correspond to the more serious and common STDs of Western biomedicine: syphilis, gonorrhea, chlamydia, and chancroid. *Siki* diseases were uniformly described as "adult diseases," meaning they are not found in children, at least before the age of intercourse. At the risk of generalization, *siki* diseases are characterized by the following symptoms in men: hot, burning urination; sores on the penis; and/or a white, milky discharge from the penis. In women, there is also hot, burning urination; sores on the genitals; and pain in the stomach. These diseases are usually said to be more common in men than women.

As a few older healers suggested, the term *siki* may derive from the

English "sick" and may have been borrowed from the Shona of neighboring Zimbabwe where English is the official language. Such derivation might lend credence to the local belief (found elsewhere in Africa) that syphilis and gonorrhea were first introduced by Europeans. Indeed healers claim that these diseases originated with Portuguese soldiers having sexual intercourse with horses, then sleeping with African women thereby introducing the disease to the local area. One healer with an etymological bent suggested that another STD term used across several local dialects, *keni,* comes from the English "watering can," since the term refers to "holes in the penis" that resemble the pouring end of a watering can. (Note that symptoms of "holes in the penis" were described in Liberia and Swaziland as well.)

*Siki* diseases are not associated with causal concepts usually found in traditional African ethnomedical thought, namely imbalance or strife from violation of social norms, pollution, sorcery or witchcraft, or evil or avenging spirits. Instead they are believed to be caused by a common invisible, microscopic agent (*khoma*), or by direct contact with pus or other genital discharges that contain *khoma.* Different diseases are carried by different *khomas,* so the word must be regarded as generic, similar to the bacterium of biomedicine. *Khoma* was sometimes translated into Portuguese as *bichinho,* a small animal or insect (Swazis and Zulus call this *liciwane*). At least one healer conversant in biomedical concepts explained that *khoma* was like a microbe.

Manica healers are allopaths when it comes to *siki* treatment: they introduce an alien element into the body to kill the specific disease-causing *khoma.* Special herbs are boiled, the decoction cooled down, and then given to drink in the morning before eating. In another type of medicine, certain leaves are crushed or ground, then the resulting juice is drunk. There are also medicines applied directly to genital sores. Treatment takes about one week and is usually accomplished in the patient's own home.

*Siki* diseases are believed to be preventable in two ways, medicinal and behavioral. There are different preventive medicines for men and women, and they are said to always work if taken before intercourse with someone carrying the disease. Several healers observed that *chimanga* and other local STDs are more difficult to prevent these days because security considerations make it difficult or impossible to travel to places to obtain the necessary plants. *Siki* diseases can also be prevented by abstaining from sex, by choosing partners unlikely to have a *siki* disease, and by refraining from sex during treatment.

A few healers thought that some *siki* diseases, such as *chikazamentu,* are really precolonial diseases that are related to the "*nyoka*" attempting to rid a person's body of impurities by "evacuating" them in pus discharge, feces, vomit, and bad smells (see below). But for the great majority of healers, *siki* diseases appeared to be understood in a naturalistic manner bearing some obvious similarity with the biomedical view.

### *Nyoka-Related Diseases*

The word *nyoka* means snake in several Bantu languages, but it has a special meaning in connection with health in Manica. Healers described the *nyoka* as a guardian or spirit-protector of the body. This guardian demands that the body it inhabits be kept free of impurities or contaminants lest it react with displeasure, causing pain and discomfort. It is referred to as if it has a personality somewhat independent of the body it inhabits; for example it may be angry or calm. In Western biomedical terms, *nyoka* may be thought of as a symbolic expression of the need to respect the human body—even as a personified immune system. A useful English translation might therefore be Guardian of Health or Guardian of Bodily Purity.

All people are born with a *nyoka* and it remains within the body until death. *Nyoka* can move up and down in the body from the area of the heart to the abdomen. It is not visible, even if one cuts open a body. Its existence is confirmed through bodily sensations when it is disturbed. For example, if "dirt," spoiled food or bad medicine enters the body, *nyoka* may contract and cause cramps, or it can make noises of complaint in the stomach. *Nyoka* cleanses the body by means of discharges such as diarrhea, vomiting, menstruation or pus, all of which are seen as natural bodily functions that rid the body of impurities.

Manica healers described only two diseases that use the name *nyoka* and that are sexually transmitted, *nyoka kundu,* which affects men, and *nyoka dzoni,* which affects women. However, these entail symptoms that are so diverse that the two diseases probably correspond to, or overlap with, a number of diseases or conditions in biomedical classification. Furthermore, there are other locally recognized STDs that do not use the name *nyoka* yet are based in *nyoka* ideas of pollution. Therefore, it seems useful to use the term *nyoka*-related diseases to refer to a category of illnesses whose etiologies are conceived in a more indigenous or traditional African way, compared to *siki* diseases. As with child diarrheas (Green, Jurg, and Dgedge 1991), STDs of this sort involve the idea of pollution and the role of a Guardian of Bodily Health.

A woman who has sex with a man who has *nyoka kundu* is said to contract the female disease *nyoka dzoni,* and vice versa, through the transmission of a kind of pollution (as described elsewhere, e.g., Botswana (Ingstad 1990:33). *Nyoka dzoni* can also be caught by stepping in urine or feces contaminated by at least the male disease. Healers also described congenital transmission. If a man does not treat his *nyoka kundu* with traditional medicines, not only will he remain sick but at the moment of conceiving a child with a woman, the unborn child's *nyoka* will be "contaminated." When the child is born, it will not only have symptoms of the disease *nyoka khundu,* but healers explained that it will also be susceptible to various other diseases. In biomedical terms, the child will have poor resistance, or a weak immune system. A mother also passes her illness on to her unborn daughter if she does not treat her *nyoka dzoni.*

Judging by the symptoms of *nyoka*-related diseases, a variety of seemingly less serious and apparently self-limiting genito-urinary infections and conditions may come under this category, e.g., nonspecific urethritis, yeast infections, prostate infections, and trichomonas. Among these are conditions that are almost certainly not sexually transmitted but that affect the genital area or lower genito-urinary tract and so might appear to be so. Other conditions may or may not be biomedically regarded as sexually transmitted. For example, swollen testicles are considered a symptom of the male *nyoka* disease. Local physicians believe this refers to hydrocele or other conditions of scrotal masses which relate to hernia or trauma, or which perhaps are congenital. Although hydrocele is not biomedically regarded as sexually transmitted, other scrotal masses such as epididymitis "may occur as a complication of urethritis or prostatitis (particularly gonorrheal)," according to the Merk Manual (11th ed.)

There are other locally recognized STDs that are not regarded as *siki* diseases yet are not explicitly referred to as *nyoka* diseases. Syndromes of this sort include *chitheta* (or *chiterera*), *iumanga, mugarapadima* and *sikumbe.* These are considered by healers as less serious than *siki,* and they include symptoms of menstrual irregularities, vaginal inflammations and discharges, sores in the groin or elsewhere, miscarriage, and infertility. Some of these are regarded as adult diseases but not as sexually transmitted. The etiology of at least one of these—*chitheta/chiterera*—involves the position or state of the *nyoka.* For our purposes, these gynecological and other relatively minor conditions can be regarded as *nyoka*-related. Minor in this sense refers to conditions other than those STDs known or suspected to play a role in facilitating HIV transmission.

## AIDS

Although all traditional healers had heard of AIDS (the Portuguese term *SIDA* was recognized and used in discussions), most claimed to know little about it beyond what they had heard and understood from the radio, e.g., that it is incurable, fatal, and sexually transmitted. A second source of information was "other people." A majority believed they have neither seen nor treated this disease and that it is new to Mozambique. A few healers seemed to confuse AIDS with familiar STDs—even referring to it as a *siki* disease—perhaps because they have heard that it is sexually transmitted. These healers claimed AIDS is not really a new disease—it is the old familiar disease *songeia,* or perhaps *chimanga.* Therefore, they claim, there are a variety of familiar medicines to cure or prevent the disease, a belief found elsewhere in Africa (de Zalduondo, Msamanga, and Chen 1989; Ingstad 1990:34; Staugaard 1991). At least one other healer thought that AIDS is different from traditional STDs, nevertheless there are traditional medicines to cure it. In short, *some* healers claimed they can cure—and have cured—what they believe to be AIDS cases. Healers reported that patients might come to them and announce that they have AIDS. This is contrary to the traditional diagnostic procedure carried out by the healer who is assisted by spirits.

Some healers reported that AIDS is highly contagious and is characterized by progressive weakness, sores on the body, appetite loss, prolonged diarrhea, emaciation, and coughing. However, there was little understanding of how AIDS is transmitted, e.g., there was almost no reference to blood. Several forms of casual contact were mentioned as means of transmission, such as people eating together. A few healers mentioned extramarital sex and noted its increase in recent times.

Some said it is better to prevent than try to cure AIDS. Although some had no ideas about prevention, a few mentioned the use of condoms. One healer even produced some condoms for an interviewer.

## Note on Sorcery

Other than *rikaho*—mentioned by healers only after probing—no evidence was found of sorcery or witchcraft in the etiology of locally recognized STDs. Focus group participants specifically denied that any form of *siki* could be willed or sent by enemies or otherwise ill-intentioned people. True, it may have been a shortcoming of the methods used that we were unable to elicit information about beliefs in a possible role of spirits, witchcraft or sorcery in connection with "STDs." Sorcery and related beliefs are found in the etiologies of STDs among the neighboring Shona (Gelfand et al. 1985), who speak a dialectal variation of the languages of our informants. It is also true that Manica healers are reluctant to speak of anything suggesting witchcraft or sorcery since the government in the recent past used such beliefs to denounce traditional healers and suppress traditional medicine. Nevertheless, I feel safe in concluding that *siki* diseases are perceived in predominantly natural terms, and these are the STDs of priority concern. AIDS is sufficiently new that it would be premature to conclude the same for this disease.

## AIDS/STDs Health Communications Strategy

From the foregoing, we may conclude that traditional healers in Manica appear to have complex nosologies based on fine distinctions between symptoms. This implies considerable skill in empirical observation and diagnosis. Interviewers encountered enough references to local *materia medica* to suggest that this is no less complex. Regarding nosology, healers appear to have no fewer diagnostic categories of venereal, gynecological, and urological diseases than biomedicine, at least as routinely practiced in Mozambique's smaller hospitals and health posts. One result of the triage conditions of Mozambique's understaffed provincial hospitals is that less-serious health problems are seldom presented at hospitals. Therefore, traditional healers in their daily practice almost certainly deal with a greater number and variety of diagnostic categories than local doctors and nurses. Considering this, the view that traditional healers need to be taught correct diagnosis appears condescending. Instead it would appear that local health workers could benefit from learning about the empirical symptom-based diagnostic practices of traditional healers.

Healers appear confident in the efficacy of their treatments for STDs. They seem to advise their STD clients to use traditional medicines and to avoid hospital medicines—or injections specifically. Healers commented that *siki* diseases are centered in the lower stomach. Traditional medicines are believed to reach this area easily, but not injections.

Since syphilis, gonorrhea, and other high-priority serious STDs fall within the *siki* rather then *nyoka*-related categories, our communication strategy was focused on the former. Such focus conformed to the priorities of the existing national and provincial AIDS/STD program that recognizes syphilis and gonorrhea as major cofactors in the spread of AIDS as well as major health problems in their own right. And unlike AIDS, which can only be prevented, syphilis and gonorrhea are curable. It seems probable that other STDs such as chlamydia, chancroid, and lymphogranuloma venereum are classed under *siki* by local healers. These are also treatable and may also be cofactors in HIV transmission.

It would appear that traditional healers' understanding and treatment of the less-serious *nyoka*-related diseases are at least noninjurious. Their preventive strategies to avoid these conditions involve maintaining bodily purity, and therefore are generally promotive of good hygiene and health. In any case, such diseases are of less public health consequence than AIDS or the systemic STD infections therefore they are not part of our strategic focus.

There appeared to be several favorable factors in developing an STD strategy for Manica healers. It seemed unnecessary to accommodate our message to complex magico-religious beliefs; in fact, *siki* diseases are thought of in much the way biomedicine understands common STDs. Furthermore, virtually all of the preventive advice given by traditional healers is biomedically sound, if incomplete: refraining from intercourse during treatment; locating and treating all recent sexual partners of a sufferer; even avoiding alcohol and spicy foods during treatment. There are other parallels with biomedicine such as recognition that STDs can infect newborn infants and that STD symptoms can become latent. Manica healers also recognize that untreated STDs, especially the disease resembling gonorrhea, lead to infertility. This was mentioned often, reflecting the traditional concern with fertility found throughout most of sub-Saharan Africa.

However, the question remains what to advise about *treatment*. Healers were convinced that only their own medicines could treat *khoma*, the causal agent of most *siki* diseases. Some healers even said that *khoma* "retreats" in the presence of hospital medicine and so may become impossible to cure. Another factor is that even if it seemed feasible to advise healers to send their patients to the hospital for treatment of STDs, hospitals in Manica province and elsewhere in the country sometimes run out of antibiotics, at least for nonlife-threatening emergencies. Assuming the availability of antibiotics in hospitals in the future, it may be possible to build upon a growing spirit of intersectoral trust and cooperation after the first workshop and persuade healers to allow at least their *siki* patients to benefit from hospital as well as traditional medicine.

One possible referral strategy would be to agree with healers that *siki* diseases are foreign, then suggest that foreign (biomedical) medicines are needed to treat them. However, short of training and supervising healers in antibiotic use—discussed below—most impact can probably be achieved in the *prevention* of both STDS and AIDS. This can be done by reinforcing existing STD preventive practices that are sound and by introducing new ones such as adopting condoms and sterilizing razor blades.

### *Concept of Latency*

Manica healers recognize latency of symptoms in STDs, therefore the biomedical concept of latency could be explained based on existing concepts. In discussion of treatment, healers gave their explanation that the *khoma* (causal agent) of *siki* "hides in the body" when a *siki* patient takes antibiotics, after which the disease may be impossible to cure. This may reflect empirical observation of patients who self-medicate improperly or who fail to take the full course of a prescribed antibiotic treatment for gonorrhea. Here healers' discouragement of laypersons medicating themselves is reinforced, and health educators could take the opportunity to explain the proper use and function of antibiotics.

We then explain how symptoms of gonorrhea and syphilis "hide in the body" yet the microbe or *khoma* is still present, in a resting state. Symptoms can disappear even if there is no treatment. In any case, a full course of treatment should be followed with either traditional or modern medicine. This would appear to be the only realistic strategy until a way is found to attract more clients of traditional healers to hospitals for antibiotic treatment—assuming the availability of effective drugs.

### *AIDS Strategy*

The topic of AIDS could be introduced without reference to scientific terms such as virus. AIDS and HIV transmission could be explained as much as possible in terms of healers' existing understanding of *siki* diseases and their beliefs about contamination. We (that is, health educators) can agree with healers that AIDS is indeed a new disease, one that is transmitted by an invisible, tiny causal agent similar in some ways to *khoma*. However, the AIDS *khoma* is not transmitted in ways the healers are perhaps familiar with. For example, it is not transmitted by touching, sharing eating utensils, sleeping under the same blanket (ideas that emerged in individual interviews), or by stepping in a sick person's excrement or discharges (by which means it is possible to become contaminated with *siki*.) Instead it is transmitted through blood, semen, or vaginal secretion contact. This means that the AIDS *khoma* can be transmitted through open wounds in the skin, especially *through the genital sores of* siki *diseases*. This also means that if one or both partners have a *siki* disease, not only can the *khoma* of the *siki* be transmitted but also the *khoma* of AIDS. Here we can remind healers that AIDS is both fatal and incurable.

Another possible opportunity for the blood of a sick person to infect or contaminate another's blood is through traditional healers' use of razor blades in vaccination or scarification. Here we say that unless new razors are used with each patient and/or used razor blades are properly sterilized, small amounts of blood—even the invisible *khoma* of AIDS—can cling to the blade and enter the bloodstream of the next person on whom the same razor is used.

There should be further research to confirm our interpretation of the indigenous concept of *nyoka* as something akin to the biomedical concept of the body's immune system. Research should be conducted with *clients* of healers as well as with healers themselves. If we are right, AIDS preventive education should draw explicit parallels between *nyoka* and the immune system. The existence of similar ethnomedical concepts should be researched elsewhere in Africa where HIV infection is prevalent. Alternative ways to approximate the concept of the immune system in communication with South African healers are presented in Chapter 7.

### *Condom Strategy*

Due to innumerable factors well documented in studies in neighboring countries, there is great resistance to using condoms on the part of Africans including Mozambicans. Our own research clearly suggested that condoms (*chibudu*, or *preservativos, camisas* in Portuguese) are held in low regard. As a means of STD prevention, traditional medicines and advice were believed far superior to condoms. Our strategy called for discovering an opportunistic entry point among traditional healers, upon which we could build a more ambitious program of condom promotion. Since healers already advise their patients with *siki* diseases to avoid intercourse during treatment, we tried to persuade healers to provide their clients with condoms to ensure compliance with the healers' own advice. Healers should find this logical and reaffirming of their current beliefs and practices. We are simply trying to add some modern technology to help them accomplish the task.

The practical, logistical strategy for condom promotion probably ought to be to promote community-based distribution in such a way that healers can earn a small profit on condom sales. Such an approach appears to be fully compatible with the condom strategy of the national AIDS/STDs program, however it remains to be elaborated.

It is further part of our strategy not to try to attempt to reduce the complexity of the traditional healer's *siki* consultation to the mere provision of a Mt50 ($.03) condom. Such consultation consists of an integrated "package," which includes diagnosis, possibly divination, preventive advice, treatment, and follow-up. Condom provision and advice can become part of this package; it is unlikely to replace it. In parallel research related to child diarrhea, we suggested the possibility that at least some Manica healers have rebelled against the government's ORS campaign (Green and Jurg 1991). To them, it may have seemed that their years of training and experience—not to mention spiritual inspiration—in understanding and treating various diarrheas had been reduced by the government to a simple treatment of sugar, salt, and water. This seems to have provoked a number of healers to advise clients to avoid any use of sugar, salt, and water in child diarrheas. In view of this, we should avoid anything that might contribute to a negative reaction by healers to the national AIDS/STDs program's condom campaign.

As discussed in Chapter 4, there is evidence that spermicides such as nonoxynol-9 kills bacteria, viruses, and parasites that cause many

STDs including AIDS. Although not a part of the Manica pilot program, these methods have a significant advantage over condoms, namely that women can initiate and have some control over them.

### *Razor Blades and Blood Contact*

Some traditional treatments—including those for STDS—may contribute to the spread of AIDS and other diseases, e.g., the use of unsterilized razor blades for traditional vaccinations or incisions for introducing medicines into the bloodstream. The same razor may be used for several patients. Although there is no clear epidemiological evidence to date that skin-piercing practices associated with traditional healing have spread AIDS in Africa (Pela and Platt 1989), potential for such transmission is sufficient that the World Health Organization inaugurated a strategy to "collaborate with member states to ensure the use of sterile needles, syringes and other skin-piercing practices in medical and other settings" (WHO 1987). Traditional healers are themselves exposed to blood and other bodily fluids in their routine practice. Some of their patients may be HIV-positive or even have AIDS, putting the healers at risk. Therefore, our strategy was to build upon a pilot program initiated by the Department of Traditional Medicine in 1989 to promote:

- use of only one razor per client when possible. This may require clients bringing their own razor to the healer;
- sterilization of razor blades used for treatment;
- healers avoiding contact with patients' blood.

To sterilize blades, we promoted locally available hydrochloride solutions such as "Javel" bleach. Each healer participating in a workshop is offered a bottle of bleach and sterilization is both explained and demonstrated. Boiling razor blades in water emerged as a less-favorable alternative for healers because healers feared razors would become blunt.

### *Traditional Ideas of Contagion*

As noted above, Manica healers associate ideas of pollution or contamination with *siki*. For example, the urine, feces and clothing of a person with *siki* are believed capable of transmitting disease by mere contact. Instead of focusing health education messages that directly contradict such beliefs, it seemed more useful to reinforce the idea that human waste can indeed carry disease agents such as those that cause cholera and typhoid. This would avoid confrontation on a minor, innocuous issue while strengthening environmental sanitation efforts and reinforcing education aimed at reducing cholera, typhoid, schistosomiasis, helminthic infections, and the like.

### *Modification of Sexual Behavior*

Among the many parallels found in Manica between traditional and modern understanding and treatment of STDs, traditional healers provide their *siki* patients with biomedically sound advice about sexual behavior. For example, patients under a healer's care for either *siki* or *nyoka*-related diseases are told to refrain from intercourse until they are free of the disease. Likewise, a few healers advise their patients to bring their husband, wife, or other sexual partner to the healer for treatment of the same disease. Healers also give considerable preventive advice to clients such as avoiding or at least being wary of sexual partners "outside the home." Healers specifically discourage relations with prostitutes and soldiers. The implication is that people should avoid relations with partners suspected or known to have had many sexual partners. Phrased in the latter fashion, this is central to our AIDS/STD preventive message. We wish to reinforce the idea that sex outside the home can be dangerous, especially during a time of population and social upheaval, particularly when a new, deadly, incurable "foreign" disease has been introduced.

Traditional healers can also influence the general public in matters relating to sexual behavior. African healers tend to be guardians of traditional codes of morality and values. Indeed, in Manica they interpret a number of diseases (other than *siki*) as *resulting* from violations of moral codes and neglect of traditions. Manica healers are in fact more conservative and restrictive than the National AIDS/STDs program in their advice about "safe sex." They adhere to a complex system of sexual prohibitions, the violation of which leads to a variety of health problems. For example, intercourse during menstruation is considered contaminating and therefore unsafe. Such avoidance under certain conditions may help prevent minor urological problems. Of more potential significance, some AIDS researchers suspect that menstrual blood—perhaps in combination with other factors—may provide a vehicle for HIV transmission (Piot and Harris 1990:12; Edwards 1992). If this proves true, healers erring on the side of greater sexual restriction may be promoting sound advice.

Other prohibitions, such as sex with a widow or with a woman who has miscarried appeared to be biomedically inconsequential and therefore no attempt was made to change them.

### *Locating Recent Sexual Partners*

Contact tracing—or partner notification and follow-up treatment—is recognized as an important tool in the control of STDs worldwide (Asuzu, Rotowa, and Ajayi 1990; Ramstedt et al. 1990). Mozambique Ministry of Health officials have acknowledged that hospitals have had little success in locating and treating recent partners of STD patients. It has been suggested that traditional healers could help hospitals in such an endeavor. The problem here is that healers feel fully competent to treat such patients themselves. We may have to settle for a short-term strategy of agreeing with healers that the full course of treatment should be followed with either traditional or modern treatment, and this includes finding and treating recent partners of *siki* patients. In any case, healers should prove relatively successful in this since they are more likely than hospital staff to know something about the social and sexual life of the *siki* patient. Compared to hospital staff, healers also have more moral and mystical persuasive power with the patient, aided by coming into regular contact with the patient.

### *Care and Support for AIDS Patients*

As AIDS cases proliferate in Africa, it is clear that national health systems will be unable to take care of even the physical needs of patients, let alone provide psychological or spiritual support. Staugaard (1991) reports a conclusion from the WHO Expert Committee Meeting in Botswana that "Healers can convey technically appropriate home care, dispense symptomatic care, treat opportunistic infections and counsel young people about control of HIV." The Mozambique National AIDS/STDs Program already recognizes this. In fact, Mozambican healers can and do help families of patients during periods of loss and trauma, including war-related trauma (Green, Williamson, and Nimpuno-Parente 1992). Such support should be recognized, accorded the value it deserves, and reinforced in a communications strategy. Chapter 7 on South Africa offers more discussion on the role of healers in care, support, and counseling for HIV/AIDS patients, as does Chapter 9 on Tanzania.

Table 5.3 summarizes the program's AIDS/STDs communications strategy for interchange and health education with traditional healers. It should be emphasized that the strategy is for communicating with traditional healers and not necessarily with clients of healers or the general public. The expectation is that healers will prove to be able to educate and motivate at least their own clients and that this will have an effect on promoting behaviors that will slow the spread of standard STDs as well as HIV infection in Manica province. It is further expected that healers will modify their own behavior in ways that decrease their risk of infection.

## The Strategy Operationalized

The communications strategy described above was operationalized in a week-long workshop held in Chimoio, Manica province in November 1991. It was sponsored by USAID. As summarized in Table 5.3, the basic

TABLE 5.3 Proposed AIDS/STDs Strategy to Promote with Traditional healers in Manica Province

| *Introduce, Promote* | *Encourage Reinforce* | *Leave Alone (But Respect)* | *Discourage* |
|---|---|---|---|
| 1. Condom use and condom education.<br>2. Steril-ization of razor blades used for treatment.<br>3. Use of only one razor per client when possible.<br>4. Avoiding contact with blood of patients<br>5. Appropriate referrals to hospital or health post.<br>6. Healers to discourage their clients from antibiotic self-treatment, and explain reasons.<br>7. Realization that shame should not prevent the sick from seeking treatment. | 1. Belief that sexual inter-course can be a health hazard (esp. if with many partners or outside of marriage).<br>2. Belief that intercourse with a person with an "STD" is dangerous.<br>3. The practice of sexual abstin-ence during STD treatment.<br>4. Belief that partners of a person with STD should be treated<br>5. Traditional healers caring for AIDS pat-ients, and providing support to family and community.<br>6. Notions of sexual morality | 1. Rituals and ceremonies.<br>2. Herbal teas, decoctions[1]<br>3. Topical remedies, ointments.<br>4. All non-dangerous treatments and preventions.<br>5. Beliefs in general, unless they lead to injurious practices. | 1. Healers having direct contact with patient blood.<br>2. Traditional vaccination if acceptable alternatives are available. |

[1]This seems both realistic and the best strategy until there is pharmacological evidence that particular decoctions may be dangerous. Indeed they may be beneficial.

workshop strategy was to identify and reinforce aspects of traditional medicine believed to promote public health, while discouraging those believed to have negative health impact. Those beliefs and practices with little or no health impact were left alone. The workshop itself consisted primarily of seminar-style discussion between peers, structured around presentations by trainers from the Provincial Health Department and by healers nominated by the group of healers. There were also demonstrations and role-playing by participants and moderators. Demonstrations included correct use of condoms and sterilization of razor blades in hydrochloric acid solutions of household bleach. From interviewing traditional healers intermittently over a nine-month period prior to the workshop and from training I provided, the trainers had become sensitized to ethnomedical beliefs and practices as well as to the approach just outlined. They had also learned how to communicate effectively with healers.

Thirty participants were invited to the workshop. In the event, eighteen traditional healers registered but one elderly man dropped out after the first day. Seventeen healers completed the workshop. The lower-than-expected turnout may have been due to internal differences within the local healers' association, to weakness in coordination on our part, or to healers' suspicion regarding government motives, given years of poor relations between the Frelimo party and Mozambique's indigenous healers. The president of the healers' association supported the suspicion hypothesis. However, both healers and government health personnel participating in the inaugural workshop were enthusiastic about the general approach of searching for the common ground between biomedical and indigenous understandings of disease. The use of indigenous disease names alone proved a great facilitator of communication, and it was taken by the healers as a gesture of respect and good intention.

It may be noted that at least one follow-up workshop for traditional healers was organized by the Manica Provincial Health Department within ten months of the pilot workshop (August 1992). At that time, healers in Manica were reported to be distributing condoms and cooperating in other areas with the Provincial Health Department. Manica is the first of six provinces in Mozambique in each of which, according to the three-year program plan, the ministry expects to conduct research on ethnomedical beliefs and behavior, develop culturally sensitive health education strategies for local healers, and conduct workshops for the exchange of information between biomedical and indigenous practitioners.

In a review of the challenge of AIDS prevention in Africa, de Zalduondo, Msamanga, and Chen (1989:165) conclude that "the complex nature of AIDS points to the need for small-scale projects geared toward culturally homogenous communities where trained staff can translate the information into locally meaningful terms." This is what was attempted in Manica. While some might feel our "translation" efforts could impede acceptance of scientific thinking by perpetuating magical thinking (Asuni 1979), I believe that traditional healers are unlikely to abandon their way of interpreting STDs and other diseases as a result of any health education resources currently available to African health ministries, at least those that directly confront existing beliefs. Biomedicine must make some accommodation to the beliefs of indigenous healers—and their clients—in order to modify significantly well-established health beliefs and behavior. I believe my colleagues and I accomplished this in Manica without compromising the principles of public health.

Assessment of the effectiveness of this approach must await evaluations planned for the third year of the project, although there will be ongoing monitoring of all aspects of the program through less-formal means. Further research in Africa is also needed to shed more light on the efficacy of AIDS control through the prevention and treatment of common STDs (Mhalu 1990).

Finally, my colleagues and I developed and submitted a proposal for a pilot program that would involve traditional healers in treating certain STDs with oral antibiotics. This is discussed in Chapter 9.

## Notes

1. This chapter represents an expansion of material that appeared in Green, E. C., A. Jurg, and A. Dgedge, "Sexually Transmitted Diseases, AIDS and Traditional Healers in Mozambique" *Medical Anthropology* Vol. 15, No. 3, Spring 1993, pp. 261–281.

# 6

# The Relevance of Family-Planning Programs

The immediate relevance of child-spacing or family-planning programs to AIDS/STDs efforts is that both rely partly on barrier contraceptive methods such as the condom, sponge, and diaphragm. Spermicides are also promoted for family planning and are lately thought to provide protection against STDs and AIDS, at least when used in conjunction with male or female barrier methods. Both AIDS/STD and family-planning programs also attempt to modify people's sexual behavior in similar ways. And not only are some of the solutions shared; the problem areas of excessive fertility (lack of responsible child spacing) and HIV/STD transmission are themselves linked. For example, infertility may result from STDs, and when both STDs and infertility are widespread, there may be greater resistance to child spacing and more pressure for women to have more children more quickly. To the extent that traditional healers are enlisted in collaborative family-planning programs, the impact on HIV and STD transmission as well as child spacing should be positive and, I think, significant.

Another way to look at the relevance of healers' involvement in family planning efforts to AIDS programs is to think of what the level of impact would be if U.S.-funded AIDS programs devoted some percentage of their training funds for Africa—say, 10 percent—to involving traditional healers in AIDS/HIV prevention. There would be about three times that impact if the same level of training funds allocation were spent to involve healers in family planning, quite apart from the beneficial impact such involvement would have on maternal and child health and survival, the growth of Africa's economies, etc. (In FY 1992 AID obligated some $326 million for population programs versus about $95 million for AIDS programs.)

The questions to be raised in this chapter are: Can traditional healers be recruited to become involved in child spacing programs in spite of Africa's celebrated "pronatalism" and healers' alleged preoccupation with assisting clients in having *more* children? Can collaborative programs successfully combine child spacing and AIDS/STDs goals and objectives? Can healers successfully promote barrier methods and spermicides, and if so, how?

## Problems of Fertility and Its Regulation in Africa

Africa has become the priority region for contraceptive programs funded by AID's Office of Population, and the approach currently emphasized—as reflected in the mandates of several recently initiated centrally funded (meaning they have global scope) family-planning projects—is to work through the private sector as much as possible, especially the for-profit or the commercial/industrial sector. This is because public sector programs have had little success in even meeting existing "demand" for contraceptives, let alone in motivating Africans to want to space births through use of modern contraception. By working through the private sector, it is hoped that many problems of cost effectiveness, humanpower development, commodity resupply, and especially escalating recurring costs can be circumvented, and the creative potential of profit-motivated entrepreneurs in the private sector can be tapped. A problem with the private-sector approach in Africa is that the commercial or industrial sectors are small and relatively undeveloped. In order for population programs to have significant impact, conventional definitions of this sector must be modified and expanded.

Traditional healers are in fact among the most successful entrepreneurs and businessmen in Africa today. The role of the African traditional healer is complex. He or she is often part health care provider, part spiritual adviser, part ritual specialist and priest, part empirical scientist, part psychiatrist, and part family therapist. Outreach with the urban poor and the rural masses is unrivaled, meaning that if the traditional healer can be persuaded to cooperate with family-planning agencies or associations, he or she can become an exceedingly effective distributor of contraceptives, as well as a contraceptive motivator—if convinced that family planning is worthwhile.

As observed in previous chapters, traditional healers are accessible to all Africans—wherever they live or whatever their circumstances—they are culturally appropriate, and they are affordable. They have credibility as well as respect and prestige in local African communities—otherwise clients would not seek their advice and pay for their services—therefore they can do much to stimulate interest in and demand for family-planning services. As guardians of the traditional moral order, they can help overcome pronatalism and resistance to efforts aimed at promoting child spacing and reduced fertility rates, which are deeply rooted in African culture.

Cultural factors that tend to reinforce pronatalism in sub-Saharan Africa have been much discussed in the literature; these include unilineal kinship descent, ancestor veneration or the "cult of the ancestors," traditional land tenure, the economic value of children, early marriage, female subordination, ethnic or "tribal" rivalries, political insecurity, bride wealth, high infant mortality, religious traditions and teachings, lack of education, poverty, rural residence, filial piety, and patterns of subsistence agriculture dependent upon woman and child labor (Green, 1982; Caldwell and Caldwell 1985, 1987; Dyson and Murphy 1985; Frank 1985; Golliber 1985). There are also culturally influenced behavioral patterns that affect fertility such as widespread abandoning of postpartum abstinence from intercourse and a decline in breastfeeding. Indeed, there are *medically* influenced factors such as reduced incidence of diseases causing sterility or subfecundity.

The complexity and sheer weight of relevant cultural and other factors make prospects for lower fertility in Africa appear remote at best. An expert on African population issues concludes:

> In sum, African parents have large families because they want them and perceive them to be in their economic and personal interest. In combination with an unpromising economic outlook and slow social development, the prospects are that fertility and population growth rates will remain high for the foreseeable future (Goliber 1985:34).

The ubiquity and power of pronatalism is well understood by African leaders, about whom the Caldwells note:

> . . . politicians, civil servants and political activists all feel that (contraceptive) programs may run counter to the basic spiritual beliefs and emotions of African society. They feel that there is little public demand and are conscious of the threat of grassroots opposition. Furthermore, they are unwilling to be too closely identified with activities which may be culturally doomed to failure (Caldwell and Caldwell 1985:26).

Where does this leave family-planning programs? Such programs are often discussed in terms of supply and demand. In fact, there is little demand for modern contraception, yet the bulk of effort goes into the supply side. This is probably because it is easier. We understand and have experience in commodity distribution systems and we're used to measuring program success in terms of commodities used or at least delivered. Demand takes us into the elusive, opaque, and complex areas of the psychology of tribal and peasant peoples, exotic religions and social organizations, and economic rationalities that don't seem rational to us—in short, into African culture. Motivation or demand relates to things over which we may have little influence namely, economic development, educational opportunities, land tenure systems, and the status and power of women.

## Background to the Nigerian Projects

In 1985, I participated in a brainstorming session at the Population Crisis Committee (PCC, renamed Population Action International in 1992) on ways to reduce Africa's excessively high fertility. During the discussion I proposed that traditional healers might promote both family planning practices and contraceptive technology if some effort were spent educating healers about the value of "modern" family planning health-related objectives, and about the effectiveness of contraceptive technology. After considerable discussion, PCC expressed an interest in seeing if traditional healers could be enlisted in family planning efforts in Nigeria. Given Nigeria's population of some 110,000,000 as well as the sheer magnitude of its development problems, there was agreement that any amelioration of problems in that country would be watched with keen interest by Africans and donors everywhere. PCC was particularly interested in low-cost, sustainable approaches to family planning that would not have to rely on government funding and that would be sensitive to the many and diverse cultural factors that have been shown to largely determine the success or failure of family planning efforts in Africa (Green 1982; Caldwell and Caldwell 1987).

A pilot project did develop in Lagos and Benue states, Nigeria. These states were chosen because both had prior experience with collaborative programs, Benue involving TBAs in midwifery and Lagos involving traditional healers in primary health care (the latter supported by UNICEF). In 1987 Lagos State had a population of over 7 million while Benue's was over 4.2 million. The maternal mortality rate was 70 deaths per 100,000 live births. The infant mortality rate was somewhat better at 50 deaths per 1,000 live births. Contraceptive prevalence was no higher than 3 percent to 4 percent, and total fertility rates were between 6 percent and 7 percent.

The Lagos/Benue projects were initially supported by PCC and later by USAID population funds administered by the Pathfinder Fund. The experience is described in this chapter. Details of certain sections of a baseline survey conducted for this project are presented not only because of their relevance to family planning and AIDS issues, but because they also shed light on more general questions relating to collaborative programs.

The basic idea behind what became known as the Traditional Sector Family Health (TSFH) projects in Lagos and Benue states was to harness the potential of traditional healers in family planning motivation—

or "demand" creation—as well as in service delivery. A fundamental premise was that it makes more sense to rely on existing health practitioners—some of whom may already be promoting traditional methods of child spacing—than to attempt to create new family-planning service providers from the ranks of local community "volunteers," as in more conventional community-based distribution (CBD) programs (cf. Jancloes 1984; Skeet 1984). Our hypotheses were that Nigerian healers could accomplish some or all of the following:

- help overcome pronatalist attitudes and opposition to modern contraceptives;
- persuade their clients or patients to adopt or at least try modern contraceptives;
- serve as male motivators (a deliberate effort was made to recruit male traditional healers for TSFH project participation);
- deliver contraceptive services in areas unserved or underserved by biomedically trained health personnel;
- quickly learn and then put into practice principles of modern family planning. As practitioners with established patient caseloads, traditional healers might already be advising their clients to use indigenous methods of birth control;
- successfully carry out the entrepreneurial aspects of community-based distribution programs, since traditional healers are already entrepreneurs by profession—and often successful ones. Because healers are already financially self-supporting, they are not forced to subsist on the usually meager profits from contraceptive sales alone;
- refer various types of clients to modern health facilities, since some African healers (and traditional birth attendants) are already doing this;
- motivate potential acceptors and deliver services in ways that are culturally appropriate and persuasive.

We recognized that given the resistance to family planning in Africa, it would probably be best to initiate programs in the traditional sector that combined primary health care, and in particular child survival technologies, with family planning. As to how to assess interest on the part of healers in "modern" family planning and child survival—and in working cooperatively with the modern sector—it seemed unnecessary to conduct a formal needs assessment survey. Informal discussions with the (national) Nigerian Association of Medical Herbalists, the Lagos Board of Traditional Medicine, and the Benue Traditional Medical Practitioners Association, and with a number of individual traditional healers in

Benue and Lagos states provided ample evidence that healers in at least the two states chosen for pilot projects were motivated to learn about contraceptive technology and primary health care, and to cooperate with the formal health sector as community-based distributors. However, funds were made available to spend a day prior to the opening of the workshop conducting a baseline knowledge, attitudes and practices survey of healers.

## Nigerian Baseline Survey

### *Research Methods*

Originally, the Central Office of Statistics (COS) was to provide experienced interviewers to serve as interviewers for the surveys in Lagos and Benue states. There had been some discussion about the relative advantages of COS interviewers and public health nurses for the job at hand. As is often the case, there were advantage trade-offs with both. Public health nurses would be familiar with the subject matter of the interviews, which meant they could clarify misunderstandings on the part of the interviewer and they could probe effectively for additional information. On the other hand, the presence of nurses might influence respondents to give answers they might think the nurses would want to hear. COS interviewers, who would probably have no particular background in public health, would have the disadvantage of not being familiar with the subject matter but the "correct answer" syndrome might be less of a problem with them. In the end, a decision was made for us because the federal and state COS offices proved unable to organize themselves quickly enough to provide the required official permission for COS employees to work on the surveys.

In early February 1988 I met with some twenty-five public health nurses in Lagos and Benue states who would serve as trainers and I provided a general orientation in all aspects of the survey, including the administration of the interview schedule (hereafter, "questionnaire"). The questionnaire was based both on experience interviewing traditional healers elsewhere in Africa and on our particular project needs. It was pretested by each nurse/trainer with at least two traditional healers who were not participating in the projects. As a result of the pretest, there were some adjustments in response categories and in phrasing of questions.

Healers were chosen for participation in the TSFH Projects by local (state and district) branches of traditional healer associations. In Lagos State, where there had been very small-scale training of healers in the recent past and where there were known to be male specialists in midwifery and gynecology, special efforts were made to select healers of this sort. Somewhat different criteria were used by leaders of the Benue healers association, probably with differences in selection criteria and procedures between districts and ethnolinguistic groups within that state. The point is that healer associations themselves assumed the responsibility of selecting workshop participants. It is well they did so, because it became apparent in the early design stages that the "demand" for training was far greater than the "supply" of training resources. Selection for training appears to have been highly political in the sense that various factions within and between groups and branches of healer organizations probably did considerable lobbying and jockeying for inclusion of certain healers in the training programs.

We decided to administer the baseline questionnaire to a group of healers that would not undergo training so that they could serve as a control group when we conducted a posttest at some stage following training. One advantage of the high demand among Nigerian healers for training was that the problem of how to obtain a control group was easily solved. Project staff simply requested the presence during workshop opening ceremonies of more healers than could be trained during in the first project year. Healers not selected for initial training were promised that their participation in the survey—which took over an hour of the healer's time not including other time, transportation, and opportunity costs to the healer to be present at the training site—would put them in a priority position to be selected for training when and *if* the projects were extended to a second or subsequent year.

Selection of both the training and control groups was clearly far more political than scientific, and no claim can be made that the resulting "samples" were randomly chosen nor that they are projectable to a universe of Nigerian healers. For one thing, there was doubtless a selection bias in favor of healers interested in modern-sector training, which might suggest a bias toward healers who are somewhat more "progressive" or more open to outside, modern, or urban influences than other healers. On the other hand, as noted already, a number of surveys in various parts of Africa have shown that interest in modern sector training is not atypical; clear majorities among more randomly selected healers claim to be interested in undergoing training.

There may also be selection biases in favor of herbalists and healers who specialize in ob/gyn and related areas such as prenatal care. With these selection biases in mind—and some were deliberate since purposeful selection served project ends—it seems reasonable to assume that the healers selected for participation in the Lagos and Benue programs are at least fairly representative of the universe of healers in those states.

### Characteristics of Respondents

Of the 399 respondents, 259 (64.9 percent) were from Lagos and 140 (35.1 percent) were from Benue. The training group consisted of 210 healers and the control group of 189. The distinction between the groups only assumes significance when and if a follow-up survey is conducted sometime after training, when the availability of control groups can help isolate the independent effects of project training efforts. In the analysis of the present survey, the 399 respondents are treated as one group or sample.

The sample can be divided on the basis of sex: 75 percent male and 25 percent female; on the basis of ethnolinguistic group or "tribe": 56 percent Yoruba, 14 percent Idoma or Igede (these two groups are closely related and come under a single traditional ruler), 12 percent Igala, 8 percent Tiv, and 11 percent "other"; and literacy: 60 percent claimed to be literate, while 39 percent claimed otherwise. Fifteen percent were under the age of twenty-five, 32 percent were between twenty-five and thirty-nine, 38 percent were between forty and fifty-three, and 15 percent were fifty-four and older. Respondents' formal educational achievement is presented in Table 6.1. On average, healers in the present sample have had some degree of primary education.

Since formal education is often a potent predictor variable in surveys that measure levels of health awareness and knowledge, we looked for educational differences among different types of healers. There proved to be significant differences by ethnolinguistic group, as shown in Table 6.2. The Yoruba, most of whom inhabit the relatively urbanized and densely populated southwestern coastal area of Nigeria, proved to be the group with the second highest level of formal education; while the Idoma/Igeda, who are found in a rural, relatively sparsely populated region of Benue State, seem to be the least well educated. It was not known why the Tiv had the highest level of education of the participating ethnic groups. In any case, it is important to remember that these educational differences exist as we encounter significant differences in answers based on ethnic group; ethnicity may be a proxy for formal education. Likewise

TABLE 6.1 Respondents' Level of Formal Education

| | *Frequency* | *Percent* | *Cumulative Percent* |
|---|---|---|---|
| No formal education | 158 | 39.7 | 39.7 |
| Some primary | 49 | 12.3 | 52.0 |
| Completed primary | 59 | 14.8 | 66.8 |
| Some secondary | 55 | 13.8 | 80.7 |
| Completed Secondary | 66 | 16.6 | 97.2 |
| Above secondary | 11 | 2.8 | 100.0 |

TABLE 6.2 Level of Formal Education, by Ethnolinguistic Group

| | *No Formal Education* | *Some or Completed Primary* | *Some Secondary or Above* |
|---|---|---|---|
| Yoruba | 30.6% | 29.7% | 39.6% |
| | (68) | (66) | (88) |
| Tiv | 20.0% | 30.0% | 50.0% |
| | (6) | (9) | (15) |
| Igala | 65.2% | 19.6% | 15.2% |
| | (30) | (9) | (7) |
| Idoma/Igede | 68.5% | 20.4% | 11.1% |
| | (37) | (11) | (6) |
| Other | 32.6% | 30.2% | 37.2% |
| | (14) | (13) | (16) |

Chi-square = 47.69 (D.F. = 8, p = less than .0001)

with literacy: over 60 percent of Yoruba healers described themselves as literate, compared with 37 percent of Igala, or 31.5 percent of Idoma/Igede. Highest in literacy were the Tiv, at 72.4 percent.

Sixty-six percent of healers identified themselves as herbalists, 9 percent as diviner-mediums, and 23 percent as combinations of herbalist and diviner-medium (2 percent did not provide information). Ninety-two healers identified themselves as specialists of some sort: 38 percent specializing in midwifery and problems associated with childbirth; 27 percent in infertility, impotence or sterility; 14 percent in malaria, fever, or convulsions; 12 percent in meningitis or yellow fever; 10 percent in diarrhea, dysentery or dehydration; 10 percent in mental illness; 7 percent in gonorrhea, pain in urination or STDs; 7 percent in broken bones or accidents; 7 percent in general witchcraft, poisoning, or sorcery; and 5 percent in worms or other parasites (some identified more than one specialty). Most (70.4 percent) identified themselves as full-time healers. The number of clients seen during an average week is presented in Table 6.3.

TABLE 6.3 Number of Patients Seen per Week

| *Patients* | *Frequency* | *Percent* | *Cumulative Percent* |
|---|---|---|---|
| 1–10 | 152 | 38.6 | 38.6 |
| 11–20 | 77 | 19.5 | 58.1 |
| 21–30 | 52 | 13.2 | 71.3 |
| 31–40 | 33 | 8.4 | 79.7 |
| 41–50 | 26 | 6.6 | 86.3 |
| 51–60 | 12 | 3.0 | 89.3 |
| 61–70 | 8 | 2.0 | 91.4 |
| 71–80 | 12 | 3.0 | 94.4 |
| over 80 | 22 | 5.6 | 100.0 |

The average healer has been practicing about thirteen years and sees about 21 clients per week, or about 1,092 per year. There were significant differences by ethnic group. Fifty percent of Yoruba healers saw more than 31 clients per week; 18.2 percent saw more than 51 per week. If we conservatively assume that the number greater than 31 is 35, then the average Yoruba healer sees 1,820 clients per year. Of course, a significant number of these might be repeat clients. The group with the lowest client "caseload" is the Igala, only 2.2 percent of whom reported seeing more than 51 clients per week. There was also variation in the catchment area from which clients come, as shown in Table 6.4.

The Yoruba, followed by the Idoma and Igeda, are the most likely to practice throughout their states and beyond: 62 percent of Yoruba and 50 percent of Idoma and Igeda reported practicing in the largest catchment area.

### *The Relative Efficacy of Traditional and Modern Medicine*

In programs designed to challenge and change basic health beliefs, knowledge, and behavior, it is important to understand attitudes healers may have already developed toward scientific or "modern" medicine. Changes in traditional beliefs and behavior ought to be easier to bring about if the competing system of healing is already admired and emulated rather than if it is mistrusted and generally held in low esteem. With this in mind, a series of questions were asked to assess attitudes toward modern biomedicine and toward biomedicine in relation to traditional medicine, beginning with, "Do you believe that traditional medicine can be more successful than modern medicine in certain cases or circumstances?"

Only 8.6 percent of healers answered no. Belief in the superiority of traditional medicine rises to 97 percent among the Tiv, who are the best educated among the groups participating in the projects. Only 83 percent of Igala held this belief. Perhaps contrary to expectation, there is a small but significant ($p = .03$) direct relationship between the belief in the supe-

TABLE 6.4 Patient Catchment Area

| | *Frequency* | *Percent* | *Cumulative Percent* |
|---|---|---|---|
| Healer's village only | 73 | 18.3 | 18.3 |
| Surrounding villages | 49 | 12.3 | 30.7 |
| Throughout local government area | 54 | 13.6 | 44.2 |
| Throughout state | 78 | 19.6 | 63.8 |
| Also beyond state | 144 | 36.2 | 100.0 |

TABLE 6.5 Belief That Traditional Medicine Can Be More Successful than Modern Medicine

| | *Frequency* | *Percent* | *Cumulative Percent* |
|---|---|---|---|
| Yes | 341 | 85.9 | 85.9 |
| No | 34 | 8.6 | 94.5 |
| Both equal | 22 | 5.5 | 100.0 |

riority of traditional medicine and formal education, where we see that 83 percent with no formal education hold this belief, rising almost steadily to 91 percent among healers with education above the secondary level.

For those answering yes to the last question, we next asked for specification of cases in which traditional medicine could be more successful than modern medicine. Answers in almost all cases were phrased in terms of illnesses or related conditions or medical specialties, and such a range and variety of these were given that it defied simple categorization. The commonest responses, in order of frequency, were madness, midwifery, and problems associated with childbirth, witchcraft and sorcery, sterility and impotence, fractures and bonesetting, sexually transmitted diseases (including symptomatic descriptions such as "pain in urination"), snakebite, malaria and other fevers, and diarrhea. Fourteen percent of the total could not or would not specify a condition or illness, yet held traditional medicine to be superior.

One of the problems of obtaining information of this sort through survey research is that healers do not use the same nosological categories or disease classifications as the interviewers, especially since our interviewers were nurses. In formal interview situations healers tend to translate what they have in mind into categories and classifications that they think will be understood and acceptable to interviewers, who are usually more educated and have a greater modern-sector orientation than the healers. The result is that illnesses and ideas related to witchcraft and sorcery tend to be underreported, traditional disease categories are glossed or approximated by a modern disease category that the healer might not understand well, and there may be other distortions due to attempts at cultural translation. It obviously would be useful to probe responses to questions such as the foregoing by in-depth interviews conducted by someone familiar with ethnomedical systems of the Tiv, Yoruba, and other groups represented in the survey.

We next turned the question around, asking "Do you believe that modern medicine can be more successful than traditional medicine in certain cases or circumstances?" There were statistically significant differences between ethnic groups, as shown in Table 6.7.

TABLE 6.6 Belief That Modern Medicine Can Be More Successful than Traditional Medicine

| *Response* | *Frequency* | *Percent* | *Cumulative Percent* |
|---|---|---|---|
| Don't know | 9 | 2.3 | 2.3 |
| Yes | 244 | 61.5 | 63.8 |
| No | 122 | 30.7 | 94.5 |
| Both equal | 22 | 5.5 | 100.0 |

(missing cases=2)

Perhaps contrary to expectation, the most urbanized group and the one with the most opportunity for contact with modern health practitioners (the Yoruba) appears to be the group *least* likely to credit modern medicine with curative capability.

As shown in Table 6.8, there is a small but significant (p = .05) inverse relationship between the belief in the superiority of modern biomedicine and formal education, where we see that 71.3 percent with no formal education hold this belief, decreasing to 58.3 percent among those with primary education, and finally to 52.7 percent among those with secondary education or higher. In other words, contrary to what one might expect, there seems to be less faith in modern medicine the more formal education a healer has.

### *Patterns of Patient Referrals*

The degree to which patient referrals occur between traditional and biomedical practitioners can provide a quantifiable measure of intersectoral cooperation and indicate attitude differences if referrals occur more in one "direction" than another. 56 percent of all healers claimed to at

TABLE 6.7 Belief That Modern Medicine Can Be More Successful than Traditional Medicine, by Ethnolinguistic Group

| | *Don't know* | *Yes* | *No* | *Both equal* |
|---|---|---|---|---|
| Yoruba | 4.1% | 47.3% | 44.6% | 4.1% |
| | (9) | (105) | (99) | (9) |
| Tiv | 0.0% | 83.3% | 16.7% | 0.0% |
| | (0) | (25) | (5) | (0) |
| Igala | 0.0% | 87.0% | 13.0% | 0.0% |
| | (0) | (40) | (6) | (0) |
| Idoma/Igeda | 0.0% | 94.3% | 5.7% | 0.0% |
| | (0) | (50) | (3) | (0) |
| Other | 0.0% | 51.2% | 18.6% | 30.2% |
| | (0) | (22) | (8) | (13) |

Chi-square = 119.8 (D.F. = 12, p = less than .0001)

TABLE 6.8 Belief in the Value of Modern medicine, by Level of Formal Education

| | *Can't Say* | *More Valuable* | *Less Valuable* | *Both Equal* |
|---|---|---|---|---|
| No formal education | 1.9% | 71.3% | 22.3% | 4.5% |
| | (3) | (112) | (35) | (7) |
| Some or completed primary | 1.9% | 58.3% | 35.2% | 4.6% |
| | (2) | (63) | (38) | (5) |
| Secondary or higher | 3.1% | 52.7% | 36.6% | 7.6% |
| | (4) | (69) | (48) | (10) |

Chi-square = 12.2 (D.F. = 6, p. = .057)

least occasionally make patient referrals to doctors or nurses; 44 percent said they never do. There were significant differences by ethnic group, reflecting a pattern already referred to: 93 percent of Idoma/Igede (perhaps the most rural of the groups involved in the projects), 70 percent of Igala, and only 44 percent of Yoruba make referrals, as seen in Table 6.9. Again we see an apparent inverse relationship between intersectoral cooperation and urbanization or opportunities for intersectoral contact. There is also an inverse relationship between intersectoral cooperation and level of formal education, as evident in Table 6.10.

Why should there be an inverse relationship between the tendency to refer patients and degree of population density and urbanization? It may be that with little opportunity for intersectoral contact, there is also less opportunity for intersectoral conflict and competition. Rural-based healers in Benue made comments to the effect that they rarely see doctors or nurses. Perhaps in such situations, patient referrals are not expected. But when a traditional and a modern practitioner practice within meters of one another in an urban area, the absence of referrals may be interpreted as a deliberate snub. Moreover, there may be direct competition for

TABLE 6.9 Patient Referrals by Healers to Doctors, by Ethnic Group

| | *Refers* | *Does Not Refer* |
|---|---|---|
| Yoruba | 43.9% | 56.1% |
| | (98) | (125) |
| Tiv | 53.3% | 46.7% |
| | (16) | (14) |
| Igala | 69.6% | 30.4% |
| | (32) | (14) |
| Idoma/Igede | 92.5% | 7.5% |
| | (49) | (4) |
| Other | 65.1% | 34.9% |
| | (28) | (15) |

Chi square = 46.78 (D.F. = 4, p. = less than .0001)

TABLE 6.10 Referral of Patients to Doctors, by Level of Formal Education

| | *Refers Patients* | *Doesn't Refer Patients* |
|---|---|---|
| No formal education | 63.1% | 36.9% |
| | (99) | (58) |
| Some or completed primary | 56.5% | 43.5% |
| | (61) | (47) |
| Secondary or higher | 48.5% | 51.5% |
| | (64) | (68) |

Chi-square = 6.19 (D.F. = 2, p. = .045)

patients in an urban setting, with the resulting possibility of mutual distrust and antagonism.

But why the inverse relationship between referrals and educational level? It might be expected that formal education, which would include a certain amount of scientific and specifically health-related education, would challenge and therefore weaken a healer's faith in traditional healing and in the magico-religious belief system that forms its basis. Instead, it may be that a certain amount of formal education provides a Nigerian a measure of self-esteem and self-assurance that is manifest partly as faith in Nigerian traditions, including medicine. Another interpretation might be that modern medicine, held in awe by those with little education or opportunities for first-hand contact with its practitioners, holds less mystery for those with greater education and contact with doctors.

Of course, the possibility exists that there are cultural or ethnic group-specific reasons that account for the relative lack of respect for modern medicine on the part of particular groups such as the Yoruba. In a follow-up to the question on patient referrals to the modern sector, healers were asked *why* they sometimes referred patients. The Yoruba were the least likely among the four ethnolinguistic groups to concede that there are times or situations when traditional medicine is less effective than modern medicine. However, we still do not know whether this pattern of differences is due to cultural factors, to some sort of reaction to greater opportunities for contact between the two types of health practitioners, to other factors related to urbanization including the important one of education, or to still other unidentified factors.

In response to the question about why those who do make referrals, make them, 39 percent said they refer cases in which traditional medicine is ineffective, or the patient is not responding to treatment or healers simply cannot cope with the situation; and 18 percent said they refer when the treatment requires modern technology such as operations, blood transfusion, sutures, IV drip, etc. Answers to this question are obviously related to beliefs expressed earlier in the survey that there are occasions when modern medicine can be more justified or effective than traditional medicine.

In another question in which healers were asked why they did *not* refer patients to the modern sector, Yoruba healers were the most likely to give as an answer that they are capable of treating all cases they are presented with, or are at least as capable as modern medical practitioners.

Healers were next asked if modern health practitioners ever refer patients to them; 46 percent said yes and 54 percent said no. This would indicate that according to healers, there are 10 percent more healer-doctor referrals than doctor-healer referrals. Some respondents expressed bitterness in answering this question, such as the young Katsina Ala (Benue) herbalist who commented, "Doctors think they know better than us. . . . They think they are perfect . . . but modern medicine has never understood us. Maybe this project is the beginning (i.e., of a new understanding)." Another observed, "Some doctors do not refer because they are protecting their profession according to a colonial mentality." It should be noted that some healers have a "mentality" of certainty themselves that prevents them from referring patients to doctors, such as the ob/gyn specialist from Lagos who heals according to the dictates of the Ifa Oracle and who noted, "What we (Ifa initiates) cannot do is beyond the power of doctors."

Modern practitioners are said to sometimes refer patients in unspecified cases when modern medicine proves ineffective, in cases of infertility, witchcraft or poisoning, or bonesetting, or madness, in that order of frequency. There were no differences in responses based on several characteristics of the healer. However, there were significant differences based on ethnic group, and on formal educational achievement.

### *Use of Modern Medicines*

It is believed by some observers that traditional healers do not use any medicines other than those considered traditional, that there might even be a taboo against such use or at least a loss of prestige or credibility on the part of healers using modern medicines. The present survey shows that 59 percent of all healers in all regions use some form of modern, manufactured, patent medicines. Fifty-eight percent of this group use such medicines on themselves and their family members, and 41 percent use them on their patients. Analgesics such as aspirin and Panadol are the most commonly used medicines (38 percent of total). Far less commonly cited were malarial drugs (8 percent), antibiotics (3 percent), and "stomach medicines" (1 percent). A few healers commented that it might be easier to use modern than traditional medicine in some cases, such as when they are away from home and they lack the time and facilities to prepare traditional medicines. (See Chapter 7 for comparable findings from South African healers.)

### *Age for Women to Begin Childbearing*

Traditional healers were asked the age at which women should get married and begin to have children. Perhaps surprisingly for a country in which marriages can occur at ages as young as twelve to thirteen, especially in the predominantly Muslim north, a plurality of respondents thought between sixteen and eighteen was the best age category for marriage, and nineteen to twenty-one were the best ages for beginning childbearing. In fact, only 32 percent of respondents thought women should begin childbearing before age nineteen, while nearly 24 percent thought the age should be over twenty-five. Most healers (more than 82 percent) were able to state reasons why childbirth at earlier ages led to various problems, such as difficulties in delivery (36 percent), the woman is not sufficiently mature or her pelvic bones are not fully formed, or she has "an immature womb" (26 percent). Other reasons given were that the woman will age prematurely; a young woman will not be sufficiently secure financially before the age of twenty to twenty-two to look after a child; and/or the woman will suffer from anemia.

There are significant differences among answers to this question based on sex of the respondent ($p < .0001$). A plurality of female healers thought twenty-two to twenty-four were the best ages for women to begin childbearing; and only 9.1 percent recommended ages less than nineteen. There was also a direct relationship between level of formal education and the belief that women should start childbearing in somewhat later years, as indicated in the next table.

### *Proper Family Size*

Healers were asked how many children they considered is "enough" for a woman to have. Answers ranged from two children to "as many as God wills." Some healers expressed characteristic pronatalist attitudes

TABLE 6.11 The Age at Which Women Should Start Childbearing

| *Age* | *Frequency* | *Percent* | *Cumulative Percent* |
|---|---|---|---|
| Below 13 | 5 | 1.3 | 1.3 |
| 13–15 | 18 | 4.6 | 5.9 |
| 16–18 | 102 | 26.0 | 31.9 |
| 19–21 | 133 | 33.9 | 65.8 |
| 22–24 | 81 | 20.7 | 86.5 |
| 25 and above | 53 | 13.5 | 100.0 |

TABLE 6.12 Correct Age to Start Childbearing, by Level of Formal Education

| | *-13* | *13–15* | *16–18* | *19–21* | *22–24* | *25+* |
|---|---|---|---|---|---|---|
| No education | 2.6% | 8.6% | 30.9% | 32.9% | 13.8% | 11.2% |
| | (4) | (13) | (47) | (50) | (21) | (17) |
| Some primary | 2.0% | 2.0% | 34.7% | 42.9% | 16.3% | 2.0% |
| | (1) | (1) | (17) | (21) | (8) | (1) |
| Completed primary | 0.0% | 5.1% | 16.9% | 39.0% | 18.6% | 20.3% |
| | (0) | (3) | (10) | (23) | (11) | (12) |
| Some secondary | 0.0% | 0.0% | 25.9% | 24.1% | 31.5% | 18.5% |
| | (0) | (0) | (14) | (13) | (17) | (10) |
| Completed secondary | 0.0% | 1.5% | 18.2% | 34.8% | 28.8% | 16.7% |
| | (0) | (1) | (12) | (23) | (19) | (11) |
| Above secondary | 0.0% | 0.0% | 18.2% | 27.3% | 36.4% | 18.2% |
| | (0) | (0) | (2) | (3) | (4) | (2) |

Chi Square = 44.53 (D.F. = 25, p. = .0009)

already well documented among traditional Africans, such as the forty-year-old Katsina Ala healer who observed, "Our Tiv traditional belief is that not all the children will be healthy, so a woman should have as many as the husband wants so that at least some will be good out of the many. Also many children die early in life so many will (be needed to) replace the dead ones."

However, a plurality suggested women have four children and over two-thirds (71.4 percent) answered in the 4 to 6 range. While this still may seem high to Westerners, the actual total fertility rate in Nigeria is estimated at 7.2, so that Nigerian healers—even before being exposed to workshops or seminars that promote Western-influenced views regarding child spacing—appear to be in favor of "smaller families" than those actually found in Nigeria. Healers with some formal education are even likelier to favor women having fewer children ($p < .0001$), and there is an equally strong association based on the sex of the healer, with female healers favoring smaller families.

### *Awareness of Child-Spacing Methods*

Most fertility regulation in Africa today is not by means of modern contraception; it results from what might be termed traditional mechanisms. These may be conscious behaviors, such as coitus interruptus or using herbal medicines for contraception, or they may be nonvolitional and operate at broader levels, such as polygamy (polygyny) or diseases such as STDs that cause infertility. Most of these mechanisms operate differently today compared with the past. For example, breastfeeding is less prolonged, postpartum abstinence is being abandoned, and the incidence of infertility-causing diseases that was decreasing through better health care, now seems to be on the rise due to increase in STD incidence. The net result has been a rise in total fertility that is not being offset by use of modern contraception. In this section we are concerned with conscious mechanisms for fertility control.

Just over 73 percent of healers claim to know one or more traditional or at least indigenous methods used to avoid pregnancy; 26.8 percent claim they did not. Allowing for multiple answers, the methods most frequently cited were herbal decoctions (sometimes specified as herbs, roots, leaves, etc.) (56 percent); a special ring worn by women (54 percent); special medicines administered by cuts or incisions by razor or similar object (21 percent); a special belt, rope or bracelet worn by the woman (20 percent); other magical talismans (5 percent); abstinence or avoidance (2 percent); and medicinal douches or vaginal implants (1 percent). When asked which of these methods was considered effective in avoiding pregnancy, 47.4 percent said the ring; 41.4 percent said herbal decoctions or teas; 14.5 percent mentioned razor incisions, and 11.5 percent cited the belt, rope or bracelet. Other methods were mentioned less frequently.

Healers were next asked if they knew of any methods used by doctors or nurses to avoid unwanted pregnancy; 52.1 percent said yes and 47.4 percent said no. Among those answering yes, methods most commonly cited were the pill (36.6 percent); condom (24.3 percent); injection (20.3 percent); IUD (12.5 percent); sterilization or tubal ligation (8 percent); spermicides or vaginal tablets (7.3 percent); and diaphragm (2 percent). As might be expected, there was a direct relationship between level of formal education and awareness of modern family-planning methods, as shown in Table 6.13. This is also reflected in ethnic differences: the most educated groups, the Tiv and the Yoruba respectively, also show the highest awareness levels in regard to modern contraceptive methods.

When healers were asked which of these methods they considered effective or most effective, there was little evidence of great confidence in modern family-planning methods. Fully 64.4 percent of all healers felt that no modern methods were effective. Only 14.5 percent cited the pill;

TABLE 6.13 Awareness of Modern Family-Planning Methods, by Level of Education

| | *Aware* | *Unaware* |
|---|---|---|
| No formal educ. | 36.9% (58) | 63.1% (99) |
| Some primary educ. | 53.1% (26) | 46.9% (23) |
| Completed primary | 54.2% (32) | 45.8% (27) |
| Some secondary | 65.5% (36) | 34.5% (19) |
| Completed secondary | 72.3% (47) | 27.7% (18) |
| Above secondary | 72.7% (8) | 27.3% (3) |

(Missing cases = 3)
Chi-Square = 31.03 (D.F. = 5, p. = less than .0001)

TABLE 6.14 Awareness of Modern Family-Planning Methods, by Ethnolinguistic Group

| | *Aware* | *Unaware* |
|---|---|---|
| Yoruba | 55.9% (124) | 44.1% (98) |
| Tiv | 66.7% (20) | 33.3% (10) |
| Igula | 26.7% (12) | 73.3% (33) |
| Idoma/Igede | 53.7% (29) | 46.3% (25) |
| Other | 48.8% (21) | 51.2% (22) |

(Missing cases = 5)
Chi-Square = 15.71 (D.F. = 4, p = .003)

11 percent cited injections; 9.5 percent cited condoms; 4.8 percent cited sterilization; 3.3 percent cited the IUD; 2.5 percent cited spermicides or vaginal tablets; and 0.5 percent cited the diaphragm.

In order to probe knowledge of modern methods further, healers were asked if there are any modern family-planning methods that should not be used by certain women or in certain circumstances. 24.8 percent said yes, 14 percent said no, and 61.2 percent did not know. For those very few able to express opinions about the circumstances under which certain modern methods should not be used, the commonest answers were that pills may not be indicated or appropriate for certain types of women or women with certain characteristics; teenagers or certain other categories of men or women should not use contraception for moral reasons; certain methods cannot be reversed for those wishing to become pregnant at a later time, or women who have difficulty in becoming pregnant in the first place should not use contraception. Very small numbers of respondents mentioned miscellaneous reasons such as: contraception going against tradition or being considered unnatural; one or more methods are believed to harm the unborn baby; women who have never conceived before should avoid one or more specific methods; and nursing women should avoid one or more specific methods.

Healers were next asked the important normative or attitude question of whether or not they thought it was right for women to seek advice or medicines to avoid unwanted pregnancy: 68.4 percent thought it was and 29.8 percent disagreed. There were significant differences by ethnic group, with the more urbanized and densely populated Yoruba leading those in agreement with 84.3 percent agreement, as shown in Table 6.15. There was also a tendency for healers with more formal education to agree with the above statement (p = .06).

The minority in disagreement commented that contraception transgresses or circumvents the husband's authority, or it might prevent future childbearing, or it is unnatural or "against religion." A number of comments supporting the right to contraception were also made, such as contraception can "save a woman's life"; "a woman must have enough strength to care for her children"; "both the husband and wife must make the decision"; and comments to the effect that lack of contraception may lead to dangerous abortions.

### *Healers' Involvement in Provision of Contraceptive Services*

After a series of relatively impersonal questions about traditional and modern contraception, healers were asked if they themselves are sometimes approached by clients seeking advice or actual services (i.e., therapies or medicines) relating to the avoidance or postponement of pregnancy. More than 2/3 (69 percent) of all healers reported that either men, women or couples sometimes visit them seeking advice or medicines to postpone or avoid pregnancy. This is a significant and perhaps unexpected finding for any region of Africa where "demand" for family-planning services is thought to be extremely low. What family-planning surveys usually fail to measure—or even consider—is demand in the traditional sector, that is, demand for services from traditional health practitioners as distinct from doctors, nurses, or family-planning clinics.

The finding of the present survey is influenced by the large number of Yoruba healers in the survey and by the fact that Yorubas practice in more urbanized areas where interest in avoiding pregnancy is relatively high, as well as by the fact that many Yoruba healers participating in the project specialize in midwifery and gynecology and are therefore likelier to be approached by those seeking contraception than, say, healers who specialize in madness or bonesetting.

There were some significantly different answers to this question based on healer characteristics. Regarding ethnicity, for example, 91 percent of Yoruba healers claimed to be approached compared to 40 percent of Tiv healers, 43 percent of Idoma/Igede healers, and only 13 percent of Igala healers. Related to this, Lagos healers were far likelier to be approached for family-planning advice or services than Benue healers ($p < .0001$) and female healers were likelier to be approached than male healers

TABLE 6.15 Agreement that Women Have Right to Avoid Unwanted Pregnancy, by Ethnolinguistic Group

| | *Agree* | *Don't Agree* | *Don't Know* |
|---|---|---|---|
| Yoruba | 84.3% (183) | 15.2% (33) | .5% (1) |
| Tiv | 53.3% (16) | 46.7% (14) | 0.0% (0) |
| Igala | 39.1% (18) | 54.3% (25) | 6.5% (3) |
| Idoma/Igede | 59.3% (32) | 37.0% (20) | 3.7% (2) |
| Other | 40.5% (17) | 57.1% (24) | 2.4% (1) |

Missing cases = 20
Chi-Square = 68.96 (D.F. = 8, p = less than .0001)

(p < .0001). Literate healers and those with more formal education were also likelier than nonliterate and less-educated healers to be approached for family-planning advice or services (p < .0001 and < .0008 respectively).

Characterizing those seeking advice or services, 43.2 percent of healers said they were usually approached by women, 21.6 percent said by couples, and 3.5 percent said by men. When healers were asked how they respond to those seeking advice or services about avoiding pregnancy, only 11.3 percent failed to answer the question because it was not applicable, suggesting that an even higher number of healers might be approached than reported in the previous question. Responses to the last question are summarized in Table 6.16.

Fully 54 percent of all healers claim they administer traditional means of avoiding pregnancy, citing methods such as the ring, herbal decoctions, and the magical belt referred to in earlier answers. Only a few healers expressed strong negative attitudes toward contraception, such as the fifty-three-year-old Tiv healer from Benue who said, "God said we should bear children and fill the world. So when such women or men come (for contraception) I will take them to the police. . . ." Another healer reported providing contraceptive services but explained that the water spirit that guides and empowers him in contraception allows him to use the magical waist belt with only three people in a year. This limitation suggests that avoiding pregnancy is regarded as something that at least to some extent transgresses community norms and traditional values. In other words, avoiding pregnancy is not regarded as the same as preventing or treating something like snakebite or diarrhea.

It may be noted that there were two references to abortion. Since the project's mandate—and indeed current AID regulations—do not support

TABLE 6.16 Responses to Requests for Family-Planning Advice or Services

| | *Frequency* | *Percent* | *Cumulative Percent* |
|---|---|---|---|
| Administers traditional FP methods | 214 | 53.9 | 53.9 |
| Could not/did not say | 91 | 22.9 | 76.8 |
| Counsels about alternatives | 14 | 3.5 | 80.3 |
| Refers patients to FP or other clinic, doctor, etc. | 10 | 2.5 | 82.8 |
| Does not help or advise | 11 | 2.8 | 85.6 |
| Administers or refers for abortion | 2 | 0.5 | 86.1 |
| Administers modern FP methods | 2 | 0.5 | 86.6 |
| Miscellaneous | 8 | 2.0 | 88.6 |
| Not applicable | 45 | 11.3 | 100.0 |

abortion in any way, there were no specific questions about abortion and no probes or follow-up questions when abortion was mentioned.

There were other survey sections of relevance to fertility regulation, such as those relating to breastfeeding, and other sections relating to maternal and child health. The interested reader is referred to the full report (Green 1989a).

### Conclusions from the Baseline Survey in Nigeria

First of all, the Nigerian healer emerges as someone quite different from the stereotypic, conservative "guardian of the traditional order" of pronatalism and female subordination, who is quick to treat any condition that inhibits fertility while condemning family planning as un-African and perhaps unholy. In fact, Lagos and Benue healers often have respect for Western-style medicine and they may use it themselves; they believe women should be in the nineteen- to twenty-four-year-old range in order to bear the healthiest children with the least danger to the mother; they support spacing births two to three years apart; they are often approached for assistance in postponing or otherwise avoiding pregnancy and they usually respond by providing traditional methods of birth control; and they believe that women should not have more than four to six children. In short, they are by African standards already relatively knowledgeable and progressive when it comes to human fertility and its regulation, even in the absence of modern-sector programs designed to influence knowledge, attitudes, and practices.

In the presence of such programs, healers' predisposition may be presumed to combine with motivational and other factors to result in significant change in healers' knowledge, attitudes, and practices related to fertility regulation. Both the nature of responses and project experience with selecting and interviewing healers reinforce the conclusion that healers are not only educable with regard to modern-sector health, family planning, and community-based contraceptive distribution, but that they appreciate the intrinsic and economic value of such modern-sector knowledge and are generally enthusiastic about prospects for cooperating with the modern health sector.

During analysis of the foregoing data, I conceived a simple behavior (knowledge, attitude) change model, which in schematic form was:

$$P + M + D = BC$$

In other words, *Predisposition* (healers are relatively "progressive" in areas of fertility regulation) plus *Motivation* (to learn about modern medicine, cooperate with modern health sector, achieve greater social recognition and respectability) plus rising *"Demand"* for family-planning advice and services on the part of consumers (due to socioeconomic factors, child-spacing education, and direct motivation from credible health opinion leaders such as traditional healers), will lead to *Behavior Change* (defined as "trained" healers promoting modern contraception, although not necessarily to the exclusion of traditional contraception).

The model as expressed simply ignores intervening variables that may impede behavior change, for example healers knew little about modern, biomedical methods of birth control; they had considerable faith in the efficacy of their traditional fertility-regulating methods (just as African healers do in most areas of their STD treatments); and they tended to lose respect for, and become less cooperative with, modern-sector health practitioners when there were more opportunities for intersectoral contact.

It has been reported elsewhere in Africa that healers may be called on to help women or couples avoid unwanted pregnancy. For example, Swantz (1990:125) reports that this appears quite common in Dar es Salaam, although "... interviews revealed that more clients seek medicine in order to conceive than for preventing pregnancies."

## Implementation of Workshops

Between February and July 1988, regional workshops were held in Local Government Areas in Lagos and Benue states for the purpose of "training" traditional healers and exchanging information about fertility regulation and related subjects. A total of 320 traditional healers attended two-week long workshops, 200 in Lagos and 120 in Benue. Discussion and training focused on indigenous and "modern" fertility regulation, community-based distribution (CBD) of contraceptives, and aspects of child survival such as breastfeeding, ORT, immunization, and infant nutrition that seem complementary to child spacing when considering maternal and child health. There was a small component concerned with diagnosing certain sexually transmitted diseases and making appropriate referrals to clinics and hospitals. In the CBD component, healers earned a 25 percent commission on sales of contraceptives; remaining funds recovered from sales were returned to the project to offset administrative and other costs.

Workshops consisted of presentations by facilitators (mostly nurses), demonstrations of how to use modern contraceptives, some role-playing and much seminar-style discussion. There was practice in recording important details of contraceptive sales (the number and type of contraceptives sold; the age and sex of clients, etc.) on pictographic record forms designed for use by non-literates. During a spot check of these forms five months after training, one Lagos state healer reported selling 100 condoms to men and 25 foaming tablets to women during the previous month. All clients were new adopters and the form had been correctly filled out. However, there were problems overall in the collection of these forms.

Workshop facilitators were given the latitude to be creative and develop approaches they thought useful in their own areas. As an example, healers in some areas were taken to the local market to gain actual experience in selling contraceptives, since CBD was an important part of how the workshop experience was to be operationalized. (It was recognized that healers would not ordinarily be selling at markets. Instead, sales and advice regarding contraceptives would become a regular part of their ongoing healing practice with an established clientele in their own communities.)[1] This exercise led to realization that healers could be harassed by police for selling "drugs" (condoms and spermicides) without a license. This in turn led to the issuing of ID cards from the Planned Parenthood Federation of Nigeria to mollify local police.

As expected, facilitators found that healers were more convinced by the maternal and child health reasons for child spacing than by ecological or macroeconomic arguments that relate to resource depletion, environmental degradation, political stability, infrastructural costs, or constraints to economic development. However, the relationship between population growth and social problems such as teenage pregnancy and unemployment was understood and appreciated.

At the end of each workshop, healers were provided a "commodities kit" consisting of an initial supply of contraceptives, ORS packets, bandages, and other basic supplies.

A local leader "awareness seminar" was held in each area for local chiefs, district and clan heads, and other traditional political authorities. This effort was undertaken to preempt possible opposition from traditional authorities and to try to gain some measure of their support. Traditional authorities were also enlisted to preside at workshop opening or closing ceremonies, where they gave speeches and (in the case of the latter) handed out training certificates to healers. Over 500 such leaders attended awareness seminars and/or participated in workshop opening or closing ceremonies.

The Lagos State project was administered by the Lagos State Ministry of Health (Board of Traditional Medicine) while the Benue State project was administered by the Planned Parenthood Federation of Nigeria (PPFN). One of the objectives of the Nigerian effort was to assess whether donors like USAID would do better to channel funds for such projects though public or private sector organizations.

## Activities After the First Year

It was expected that funds would be found to support a post-test several months into the life of both projects in order to actually measure changes in knowledge, attitudes, and practices (including CBD) on the part of trained healers, and to compare this with the control groups of non-trained healers. Of the two projects, I predicted that the one based in Lagos had somewhat more potential for results, as measured in such quantifiables as contraceptive sales and "couple years protection," because: (1) there was greater population density in Lagos than in Benue and there was higher existing demand for family-planning services; (2) Lagos healers saw more clients than did their counterparts in Benue; and (3) Yoruba healers specialize in ob/gyn (while this was absent or at least rare in Benue), therefore they already had clients requesting means to avoid unwanted pregnancies. It seemed that Lagos healers were in a position to motivate more clients more easily than Benue healers, resulting in higher contraceptive sales. However, the Benue State project also had potential, plus there was probably greater need for such a project in Benue, considering the relative lack of family planning and other health facilities and services in that largely rural state—conditions that are more typical of the whole of Nigeria and indeed Africa.

However, in 1988–1989 there was a restructuring of AID's financing of family-planning programs in Nigeria, which resulted in the consolidation of all such programs through one consortium of so-called cooperating agencies (private voluntary organizations, universities and for-profit consulting firms). Somehow, the traditional healer collaborative programs in Lagos and Benue were lost in the bureaucratic shuffle, and to my knowledge they received no AID funds after the first year. This was through no fault of AID; rather it was through apparent benign neglect on the part of the consortium that won AID's contract for family-planning programs for the next five years.

In 1990 the Pathfinder Fund expressed interest in evaluating the projects with a view toward possibly continuing them. But more than two years later, nothing had come of this.

## Notes

1. It was also discovered that people felt embarrassed about buying contraceptives in the public marketplace; they preferred to make private arrangements to meet the healers at night.

# 7

# Developing Roles for South African Traditional Healers in HIV/AIDS Prevention and Management

### Background to USAID-Funded Program

In South Africa, two USAID-funded projects, AIDSCOM (AIDS Communication) and AIDSCAP (AIDS Control and Prevention) collaborated as a joint program between 1991 and 1993. The USAID program in South Africa operates under antiapartheid legislation from the U.S. Congress, which means that assistance must be through nongovernmental channels, specifically through "progressive," antiapartheid organizations. The joint program's experience in AIDS prevention during the first year convinced AIDSCOM/AIDSCAP of the importance of traditional healers in HIV/AIDS and STD control in South Africa. I was asked to assist in designing a pilot project for traditional healers, conducting baseline/formative research, facilitating a preliminary workshop for healers, and evaluating the overall effort.

One decision had been made prior to my arrival in South Africa, namely to turn over most the responsibility for selecting workshop participants to five traditional healers associations that claimed national membership: (1) the Traditional Doctors AIDS Project [TRADAP] with headquarters near Johannesburg; (2) the Traditional Healers Organization of South Africa [THOSA] with headquarters in KwaXuma; (3) the Professional Herbal Preparations Association of Inyangas [PHPAI], with offices in Johannesburg, Qwa-Qwa and Bergville; (4) the Traditional Healers Organization of Africa [THOA], headquartered in Siteki, Swaziland, but said to have two branch offices in South Africa; and (5) the African Natural Healer's Organization [ANHO] with offices in Johannesburg. On the donor side, we provided some selection criteria in order to ensure gender and geographic balance, but the five healer associations did the actual selection. Virtually every major region of South Africa was represented in the final roster of participants.

The original and ideal plan of this project was to train thirty healers as trainers-of-trainers skilled in HIV/AIDS prevention during the first workshop. These thirty were to train thirty additional healers within six months of the workshop, in addition to incorporating the learning into his/her healing practice with patients. The former group of healers were referred to as the first generation, and the latter, the second generation. It was anticipated that the second generation would be trained in special workshops although it was recognized that informal or nonworkshop sharing of AIDS knowledge would also occur, for example between trained healers and their initiate-apprentices (Zulu: *amathwasa*). AIDSCOM/AIDSCAP would help defray the costs of workshops held by first-generation healers, although it was hoped that healer associations would also make in-kind contributions to defray costs. In addition, the project would provide materials and technical assistance for those workshops.

After six months, the original group of 30 healers would be reconvened by AIDSCOM/AIDSCAP for an assessment. It was hoped that some 900 healers would by then have been exposed to AIDS/HIV training. There would be an evaluation of the second generation of healers, and plans for training a third generation would be developed based on lessons learned to date. If the 900 healers of the second generation would each train 30 more healers in AIDS prevention within the same time frame, some 27,000 traditional healers could be trained a year from program start-up. Such was the ideal plan.

The number of healers' *clients* who could be reached potentially were even more impressive. Our baseline survey of healers participating in the first workshop suggested these healers saw an average of 2,000 clients per year. Even allowing for half that number to be repeat (as distinct from new) clients, that is still 1,000 clients or patients per year. That means that 27,000 healers potentially could reach 1,000 clients each with HIV/AIDS/STD preventive education—27,000,000 South Africans. Of course, second- and third-generation healer-trainees might not see as many clients as the group in the first workshop, and not all clients (some of whom are children) would be exposed to AIDS education. But still the potential seemed there for South African healers to quickly reach large numbers of people with AIDS- and STD-related information.

The preliminary workshop for South African healers was held between November 22 and November 27, 1992 at the Tzitzikama Forest Inn, 160 km from Port Elizabeth. Due to last minute changes and confusion over the stipulation that all participants had to be traditional healers—not just members of healer associations—twenty-eight rather than thirty healers actually attended. The AIDSCOM/AIDSCAP Resident Adviser and the Deputy Programme Officer served as workshop facilitators, assisted by a representative from SABSWA (South African Black Social Workers Association), from PPHC (Progressive Primary Health Care), and from the ANC Health Department. As an AIDSCAP consultant from Washington, I also served as a facilitator. Plenary sessions were conducted in English, while small group work was conducted in Xhosa, Zulu, Pedi, Sotho, Tswana, Venda, and Tsonga.

## The Baseline/Formative Survey

Unlike in Mozambique, funds were not available for ethnomedical research prior to the workshop in South Africa. However, immediately prior to the workshop, a knowledge, attitudes, beliefs, and practices (KABP) survey of participating healers was conducted for both formative and baseline purposes. Although the twenty-eight healers constitute a small and a nonrandom sample, the week-long workshop also served as an extended focus group that complemented and illuminated the survey-derived information. Furthermore, I had some opportunity for in-depth, follow-up interviewing during and after the workshop. The combined "survey" and extended discussion group obviously had little value as a quantitative research tool by which to measure expected patterns. However, it proved quite valuable as a qualitative research tool by which basic—sometimes unanticipated—patterns emerged.

According to our findings, the mean age of participants was 44.2 years, with a range of 24 to 69. There were sixteen female and twelve male healers. The "home" or first language of healers was as follows: Xhosa (eleven), Zulu (seven), South Sotho (three), Tsonga (three), Swazi (two), North Sotho (one), and Pedi (one). Literacy was supposed to be a general criterion for participation in the workshop, however four of the twenty-eight described themselves as nonliterate. The (modal) average level of formal education for the twenty-four literate healers was six years.

Bearing in mind problems inherent in classification and the overlap of healer roles in Africa, nineteen healers described themselves as primarily diviner-mediums (*sangoma, ixhwele*, or *ngaka*); the other nine described themselves as herbalists (*inyanga*) (all terms are in the singular form). All but one healer regarded herself as a specialist. The specialties identified (allowing for more than one) were sexually transmitted diseases (fourteen), mental illness (eleven), epilepsy (eight), high blood pressure (seven), childhood illness (six), barrenness or fertility (six), diarrhea (two), and evil spirits (two). Other specialties mentioned include tuberculosis, stroke, diabetic sores, arthritis, bone problems, hiccups, heart disease, ulcer, unemployment, blood purification, counselling, oedema, whooping cough, luck medicine, pneumonia, breached birth, headaches, swollen feet, traditional birth control, female bladder complaints, warts, and training other healers. Treatment of STDs was the most common specialty, which of course is entirely appropriate for an AIDS workshop and, in fact, probably should have been a criterion for selection of participants.

### *The Relative Efficacy of Traditional and Modern Medicine*

Here we posed a group of questions I asked previously in Swaziland and Nigeria. In response to the first, twenty-three healers (82 percent) said they believe traditional medicine can be more successful than modern medicine in treating certain types of disease; three—perhaps diplomatically—said they thought both equally effective, while two preferred not to answer. We next asked for specification of cases in which traditional medicine could be more successful than modern medicine. The most common responses, in order of frequency, were sexually transmitted diseases (fifteen), mental illness (nine), epilepsy (five), and high blood pressure (three). There were various infrequent mentions such as midwifery and problems associated with childbirth, witchcraft and sorcery, fertility, heart failure, and cancer.

We next turned the question around, asking whether healers believe modern medicine can be more successful than traditional medicine in treating certain types of disease: eighteen (64 percent) said yes, seven said no, and once again three said that both were equally effective. Some answered in a more qualified way than others ("sometimes," "occasionally"). For those answering yes to the last question, we next asked for specification of cases in which modern medicine could be more successful than traditional medicine. The most common responses, in order of frequency, were TB (ten), X-rays (seven), "shortage of blood" requiring transfusion (five), "shortage of water" (four), dehydration (four), and various other less frequently mentioned conditions such as cancer, AIDS, asthma, bone setting, anemia, and open wounds. One healer mentioned that traditional herbs dehydrate patients, therefore excessive use of herbs might require that a patient go to the hospital to overcome shortage of water.

All twenty-eight healers claimed they at least occasionally refer some of their patients to a Western-trained doctor or medical facility, most often in cases of TB (thirteen); X-rays (nine); "shortage of blood" requiring transfusion (five); "shortage of water" or "need the drip" or dehydration (eight); when "technology" or drugs are needed (four); complications of childbirth (four); or simply "when I cannot cure or understand the disease" (three). On the other hand, when healers were next asked if modern health practitioners ever refer patients to them; nineteen (68 percent) said no and only nine (32 percent) said yes.

### *Sexually Transmitted Diseases*

We asked what diseases the healers treat that are related to sexual intercourse, inviting them to use local disease names. We also asked about causes and treatments. Keeping in mind that respondents represent five to six Bantu-speaking groups, Table 7.1 summarizes our findings.

TABLE 7.1 Sexually Transmitted Diseases Recognized by South African Healers

| | *Cause* | *Treatment* |
|---|---|---|
| "Drop" | (1) many sexual partners, his/her blood gets dirty; (2) failure to practice safe sex; (3) sex with someone who has had an abortion | (1) prepare special medicine, then give as enema; (2) herbal tea only—no referral for injection; (3) special herbs cooked—drink 6 am and again at 6 pm; (4) enema, douching (5) "I prefer to treat two partners if one approaches me. I tell my patients to stop sexual action." |
| Gcushuwa | (1) many sexual partners; (2) use of herbs, i.e. *intando* | (1) clean infection, *muti* treatment |
| VD—unspecified | (1) having sex with person with STD; (2) sexual contact with person with bad blood | (1) hot vapors; (2) enemas; (3) give drinking medicine and powdered medicine |
| Syphilis | (1) transmitted by sexual intercourse | (1) give traditional medicine for drinking, washing and application; (2) application on genital sores, herbal tea enema, or refer patient to a medical doctor |
| Gonorrhea | (1) transmitted by sexual intercourse | (1) prepare medicine for drinking, wash septic areas and apply powder |
| Sores (or genital sores), burning urine | (1) having many sexual partners; (2) having sex with a widow(er); (3) mixing blood from different sex partners; (4) sex with woman who has aborted, dirty genitals, bad hygiene | (1) herbal drink, steam the vagina with herbs; (2) send patient to doctor for injection, then treat sores on penis |

(*continues*)

TABLE 7.1 (*Continued*)

| | | |
|---|---|---|
| Prolonged menstruation | (1) sexually transmitted | (1) hot vapor |
| Lombu (back, stomach, testes, bladder, kidneys, headache) | (1) sexual practices; Sex with STD-infected person | (1) traditional medicine (herbs), 1–3 day treatment |
| Grey-horse (Thosula) | (1) many sexual partners, blood gets dirty | (1) Prepare special *muti* and cook and later spade (enema?) the patient |
| Genital warts | (1) intercourse | (1) poultice, herb tea |
| Bhajiwe | (1) many sexual partners; (2) sex with a widow | (1) herbal decoction; treating with my own methods |

Some mentioned antibiotics as a modern treatment during group discussion, but these were said to not work as quickly as traditional STD treatments, or not to clear up symptoms permanently. We elicited the following symptom and cause descriptions from group discussion:

Drop [gonorrhea?]

- oozing genital pimples, sores
- discharge, bad odor
- headache, abdominal pain
- burning urine
- clear facial complexion
- itching urination
- if untreated, leads to infertility; babies will have eye problem, intercourse is painful for men.

"Cauliflower": (*ihashe elimhlophe, chovela, jovela*)

- swelling, white sores which grow and cover the genitals as the sores multiply
- urine can't get out

*Ukubajwe* or *Likhubalo*

- like "drop," but symptoms are immediate
- a jealous husband "protects" wife from infidelity
- a type of sorcery

*Gcushuwa* or *Gcunsula*

- greenish, thick discharge
- sores, boils
- walking like a duck

- blood in urine
- burning during urination
- miscarriage, fetus has greenish patches and pus
- pregnancy hard to determine

Locally recognized STDs were said to be preventable in much the same way: using a condom (thirteen mentions), taking traditional medicine, usually orally before engaging in risky sex (nine), sticking to one, or few, sexual partners (six), and avoiding sex with risky partners (specified were those who have had sex with many other partners and "strangers") and sex with a woman who has aborted (two).

Other preventive measures included healers counseling their clients on the above; strengthening the individual and family; sexual abstinence if the client is sick; avoiding sex with menstruating or infected women; avoiding sex with widows; and avoiding breaking taboos such as those against adultery.

***Use of Antibiotics for STD Treatment***

We asked if healers themselves ever use any modern medicines of the sort "sold in pharmacies and used by scientifically trained doctors or nurses." Twenty healers (71 percent) said they did, although three said they only used such medicines for themselves or their families. Eight healers claimed they never used modern medicines. Some of the latter commented that traditional and modern medicines cannot be mixed, at least for their patients. But note that a majority answered yes, a finding comparable to the 59 percent of a much larger sample who answered yes to the same question in Nigeria.

When we next asked which medicines are used, nine of the twenty healers answering yes to the last question felt uncomfortable about specifying medicines. Those who provided answers mentioned common analgesics, eye drops, "stomach medicine," vitamins, treatment for pregnancy, and injections. Several healers mentioned using "Flowers of Sulphur" (sulfa powder) for any disease that produces pus, that is, for infections. Some said this was used only for STDs, including sores on the skin caused by STDs. From follow-up questions after the workshop, I was told that sulfa powder is known locally as *loro* or *ndonya* (in Xhosa, Zulu). The cost of *ndonya* at a Johannesburg pharmacy was R1.49 (US$.50) for a 50-gram bag. Some healers said they mixed the powder with raw honey for STD treatment. In any case, the sulfa is usually or always mixed with herbal medicines and either served as an oral decoction, or used as a poultice, a purgative or an enema.

Since sulfa was used as a common antibiotic before the advent of penicillin, I wondered whether "Flowers of Sulphur" has any antibiotic properties. I phoned two pharmacologists employed by the product manufacturer, Allied Pharmaceuticals Ltd., and was told that sulfa powder has bacteriostatic and perhaps bacteriocidal properties. It can also kill certain parasites, at least those of the skin. I learned that Allied Pharmaceuticals also sells a sulfa ointment called Eskamel, a U.S. product more of which is said to be sold in South Africa than in the rest of the world combined. The company believes that South African traditional healers use and promote Eskamel with their clients. The company pharmacists thought it possible that the mixing of sulfa powder with herbal medicines which might already have antibiotic properties could possibly eliminate the symptoms of certain urethral infections. Sulfa products may be even more effective in the treatment of genital sores, an assessment shared by Ruben Sher, MD of the South African Institute for Medical Research (SAIMR).

These findings—very preliminary though they be—raise the possibility that some healers in South Africa may be combining over-the-counter pharmaceuticals with traditional medicines to treat at least genital sores successfully. Clearly, this should be a priority area of medical and anthropological research. It should be noted that some people are allergic to sulfa, reacting with a skin rash. For a very few, allergic reactions to sulfa are far more serious.

### *The Circumcision Factor*

A male Tsonga-speaking traditional healer from Soweto commented that he routinely advised his clients to become circumcised as a way to prevent STDs. When this was mentioned to the plenary group of healers during the workshop, several other healers—particularly women, it seemed—strongly agreed with this preventive measure and reported that they too advised their clients to become circumcised. In further discussion it emerged that a number of healers have been addressing a probable AIDS risk factor—and known STD risk factor—that is seldom if ever discussed, let alone addressed in AIDS-intervention programs, namely lack of male circumcision. These healers advise clients from non-circumcising societies (e.g., Zulu, Swazi) to become circumcised as a way to prevent STDs—and such clients apparently are complying by visiting hospitals or traditional healers to become circumcised.

In Johannesburg, after the workshop, I was given a pamphlet mass-produced by TRADAP (Traditional Doctors AIDS Project), which was one of the healers' organizations that had participated in the workshop. The pamphlet advises: "TO CIRCUMCISE IS THE BEST REMEDY TO REDUCE SEXUALLY TRANSMITTED DISEASES." I was told that TRADAP has been advising uncircumcised men to become circumcised as a way to prevent STDS since September 1991. As I was unaware of any

African or international AIDS or STD education or intervention program that promotes male circumcision, I asked how TRADAP came to learn about a relationship between lack of male circumcision and STDs, including possibly AIDS. The TRADAP president claimed that healers in her organization discovered this connection by themselves, through their own clinical experience. Specifically, they noticed that male patients who repeatedly become infected with STDs tended to be uncircumcised. Such patients were said to have rashes, "dirt," or infections under their foreskins (as we saw in Chapter 3, Swazis referred to this condition as *luhlanga*.) When I pressed further, my informant told me many rural men bathe infrequently and may not wash their penis after intercourse. She said that "stale sperm" and the blood or fluids of the woman remain under the foreskin and fester over the days into a foul-smelling "dirty something." She has seen many a penis crown with a rash due to what she called unhygienic practices. The "dirty something" was said to be passed to the next sexual partner of the uncircumcised man, thereby spreading disease.[1]

Some healers claim they have convinced parents from noncircumcising societies to have their children circumcised in order to "protect them in later life." When I asked about cultural resistance to circumcision in noncircumcising societies, the TRADAP president observed, "When tradition and the health of our people are in conflict, it is tradition we must sacrifice."

In South Africa, Xhosa (save the Bhaca and Mponda subgroups), Tsonga ("Shangaan"), and Sotho men practice circumcision traditionally, and it is healers from these groups who seem to be advising men to become circumcised. No doubt cultural values and traditional attitudes toward circumcision on the part of healers from circumcising groups play a significant part in their decision to advise circumcision. According to Xhosa informants, healers from these groups believed that circumcision helps protect against STDs long before the advent of AIDS.

I had another postworkshop interview with a female healer of Sotho origin who practices in Natal where Zulu speakers predominate. She also claimed to be advising men to become circumcised as a way to avoid STDs. She made two observations about men who become circumcised as adults: (1) they tend to not get STDs again and (2) their penises become more sensitive, therefore "they can keep their erections longer." She apparently holds these up as incentives to persuade men to become circumcised.

The TRADAP informant noted that not all Xhosa and Tsonga men are becoming circumcised these days. She believes that about 50 percent circumcise in the traditional way; 25 percent have the operation done at the hospital; and 25 percent do not do it at all. The traditional way involves a ritual circumsiser who may or may not be a traditional healer. The reason about half the boys in circumcising societies do not have the operation done in the traditional way is due to urbanization, modernization, disruption of culture, and the fear of consequences if the operation is not done properly. Ritual circumcisers are supposed to observe traditional taboos against sexual intercourse one week before and one week after performing the circumcision. When these taboos are violated, the penis of the boy being circumcised is said to swell up and the mystical transition from boyhood to manhood does not take place. The result is "a boy in a man's body." My informant lamented this decline in tradition, especially since circumcision protects against STDs.

Soon after the workshop, the (Johannesburg) *Sunday Times* (December 27, 1992) carried a page-long article about untrained "bush doctors" mutilating "scores" of Xhosa young men. It said that due to high unemployment and poverty, unscrupulous men are posing as ritual circumcisers and are doing such a bad job that in one location, thirty-nine initiates had to be hospitalized with septicemia—some even required amputation of their penises. Fennell (1991) has documented these practices and consequences in South Africa.

There needs to be empirical research to determine the extent to which men may become circumcised as a result of preventive STD or AIDS education from traditional healers. Part of the research should be to determine who performs the circumcision and whether any operations conducted outside of medical settings are safe. There should be interviews with men from noncircumcising cultures who have become circumcised as a result of a healer's admonitions. What arguments were used to convince the client? How does the client feel about his decision to become circumcised several months afterwards? Is there any ostracism from other men or women from the noncircumcising group?

We gathererd more information on this subject seven months later, as documented in Chapter 8.

### *AIDS and HIV*

Returning to the survey, all but one healer had heard about AIDS, not surprising since they were attending an AIDS workshop. Most reported learning about AIDS mostly from television, or radio (nine); hospitals, clinics, or health workers (seven); various conferences (six); AIDSCOM or TRADAP (four); AIDSCOM (four); TRADAP (three); or from patients (two). Other sources mentioned include rumors, other people, another healer, the government, and local communities. Only five healers reported they had treated any cases of AIDS or HIV.

Twenty-three of the twenty-eight healers had heard of HIV. They had heard it causes or leads to AIDS (eight); it is a virus or germ (eight); they had heard of it but they don't really know what it is (three); it reduces body's immune system (one); it is "a demon that predicts AIDS" (one); "it kills" (one); and it is "something incurable" (one). Five could give no answer. Twelve healers felt they knew "a little" about AIDS; eight said a "moderate amount"; four said "a lot"; and two said "nothing." Twenty-two thought AIDS is currently a "great" threat to the people of their area. Twenty-five thought AIDS will become an even greater problem to their people in the future.

The healers were quite knowledgeable about AIDS symptoms, mentioning (in order of frequency): weight loss, bodily sores, weakness, energy loss, skin disease, rash, diarrhea, dehydration, sweating, STDs, coughing, TB, swelling, hair loss, appetite loss, headaches, continuous fever, mental confusion, "black blood," and pneumonia. They were likewise quite knowledgeable about the cause of AIDS, citing (in order of frequency): having many sexual partners or "lack of self-respect"; sexual contact, untreated STDs, prostitution, HIV, polygamy, and "sexual dishonesty." The same is true for how the disease is transmitted. Answers included (in order): sexual intercourse, blood contact, traditional practices such as razor cuts or scarification, mother-to-child infection during pregnancy, having many sex partners, and blood transfusion. Only two said sharing a toothbrush. In answer to a separate question, all but two healers denied AIDS can be transmitted by people who share the same toilet or dishes. It is clear from these answers that these healers had previous exposure to AIDS education.

A somewhat surprising finding was that about 40 percent of this rather well-informed group of healers believed AIDS can be cured by either traditional or "modern" treatment. The remainder didn't know or equivocated in their answers; only two said AIDS cannot be cured. Eight of those believing there is a cure thought traditional medicine can cure AIDS, while three believed "modern medicine," or a combination of traditional and modern medicine, could cure AIDS. During the first day's group discussion, several opinions were given to the effect that AIDS can be cured if traditional healers can unite, or if healers and doctors can tackle the problem together. Many or most healers believe they and other traditional healers can treat some of the opportunistic infections of HIV/AIDS successfully, a conclusion shared by a recent WHO Expert Committee Meeting in Botswana (Staugaard 1991). This belief probably explains the relatively high number of healers that gave the opinion in the survey that AIDS can be cured. In another unexpected finding, a majority of healers did not know if AIDS could be prevented, a finding that should prove significant for posttraining evaluations.

Finally we asked healers what they thought their own chances were of getting AIDS. Fifteen thought they might be at risk; three thought they were not, and the rest did not know. Some among the first group thought they might be exposed to AIDS through traditional healing practices such as razor cuts or other skin piercing that results in contact with patients' blood. One remarked, "If I don't use gloves or take safety measures, I'm in danger." Some others "never thought about it." All but two healers reported using a razor in their practice. Nine healers specified that the razor is the only piercing instrument they use; six said they use needles for traditional piercing practices, but not injections. Of the former, one commented, "I've had special training in how to clean my razors." Another said, "Nowadays I change razors with every patient." Razors are used to introduce traditional medicines into the bloodstream to "protect" or "strengthen" the client, or to treat "fits," "broken leg," or "cauliflower" (chlamydia). The six needle-users said needles are used for traditional piercing practices (*kuchopa, uluxhola*) and/or for letting pus out in certain cases of swelling. None reported using syringes to give injections.[2]

### *Sexual Behavior*

We began this topic with general questions about the age at which boys and girls usually begin to experiment with sex. Boys were said to begin at about fourteen (with a range given of twelve to nineteen); girls were said to begin at about twelve (with a range of seven to fourteen). Without influencing the answer, interviewers were asked to determine what types of experimentation are typical in early stages of sexual awakening, such as masturbation, nonpenetrative intercourse, actual intercourse, heavy petting, homosexual play, etc.

Most healers specified that actual intercourse begins nowadays at about fourteen for boys and twelve for girls. There was little or no mention of masturbation, foreplay, or "thigh sex" in answering survey questions, however this emerged later during workshop discussion. Comments to this question from the survey include:

> In former times, the elders educated the boys in the bush about proper sexual behavior. They rarely do it now. . . . Our youth see sex practices on TV and then want to try them themselves. They also see (the behavior of) drunk people in shabeens (bars) and copy them. . . . Young girls are raped by older boys or men. They then continue with sex (paren. mine).

We asked specifically if any people in the healer's area engage in "thigh sex" (*ukusoma, ukufema*), or other type of intercourse where there is no penetration. Fourteen said no, ten said yes, three reported it was practiced in the past, and one did not know. Some commented that elders' advice on sexual matters is no longer given or heeded. Another commented that boys raised traditionally may still practice thigh sex.

We asked if any men in the healer's area engage in homosexual behavior. Apart from four who claimed they did not know, twelve answered yes and twelve answered no. Additional comments included:

> It happens when men are drunk. . . . It is related to drugs and booze. . . . There are rumors that it happens. . . . It occurs too much! . . . White patients may do it, but not blacks.

In response to a question about anal intercourse, twelve did not know, ten denied it occurs, and five said it does occur. One commented, "It's rare. It's related to drugs and alcohol." Only one female healer from Soweto said anal intercourse is quite common, both male-to-male, and male-to-female.

Comments from the workshop discussion helped illuminate survey findings on sexual behavior. Discussion followed an oral summary of the survey findings. First, there was some consensus that masturbation is practiced by young people, either singly or in pairs. Regarding the early rape or seduction by young boys of even younger girls, a female healer remarked, "Don't put all the blame on boys; girls reach puberty faster and they attract the boys."

Comments suggested that homosexual experimentation occasionally occurs among boys, but in adults—where it occurs—it usually results from men being deprived of normal sexual outlets when they are in prison or working in the mines. Some thought deprivation of contact with women accounts for the origin of male homosexuality.[3] One healer commented that there are men who may not be fully homosexual, but who engage in male prostitution with other men out of economic necessity.

Female homosexuality was discussed, more because of interest by male healers than because of public health concern. A female healer, with consultation from others, reported that such women may engage in foreplay, then rub vulvas together in a scissors position. They may also use a dildo together.

Bestiality was said to occur sometimes in rural areas. Herdboys may have intercourse with sheep or goats.

It may be noted that the workshop discussion proved a somewhat better way of eliciting information on sexual behavior than individual interviews. However, it was the third day the group was together, the ice was broken, and most healers felt very relaxed with each other and with the workshop facilitators, having joked, laughed, and eaten meals together.

It seems doubtful this information would have arisen in formal focus groups had they been conducted on the first day.

Returning to the survey, we asked what types of sexual behavior are forbidden, or considered bad, or dangerous in the healer's area and tradition. Six said homosexuality and another six specified anal intercourse; four said sex with a widow; and two said intercourse with a girl prior to menstruation. The frequency of answers relating to homosexuality and anal intercourse may have been influenced by the earlier questions on these topics. Other forms of prohibited sex mentioned were: sex with a woman who has aborted, sex with a married woman, sex with a widow during the first year (before she has been ritually purified), sex with strangers, oral sex, unlubricated sex, having too many partners, sex when there are sores on the genitals, sex "using too many postures," sex with partners where there is a great age difference, sex while mourning, postpartum sex, sex during early pregnancy, and having sex "from behind a woman."

We asked whether some people engage in these behaviors anyway; fourteen said yes; three said no, and ten preferred not to answer. We then asked, "If people engage in forbidden or bad sexual behaviors, can this result in health problems, or even death?" Those answering "yes" to the last question—plus some others—gave the following answers:

In case extramarital sex was not mentioned already, we next asked a

TABLE 7.2 Results of Engaging in Prohibited Sex

| *Prohibited Sex* | *Results* |
|---|---|
| Early pregnancy | cervical cancer, death after birth |
| Having sex from behind the woman | penis penetrating the woman's womb, causing pain and damage |
| Sex during menstruation | bad luck |
| Sex right after birth | leads to another unplanned pregnancy |
| Anal intercourse | causes other diseases; it is not healthy; it can cause STDs and HIV |
| Homosexual relationships | relates to unknown causes of diseases, syphilis |
| Older people having sex with younger partners | brings bitterness, unhappiness. |
| Sex with sores on genitals | can cause Makoma and Kubalo, diseases which can kill |
| Sleeping with prostitutes or with many partners, without a condom | leads to sexually transmitted diseases |
| Sex with one who has aborted | leads to the syphilis-like disease *uQuntsula* (*gcunsula*) |

group of questions about any possible health consequences of adultery between a single man and a married woman, or between a single woman and a married man. A slight minority of healers (44 percent) denied there are consequences in the first case. At least one healer denying health consequences qualified the answer by adding that the man must wear a condom. Of those believing in health consequences, two mentioned the disease *(li)khubalo* (described in the Swazi interpretation in Chapter 3)—one saying *likhubalo* is a virus like AIDS. Others commented that STDs (including *isixitho*) or simply unspecified disease can result from extramarital sex. Other healers focused more on the violation of social norms than on disease consequences, saying that it is not right or proper or that, "You've committed a crime. Divorce and mental problems will result."

A higher proportion of healers (58 percent) believed in negative health consequences if a single woman has intercourse with a married man. Again, some of those denying consequences saw use of condoms as a way of avoiding at least the health consequences of extramarital sex.

We next asked whether there are any health consequences to having many sex partners, and if so, what. The great majority (88 percent) believed there are such consequences; those denying this again specified that people can escape negative consequences only if condoms are used. Fully 93 percent of healers thought there are health consequences if the person with many sex partners is a woman; and 100 percent thought there are consequences if a man has sex with a prostitute or sex worker. Mentioned in all cases above were VD, STDs, and AIDS. One said malaria can result from sex with prostitutes.

Just over half (52 percent) said there are health consequences if a man has sex with another man. Most of the others (ten of thirteen healers) preferred to say they did not know. The three who said there are no consequences all specified—as in their responses to earlier questions—that one is safe as long as condoms are used. There was not much elaboration about the nature of the consequences. Some said "Unknown diseases can result"; some specified AIDS; one healer said male-male intercourse can damage the anus. One simply said it is taboo.

We next asked "For your male patients who are married, how common is it for them to have lovers outside the marriage?" The choices were "Rare," "Somewhat common," or "Very common." Every healer said it was "very common" for both male *and* female clients to have outside lovers.

We then asked if healers can influence the sexual behavior of their clients. Twenty-three (85 percent) said they could, by giving counseling or advice (seven), by providing sex education (four), by advising a reduction of sexual partners (three), or by the promotion of safe sex or condom use (three). Others commented, "They obey my advice. I can even see evidence of condoms in their possession," "I can warn them about STDs (to prevent AIDS)," or can give threats or threats of death."

Last in this section we asked if the healer knew of cases where a traditional healer has had sex with a patient. Twenty-one (78 percent) said yes, four said no, and two did not know. Six said it is very common; three said it is rare. Comments included:

> "Some (men) can't control their feelings when they order a patient to take off her clothes. Traditional healers—both male and female—may become sexually interested. Some even marry as a result." "(This outcome) is common for the healer who fails to respect his/her work." "It mostly happens between a male healer and a female client." "It is very wrong. It's unethical."

### *Contraceptives*

All but one healer knew what a condom is, and correctly described its uses, namely: to prevent AIDS or HIV (seventeen); to prevent (other) STDs (fifteen); to prevent pregnancy (nine); and to prevent general infections (one). Fully twenty-three healers (85 percent) said they have at some time advised a client to use a condom. Note again that these healers are certainly not representative of South African healers in regard to condom familiarity and acceptance. Several mentioned they have seen and learned about condoms from previous contact with AIDSCOM or from a clinic. Additional comments include:

> A woman must be brave to ask a man to use a condom. . . . I advise when treating my patients for STDs, AIDS. . . . I also teach them *how* to use a condom. . . . I both keep and distribute them. . . . I have advised about condoms when talking to our youth club. . . . This (condom) is to prevent my patient from infecting others. . . . I advise (clients to use condoms) to help them avoid unwanted pregnancy.

During group discussion, some important information about condoms and "entry points" for their promotion (with most African healers I would say "introduction") arose. Several healers said it is not traditional for a healer to advise a patient to refrain from intercourse while a patient is undergoing treatment for an STD or another illness. A husband may react negatively if his wife is advised by a healer to refrain from intercourse during her treatment. Intercourse with a condom is preferable to refraining from sex altogether, and a husband can understand that "bad blood" will not be transferred to him by his wife if he uses a condom. Note that healers at the workshop emphasized the notion of bad or impure blood—in fact AIDS seemed to be understood more or less accurately as a disease of bad blood, which for healers explains why people must avoid any form of blood-to-blood contact. Thus, it seems that healers can and do advise seropositive clients and their sexual partners to use a condom in order to avoid contact with the impure blood of AIDS. The notion of impure blood seems rooted in traditional ideas of the role of pollution and contamination in illness found throughout Africa. And, as the workshop healers indicated, sexual intercourse is believed to provide an opportunity for men to have contact with menstrual and other blood.

There was also some discussion of traditional postpartum abstinence from intercourse. A female healer said she believes this abstinence can be avoided if the husband uses a condom.

There are also entry points for promoting the adoption of condoms by healers themselves and their partners, a benefit of which would be that healers could speak with the authority of personal experience when recommending condom use to their clients. Female traditional healers are considered "impure" after they have intercourse with their husband or lover due to having received the man's sperm. The question arose: Is a woman healer impure after sex if her partner uses a condom? One of the most senior and respected healers at the conference said no, because with a condom there would be no contact between sperm and vaginal fluid. The other healers seemed to agree with this assessment. It was noted that a female healer cannot throw bones or divine in another manner if she is in an impure state. One woman complained that with patients coming to her urban clinic night and day for consultation—which includes divination—she is always impure and therefore cannot ever have sex. She said she was glad if she can now remain pure if her husband uses a condom when they have intercourse.

Some other healers disagreed with this conclusion or added certain qualifications. For example, when a woman is an apprentice (*lithwasa*), or she is treating children, she must be "cool," not "hot." Even sex involving use of a condom will make a female healer or apprentice healer "hot," some felt, therefore she must abstain.

## The Workshop Itself

### *The General Approach*

"Translating" modern biomedical concepts such as T-cells and immune systems into something understandable to traditional healers who lack much formal education and who embrace an African, indigenous paradigm of health and disease is a challenge in cross-cultural communication. The AIDSCOM/AIDSCAP Deputy Program Officer, a Xhosa speaker but conversant in the languages of all the participants, took the lead in such cross-cultural translation. She basically used two extended analogies with either the military or with the professional hierarchy among healers themselves. White blood cells were described either as soldiers (*amasoja, amajoni*) or as apprentice healers (*amathwasa*); T-cells were described as military commanders (*inkokheli*) or master healers (*gobela*).

Using these analogies, the explanation of how HIV invades the body was as follows: the senior officers (T-cells) are continuously being guarded by the soldiers (white blood cells.) Through unsafe sexual practices, the enemy (HIV) slips into the body and dodges past the soldier guards. This enemy kills the senior officers and tricks the soldiers into thinking they are still taking orders from the murdered officers. In this guise, the enemy orders the soldiers to let in more enemies. Soon the whole body is administered by the enemy (HIVs), and this is manifest as a full-blown case of AIDS. The traditional healers at the workshop seemed to have no trouble understanding the etiology of the disease in these terms. Indeed, the soldier/senior officer analogy was being used in print media in some other AIDS prevention programs in South Africa.

### *Methods and Topics*

Workshop training methods included lectures, small and large group discussions, role-playing, questions and answers with invited HIV-infected persons, and educational videos. Topics included epidemiology (global, regional, and local); family life in South African subcultures; care and support for HIV/AIDS patients; traditional healers' practices: (instruments traditionally used; sterilization; locally recognized STDs; beliefs about contamination; client/healer direct blood contact; variations of sexual behavior; safer sexual practices and abstinence; locating recent sexual partners); traditional practices related to death and dying in South Africa; counselling issues for at-risk populations (women, youth, sex workers); the psychological impact of HIV/AIDS on individuals, families, friends, and community; a discussion panel of HIV-positive and PWA (persons with AIDS) families and friends; sharing of record-keeping information, HIV test results, information and confidentiality; systems for recording patient contacts; translating information into practice; and the training of other healers and patients.

This is not the place to describe what transpired in each of these sections. Presented here are notes of certain sections that seem most relevant.

### *The Persons with AIDS (PWA) Visit*

Four HIV-infected adults, two with children, joined the workshop on the third day and remained until the end. The adults spoke about their condition, the rejection they had experienced by family and friends, the discrimination they faced at the workplace or their loss of employment, their need for support and love, and their hopes and fears. One spoke poignantly about how it feels to never be touched because people have misconceptions about how AIDS is spread.

After hearing these accounts, the healers had supportive comments for the visitors. In a representative remark, one healer said, "We are deeply moved by your courage. We promise to be your support group in the future." Another observed that the healers present do not understand HIV or AIDS very well, but they all feel they can treat the opportunistic infections or symptoms successfully. He suggested that healers ought to treat HIV- positive patients without charge since the healers are still learning about these infections. One of the PWAs said of the earlier comment, "As far as I'm concerned, if you can cure the infections associated with AIDS, then you can cure AIDS." Other reactions of PWAs can be found in the section on participants' end-of-week comments.

### *Counseling Persons with AIDS*

After training and discussion about counseling HIV/AIDS clients, a model counseling session was held involving a healer and one of the PWAs present. During this role play, the female healer was dealing with a repeat client whose symptoms she had been able to treat successfully, only to have new ones emerge. She interpreted these repeated (HIV) symptoms as something related to *thikolosho* (a witch's spirit familiar), which has made the client's blood "impure." During the session, the healer told the client, who was at the workshop with his wife, that both of them should remain sexually faithful lest they pass the disease to others.

The client then made some remarks about his problems of family rejection and job discrimination, whereupon the healer gave the couple positive and upbeat advice, noting that there are many people out of work nowadays and there are even handicapped people missing bodily parts who can make handicrafts and earn income in other ways. "*Thikolosho* hasn't affected your sight or your limbs so you are still able to work." The healer advised the couple to keep coming to her often: "Don't be afraid of bothering me." The male PWA, perhaps forgetting he was engaged in role play, suggested hopefully that he has carpentry skills and that his wife is able to sew and do bead work. At this point, the healer mentioned that her healer organization in fact has initiated an income-generating program for patients who are unable to work because of job discrimination due to their health status. She explained the program to her clients, who, by the end of the model session, seemed genuinely more hopeful about their situation.

During later questioning it emerged that TRADAP offers an income-generating and skills-training program for HIV-positive and other clients who are unable to find or keep employment because of health-related discrimination. TRADAP—which has branches in Johannesburg, Capetown, the Transkei, and elsewhere in South Africa—had obtained small grants from the Anglo-American Corporation, South African Breweries, King Korn Breweries, the Red Cross, and other private sector donors to provide monthly support for destitute patients while they are undergoing skills training. The money is also used to pay for materials such as beads, thread, and wool for making handicrafts.

### *Healers' Plans for Conducting Future Workshops Themselves*

By the end of the workshop, each traditional healer was committed to train thirty other healers of their own selection within six months. Each of the five healers associations was asked to develop training plans, specifying any financial or materials needs, then report them to the larger group. During the reporting, the plans varied greatly from those which were relatively "high-tech," expensive, and dependent on outside resources to those which were low-tech, self-reliant, and dependent on local materials. As an example of the latter, one organization spokesperson reported to the group, "We are used to walking or riding horses to meetings; we'll only provide bus fare for those who are coming from far away." This can be contrasted with another group which felt it needed over R12,000 (U.S.$4,000) for total workshop costs—about three times the estimate of another organization. Facilitators noted that healers seemed to like the model and materials used in the present workshop, and therefore were influenced in the direction of planning for more expensive transportation and venues.

### *Participants' End-of-Week Comments on the Workshop*

The following are verbal comments (see below for written comments) made by workshop participants on the last day of the workshop:

- "I have overcome my fear of AIDS."
- "I have learned about love, respect, caring, sharing ideas, and the importance of counseling. I have been inspired by our PWAs and our healers who came here."
- "We thought at first that you whites were after our knowledge to take it to America. This is the first time traditional healers from so many tribes have assembled under one roof. We wouldn't have done this thing without being brought together this way."

- "It is going to be Death For All by the Year 2000 if traditional healers are not involved in AIDS health education programs in South Africa."
- "We needed this information sooner. Where has AIDSCOM been?"
- From a female PWA: "I was overcome with the love of our family here at the workshop."
- "We must treat a patient with love and respect their dignity. I must reach out to patients, not just treat them with detachment."
- "I thought I knew a lot about AIDS, but now I know I didn't."
- "We didn't realize the ways we traditional healers could become infected."
- "The knowledge we have learned is not just for *us*. It is to help (all) the people. We shouldn't feel we are better than the traditional healers who couldn't be trained by AIDSCOM. We must share our knowledge with them."
- "I wish I could keep up my professional contacts with all the traditional healers I have come to feel close to here at the workshop."
- (From a male, educated PWA): "You healers are the first (people) I would turn to after my mother for counseling for my problems."
- "Traditional healers could now develop a larger congregation, like the ZCC (Zionist Christian Church). Then there would be more love between us, and the white doctors would respect us more."

A posttest evaluation questionnaire or interview schedule (depending on a healer's literacy in English) was given on the last day of the workshop. For their overall evaluation, participants and (national) facilitators were offered a four-point scale: Very useful; Useful; A little useful; Not useful. All but one participant rated the workshop as "Very useful"; the other answer was "Useful." Respondents were asked to continue using the 1 to 4 ranking for all questions, but only about half used this system. Those who did not usually provided various comments which were overwhelmingly favorable. The very few less-than-favorable comments are recorded below. These and other comments are provided verbatim, or with very slight editing to make the grammar clearer. Repeat comments are not usually presented more than once, or quantified unless this seemed significant (e.g., more than five respondents made essentially the same comment).

Regarding individual section or workshop components, Care and Support for HIV/AIDS Patients received the highest rating, followed by People with HIV/AIDS (PWAs), Traditional Healers' Practices, and Training Other Healers and Patients—all tied for second place.

On a personal note I must admit that prior to the workshop, I was

TABLE 7.3 Summary Evaluation of Workshop Topics

| | *Very useful*[1] | *Useful* | *A little or not useful* | *Not useful* |
|---|---|---|---|---|
| Epidemiology of AIDS | 13 | 7 | | |
| Condoms and condom demonstration | 11 | 8 | | |
| Family life in South Africa | 10 | 7 | | |
| Death and dying in South Africa | 8 | 6 | 1 | |
| Traditional healers' practices | 15 | 3 | | |
| Care and support for HIV/AIDS patients | 16 | 5 | | |
| Counseling issues for at-risk populations | 12 | 10 | | |
| People with HIV/AIDS (PWAs) | 15 | 1 | | |
| Role-playing on AIDS counseling and advice | 14 | 8 | 1 | |
| Training other healers and patients | 15 | 6 | | |

[1](or "very, very useful" written in)

somewhat uneasy about my colleagues' plans to teach African healers how to counsel their own clients. It seemed to me presumptuous that Americans and (black) South African nonhealers could imagine that they could teach healers about patient care, love, sympathy, understanding, and the like. There were even plans to talk about an HIV-positive client's need to be hugged. I was also uneasy about expecting healers to practice unrolling condoms over lifelike dildos procured from "adult" shops in the United States. To my surprise, healers reacted to such training and exercises as well as any group of sensitized social workers or nurses from, say, California. They learned and grew from the experience and became excited about improving patient care in their practices. Traditional healers were seen hugging PWAs as an added part of their morning greeting. One healer even said "love can work better than herbs."

In the posttest we asked, "What was the most *useful* thing you learned in the workshop?" The various responses speak for themselves:

> The role played by THs in AIDS counseling. . . . How AIDS is spread. . . . What people with HIV look like. . . . Love. . . . Cooperation and knowing each other. . . . Counseling of a client. . . . Educating people with AIDS. . . . (the relation between) STD symptoms and AIDS. . . . How to care for and love patients with or without AIDS. . . . Patient care (at least three or four said this). . . . Counseling and conflict resolution in the lives of HIV/AIDS patients. . . . The manner of approaching my clients. . . . How to treat

> patients. . . . (PWA) Philli Lutaya's courage (in an AIDS film). . . . Discovering that traditional practices could be fatal . . . . My personal conduct as a traditional practitioner. . . . Witnessing (meeting) HIV clients. . . . Family life in South Africa . . . . How to use the condom. . . . All sections. . . . The condom demonstration . . . . How to educate people about AIDS. . . . To be positive about being HIV positive and to look forward to life (this came from a PWA). . . . How the virus can be spread.

We also asked, "What was your *favorite part* of the workshop?" Responses were similar:

> What AIDS is and how it is spread. . . . The symptoms of AIDS. . . . The condom demonstration. . . . Presentation of the PWAs. . . . Counseling for PWAs. . . . Practical education in the presence of PWAs. . . . Learning about STDs and HIV. . . . Discovering that different healer organizations could have one idea (could unite in purpose). . . . AIDS and infectious diseases. . . . About living with HIV. . . . The videos. . . . (How we) can help each other. . . . AIDS epidemiology. . . . All sections were (equally) useful. . . . The introduction of AIDS and how it spreads. . . . The training has empowered me. . . . Talking with HIV patients. . . . Counseling and meeting our (PWA) guests.

The least favorite part of the workshop proved to be topics related to death and dying, as well as videos depicting this. This assessment probably was due to healers being shocked, frightened, or depressed, and probably to taboos concerning the open discussion of death. It does not necessarily mean healers failed to learn from the topic. Comments written by healers themselves (see below, this section) tend to confirm this interpretation.

Most of the eight to ten videos shown poignantly depicted suffering, dying, and loss. The videos remembered best were BORN IN AFRICA, AIDS ORPHANS, and IT'S NOT EASY. BORN IN AFRICA was the one that had been shown most recently at the time of the evaluation, therefore it may have been the one most easily remembered, whereas, IT'S NOT EASY, for example, was shown at the beginning of the week. It seemed clear that IT'S NOT EASY made a deep emotional impact on the healers, judging by comments made in group discussion immediately after it was shown and early the next morning. In comments I recorded, several healers said that their sleep or dreams were haunted by the film. Many said they now wanted to *mobilize their home communities* and teach people about AIDS prevention, how HIV can and cannot be transmitted, and how to treat PWAs with care and respect. Still others said they wanted to organize hawkers, market women, and various community groups about ways to prevent AIDS.

Some comments made in reaction to the films again speak for themselves:

> It gave me knowledge and understanding that if I don't educate the community and my family, we shall face the same situation here (as in Uganda).... It's very painful (more than one said this).... It makes me think about the problems we are facing in South Africa.... What if (the AIDS orphans) were mine?.... My own kids may be orphans.... (I admired) the determination to face death as shown by the main actor.... (I admired) the way in which the man agreed to go public and teach the people of Uganda about AIDS and HIV.... (I admired) the way Lutaya looks happy even when he knows that he was going to die.... (I admired how) Lutaya went public to educate the community about family support.... (I admired) the courage shown by this hero although he knew he was going to die....

Other comments that provide general insight into healers' thinking, reactions, and possible future actions include:

> I thought of the carelessness of how I used to heal my patients.... It was a pleasure to know how to prevent AIDS.... I was filled with fear.... It is important to educate the community in general.... We now have the knowledge about this disease and I shall use it at my surgery (and with my) family and community....

On condoms and condom demonstration:

> It was important to know how to use a condom. I shall discuss it with my husband and also teach my patients while I heal.... (Condoms) will help people in prevention.... Healers overcame their cultural shock with ease.... It was good to learn how the disease can be prevented.... (We) need more (education). This was not enough—a lot of training is needed.... The condom demonstration enables people to know how to use it.

On family life:

> It helped me understand dynamics of family life in our country.... It really answered my problem about the divorce rate and promiscuity in this country (and how this relates to AIDS and STDs) .... It strengthened my determination (to give) AIDS or sex education.... Family life was important, it reminded me of my ignorance.... (The workshop facilitators were) very sympathetic about our poor people.

## On death and dying:

It is going to be Death For All by the Year 2000 if traditional healers are not involved in AIDS health education programs in South Africa.... I was touched and told myself I am going to teach my people.... If we are not fast in spreading the gospel of AIDS, in three to five years over 3 million people will be dead.... It makes me sad to see people are dying in South Africa due to ignorance/misinformation.... (It made me) think about methods to save the world.... It was important but hurting (to discuss) .... Information on handling the deceased with HIV is very important.... (We must) involve the traditional healers in training.... Healers must also be involved in training their clients.... It was frustrating to learn of people dying of curable diseases (i.e., opportunistic infections).... It made me depressed but also I learned as a traditional healer because that is what normally happens to us and in most cases we shall be alone to face our patients' families and friends.... It prepares people to be able to understand all these stages (of AIDS).

## On traditional healers' practices:

It was a mind-opening session to learn about STDs and how they relate to AIDS.... We must be prepared to treat the STDs mentioned here.... It helped healers in understanding AIDS education from where they (already) are.... Traditional healers need not be jealous.... I realized that traditional healers are useful since they are capable of healing STDs.... It's important to learn how our practices could promote the spread of STDs.... There's a need for us to learn more on healthy storage of our drugs.... It teaches us how to cool down a person affected with AIDS, how to teach them to use a condom.... In a way we were a bit reluctant and I learned more about STD symptoms.... It helped in exposing traditional practices.... This (topic) is well understood by the healers but a lot has to be done in training.... This is good information for (workshop) organizers.... I learned about STDs.

## On care and support for HIV/AIDS patients:

It helped in promoting our caring and loving capabilities .... This knowledge is important for the care of HIV/AIDS patients.... I thought about the way they were being treated. It's (only) now that I've learned how to handle them because they need our love.... We must give love and help.... They've shown us that love can work better than herbs.... It's important to show care and love for the affected.... Traditional healers need to be supportive.... Love is needed for those people.... (I am now) determined to help the HIV+ and AIDS clients.... I was happy about this part as most of our healers are (already) doing that. They keep them (HIV clients?) as a part of their families. . . . (I learned) not to be afraid of them and to support them with love. . . . I was useful to learn how to give care and support.

On counseling:

It helped us understand the counseling of seropositive patients. . . . It was important to understand the at-risk population. . . . (I learned) counseling without any fears. . . . It's important to learn that we can be of help in referring our patients for HIV testing, with (those testing positive being) counseled. . . . It's important for practical purposes. . . . It's a very useful (topic) but (was) not well treated. . . . There's a big need. . . . They (PWAs) need love from us. . . . It will bring about change to HIV patients in South Africa.

On role-playing in AIDS counseling:

It (provided) a clear picture on how I must counsel my fellows. . . . It was a big part of what we are supposed to be doing to help families. . . . Role-playing was important to demonstrate our daily work. . . . It cleared up some myths. . . . (It was) important for reflecting on our daily practices. . . . It was a blueprint of what we were supposed to be doing to be loving such families. . . . Some introspection on daily activities was done by healers. . . . (It was) a learning experience for future counselors. . . . (It was) very educational. . . . Counseling was not good; more education is needed. . . . The healer must also counsel when consulting his client.

On the visit and participation of PWAs:

It convinced me that a healthy-looking person can be a carrier. . . . They were not afraid of meeting us. . . . Seeing is believing. . . . They look very strong and they taught us not to feel sorry (for them). I know what I need (to give) is love. . . . They made me believe that AIDS exists. . . . They were depressed when they came but O.K. when they left (the workshop). . . . They showed strength and preparedness to go on irrespective of having acquired the virus. . . . Their role is paramount in AIDS education. . . . Opening up was an experience for them. . . . (I am) appreciative and very pleased. . . . They can set a good example. . . . It made the workshop very happy. . . . They were like the heroes of Africa to stand up and show people. . . . There's a need for them to be involved. . . . They are very brave, the heroes of Africa. . . . I have made good friends among the PWAs.

On training other healers and patients:

I am highly motivated and hope to train (others). . . . (This was) to train more healers so that they can train more patients . . . . It was important for

> us to make plans which we are to implement at our places of work. . . . We are going to spread the gospel. . . . Traditional healers need to be trained more (in order to train patients). . . . It's important to feel empowered. . . . This section is more important for without the experience that I got, I was not going to face those who are not in my organization. . . . I am going to do it. . . . The different regions should implement their plans.

Perhaps not surprisingly, when we asked, "Would you be willing to go to another workshop like this one?" all said yes. Some went further and said, "Yes, next week," or "Yes, I would come running."

## Summary of Survey and Group Discussion Findings

Healers recognize and treat many STDs, and many recognize the causal connection between STDs and HIV transmission. Most could identify sound methods of STD prevention e.g., use of condoms, restricting the number of sexual partners, and avoiding sex with risky partners. Most healers felt they knew only a small or moderate amount about AIDS—a modest and rather accurate self-assessment. They proved to be quite knowledgeable about symptoms, means of transmission, and prevention of HIV/AIDS. Although only a handful of healers reported having already treated what they believed were HIV/AIDS cases, many or most felt they and other traditional healers could treat some of the opportunistic infections of HIV/AIDS successfully. HIV-infected guests at the workshop also expressed faith in healers' ability to treat infections. One male, educated patient said, "You healers are the first (people) I would turn to after my mother for counseling for my problems. As far as I'm concerned, if you can cure the infections associated with AIDS, then you can cure AIDS."

Most healers believed themselves to be at risk of HIV infection through direct contact with patients' blood. This is one of several reasons traditional healers were interested in learning the facts about AIDS. At least equally powerful was their desire to help their clients.

More evidence of male homosexual behavior including anal intercourse emerged than is usual in research of this sort in Africa. A number of healers believe these practices began—or increased notably—when men were isolated from women in mines and prisons. More types of sexual behavior are considered "forbidden, bad, or dangerous" by healers than are considered such in the industrialized West. In addition to adultery and sex with risky partners such as sex workers, healers identified sex with a woman who has aborted, with strangers, and with a widow during the first year (before she has been ritually purified) as dangerous. Healers also warned against oral sex, unlubricated sex, having too many partners, homosexuality, anal sex, sex when there are sores on the genitals, sex "using to many postures," sex with partners where there is a great age difference, sex prior to a girl's first menstruation, sex during mourning, postpartum sex, sex during early pregnancy, and having sex "from behind a woman."

In spite of conservative sexual norms, most healers reported that at least some people engage in these behaviors anyway. Every healer without exception reported that nowadays, extramarital sex is "very common" for both men and women. This however should not be taken as evidence of black South African promiscuity or hypersexuality, especially among women. A study of 2,682 men and women at a Durban STD clinic (biasing the sample strongly toward the sexually active) showed that men had had 6.4 sexual partners during the previous year while women had had 1.5 partners; 90 percent of the women had had less than 5 lifetime sexual partners (O'Farrell and Windsor 1991:1258).

Violation of norms regarding sexual behavior was said by healers to lead to a number of locally recognized illnesses (some considered fatal) as well as misfortune. Most healers said they felt they could influence the sexual behavior of their clients by counseling and providing sex education. During workshop role-play exercises with HIV-infected clients, there was evidence that healers can indeed be effective counselors.

Regarding efforts to influence sexual behavior, there seems to be a clear basis for building upon what traditional healers—if not their clients—already believe about the hazards of having sex with strangers, risky partners, or a multitude of partners. Traditional healers had strong, unequivocal and moralistic opinions on this subject. Healers had ways of describing the advantages of sexual restraint and monogamy in terms of "self-respect" and treating oneself and one's body with "dignity." Indeed some healers cited "lack of self-respect" as the *cause* of AIDS. Others cited "loss of respect" (along with adultery) as a major negative impact of foreign culture on black people. If further research shows such terms are in common use among at least healers, such language—as well as related and underlying ideas—could be usefully incorporated into HIV/AIDS preventive education messages in South Africa and perhaps the broader region. A Zimbabwean healer, reporting on a meeting between healers and local chiefs, quotes the chiefs as saying, ". . . to solve the problem (of AIDS) we would like things to be the way they were yesterday and not today. Wives and husbands must respect each other as they used to do before" (Musara 1991:32).

Traditional healers could also influence people at risk (or already HIV infected) to adopt safe, nonpenetrative sexual practices, such as thigh sex, as a safe alternative to penetrative sex. This may seem unrealistic, but some Africans will undoubtedly prefer to revive a traditional practice than to adopt condoms, spermicides, or other practices seen as non-

African and dependant on outside technology. And traditional healers are likely to be among those who prefer the time-honored, ancestor-sanctioned ways of the past. At the same time, it must remembered that there may be no tradition of nonpenetrative sexual intercourse in some parts of Africa.

Unlike healers in many or most other African countries, the healers at our workshop were relatively knowledgeable about condoms. As influential health opinion leaders, perhaps especially in matters related to STDs, their support could be crucial to the success of AIDSCOM/AIDSCAP efforts to promote the adoption and correct use of condoms on the part of sexually active South Africans. Nearly all healers at the workshop understood the functions of the condom and were already advising clients to use them. From listening to healers in discussion, strategies emerged for culturally appropriate and effective ways of introducing and promoting condoms: (1) AIDS or HIV (and perhaps some other STDs) seem to be understood as a disease of "bad blood"; (2) people must avoid contact with one another's blood; and (3) people with HIV/AIDS (or perhaps certain other STDs) and their sexual partners must use a condom in order to avoid contact with "bad" or "impure" blood. At the workshop, healers learned how to demonstrate correct condom use (including safe removal) with an artificial penis (dildo), one of which each healer was able to take home.

A number of important and indeed very unusual findings emerged in the baseline KABP survey. Several are of sufficient public health importance for AIDS/STDs prevention that further empirical field research is highly recommended. Examples are healers' promotion of male circumcision to avoid STDs if not AIDS; the provision by a national healers' association of training and start-up materials for income generation by HIV-positive clients; and the efficacy of treatment of genital sores and urethral infections with mixtures of sulfa powder and herbal medicines.

## Notes

1. It is interesting to note the parallel and apparantly independent observations made by South African healers and epidemiologists like Plummer, Moses and Ndinya-Achola (1991).

2. It was suspected by many epidemiologists and others that traditional skin piercing practices including scarification and circumcision spread HIV infection. However no evidence has been found to date to support this thesis. Exposure of razor blades and other piercing or cutting instruments to sunlight and dessication may reduce the viability of the virus (Berkeley 1991:89–91).

3. An account of homosexuality among South African urban hostel dwellers—who typically live apart from wives and girlfriends—can be found in Mark Mathabane's compelling autobiography *Kaffir Boy*, pp. 68–74.

# 8

# Evaluation of the "Second Generation" of South African Traditional Healers Trained in HIV/AIDS Prevention[1]

## Progress Since Late 1992

Between July 11 and 16, 1993 a second workshop for the original group, or first generation, of "trained" traditional healers was held in Emaweni (Northern Transvaal) for the purposes of: (1) evaluating the impact of the earlier training; (2) assessing the experience of healers who trained other healers; (3) discussing problems that arose since the first training; and (4) making plans for the future AIDS/STDs prevention activities involving traditional healers in South Africa. As at Tsitsikama, a knowledge, attitudes, and practices (KAP) type of survey was conducted to assess the impact of the earlier training of participating healers. Only nineteen of the original twenty-eight participants of the first workshop were present at the second, for reasons discussed in the second workshop report (Green, Zokwe, and Dupree 1993).

In addition to the workshop, we gathered evaluation data during July–August 1993 to assess the impact of the training of the first generation of healers on the second generation during site visits to seven representative areas throughout South Africa where training occurred. Methods and findings are presented here.

## Evaluation Research

### *Methods*

We first selected seven representative and geographically dispersed sites where training took place. We then contacted the first-generation healer-trainers from those sites and asked them to invite a sample of ten of the healers they had trained to one or more central locations where we could: (1) conduct individual, formal one-on-one interviews in private, and (2) hold an informal group discussion about various issues related to healers and training. In addition, we conducted home visits to second-generation healers when time allowed, during which we (3) had informal discussions and made direct observations. An open-ended interview schedule was used for the formal interviews; this means that response categories were constructed after reviewing all answers to a question, and were based on those answers.

We recognized that the healer-trainer might introduce a bias into the sample by tending to choose those healers who would make the best impression on those representing the funding organization. On the other hand, the trainer may not have really known which of their trainees had learned and retained the most. Furthermore, there were the practical matters of where healers lived, whether they could be reached directly or indirectly by phone, and whether they were available on a particular day. Had we randomly selected a sample of healers ourselves we no doubt would have faced problems of reaching all or perhaps even most of the sample in the short period of time available for interviewing. Moreover, it is probable that whatever our plans might be, the healer-trainer would in the end have assembled those healers reachable and available at a given time.

Thus, while it is possible that the sample interviewed might have been biased slightly toward those who would make a better impression, the costs and time and therefore money in eliminating this bias—assuming this were possible—would have been considerable.

We interviewed a sample of seventy healers, or 12 percent of the 630 so far trained. (An eight-year-old spirit medium was also interviewed at her insistence. She attended the workshop with her parents—both healers—however, due to her age, her responses are not included with the others).[2] The plan to interview ten from each area was modified somewhat in the field. Since ninety-three were trained in the northeast Transvaal, we interviewed fourteen there. We interviewed thirteen in Qwaqwa to better ensure a rural/urban balance overall. Only seven were interviewed in the Capetown area because circumstances such as bad weather and violence in local townships prevented us from reaching more trained healers within the allotted time. Thirty-three healers were from predominantly urban areas and thirty-seven from predominantly rural areas (self-governing "homelands"), although some of the latter may live in towns within the homelands.

### Respondent Characteristics

As noted in the previous chapter, the first generation of healers was selected by the leaders of five national associations of traditional healers; however, AIDSCAP itself selected the associations based on their pre-

TABLE 8.1 Sample of Healers Interviewed

| *Location* | *Number Interviewed* |
|---|---|
| Alexandra (Johannesburg) | 10 |
| Northern Transvaal (Gazankulu) | 14 |
| Eastern Transvaal (KaNkwane) | 10 |
| Soweto/Orlando townships | 6 |
| Qwaqwa | 13 |
| Capetown environs | 7 |
| Durban environs | 10 |
| Total | 70 |

sumed national membership and their reputation. Association leaders were also given selection criteria to follow, to help ensure fairness in such things as gender composition and rural/urban residence. It is interesting to note the respondent characteristics of the second generation of healers as there were no restrictions or suggested selection criteria from AIDSCAP. We see that women in their late forties predominate, and that virtually all are diviner-mediums (*sangomas* in Nguni languages). *Sangomas,* in fact, rank highest among traditional healers in Southern Africa (Christian and Muslim healers should be considered religious/faith- or "alternative" rather than traditional healers).

Six years of formal education was found to be the modal average. Of the fourteen who reported less than three years, eight healers had no formal education whatever. Three healers reported some professional training: one in nursing, one in accounting, one in naturopathy and herbalism.

There was considerable ethnolinguistic diversity among healers trained. The sample of seventy healers included twenty Zulus, seventeen Tsongas, thirteen Sothos, eleven Swazis, eight Xhosas, and one Pedi. Note that Tswanas were trained in Rustenburg, including some from self-governing Boputhatswana; however, there was insufficient time available to visit all training sites. If Tsongas seem overrepresented it is because ninety-three healers were trained (instead of the suggested thirty) by a dynamic healer (in fact a Pedi) in a predominantly Tsonga area of the northeast Transvaal, therefore her area was oversampled. Xhosas predominated among the first generation of healers. In any case, there was no complaint from any quarter that one group was favored in selection. South African traditional healers appear not to be ethnocentric in the sense of "tribal"; instead they tend to be active promoters of cultural pluralism, as discussed below in the context of *impandes.*

Regarding the number of patients seen in an average week, there was a range of 1 to 70 patients with the mean, median, and mode clustering around 14 per week. This is comparable to the number of weekly patients claimed by the first generation of healers in 1992 (mean of 20.8, mode of 10).

Almost all healers cited the AIDSCAP-supported workshop they had attended as their primary source of knowledge about AIDS. Although we lack formal baseline data on knowledge levels, informal interviews with healers provide evidence that their preworkshop knowledge about AIDS was minimal to nonexistent. Some said they had picked up many misconceptions about AIDS, having heard rumors about toothbrush sharing and transmission by other casual contact. They appeared to know nothing about the possible role of razor blades or needles, and almost certainly nothing about a relationship between standard STDs and AIDS. Most had heard only that AIDS is something that kills people. Condoms were described as something associated with commercial sex and not something one spoke about openly. A few cited newspapers, radio, and television as secondary sources of information about AIDS but several characterized the information derived from these sources as fragmented and incomplete.

We also asked healers if they ever use any modern medicines with their patients—medicines of the sort sold in pharmacies and used by scientifically trained doctors or nurses. We knew from the 1992 workshop that such a question is better explored in focus group discussion or in open-ended, in-depth interviews. In fact, we learned from such approaches that South African healers frequently use common analgesics, eye drops, "stomach medicine," and vitamins for their own use, as well as "Flowers of Sulphur" or sulfa powder (see Chapter 7). Only twelve healers in the present survey reported using modern medicines. Several healers mentioned Flowers of Sulphur, usually but not always when the product was prompted. One healer said, "Oh, that's a modern medicine?" She said she uses sulfa for treating STDs, both topically and as a tea.

Note that it is not uncommon to find former nurses among *sangomas*. Some of these may use standard antibiotics. One in the present survey commented that she obtains antibiotics from her former colleagues at a nearby clinic. Other medicines mentioned include camphor (used in a variety of home treatments), Behoedmiddel (for flatuance), Haarlemnsis (for abdominal pains), and Entress (for bad spirits).

### *AIDS and Sexually Transmitted Diseases*

All seventy healers had heard of HIV; fifty-one healers gave a fully correct definition of HIV; seven gave an ambiguous answer; and twelve gave a minimal or inadequate answer. Examples of a fully correct answer include: a virus or *(l)iciwane* (an Nguni term meaning germ or virus, and the term used in training) that caused AIDS, or one that "kills your body's soldiers (*amasoja*, the Nguni term referring to the immune system) until you have none and you can easily die of any sickness"; or a virus that "makes a patient vulnerable to all diseases"; or "a virus passed through intercourse or blood contact such as sharing needles or razors." An inadequate answer was simply that "it kills"; "it causes AIDS"; or "HIV is AIDS."

Regarding the symptoms of AIDS, sixty (86 percent) gave fully correct answers; six gave ambiguous answers; and four gave inadequate or incorrect answers. To score fully correct on the answer a healer had to mention three or more correct symptoms and none that were incorrect. For example, a healer in Qwa Qwa said the symptoms are "loss of weight, energy and appetite, diarrhea, dry skin, septic sores, swollen glands, STDs, thrush, boils, constant thirst, loneliness, self-pity, and the need to have the skin massaged." An inadequate or incorrect answer was one that had no or only one correct symptom and/or one or more incorrect symptoms such as "having a great appetite."

Sixty-five healers (93 percent) gave fully correct answers about the modes of HIV transmission; four gave correct but flawed answers; and only one gave an inadequate or incorrect answer. A fully correct answer was one that mentioned sexual transmission (because this was emphasized in all the workshops) and at least one other correct mode. Blood-to-blood contact (such as through needles) and mother-child transmission were usually mentioned in addition to sexual intercourse. One healer commented after listing correct modes, "since HIV is a devil you cannot know all the transmission modes. It's very tricky."

All seventy healers affirmed that AIDS can be prevented. As for means of prevention, fifty (83 percent) gave fully correct answers (three or more correct means of prevention); nine gave correct answers (one to two correct means of prevention); and only one gave a flawed answer (i.e., one or more correct means mixed with an incorrect one such as sharing dishes or toothbrushes). Fully correct answers usually mentioned condom use, sticking to one sexual partner, sterilization of razor blades, abstinence, thigh sex, and wearing of gloves on the part of health practitioners. One or two even mentioned the screening of blood supplies. Use of traditional herbs was not counted as a correct method of prevention for our purposes. Some healers mentioned the need for education in the wider community, or for community mobilization. One healer mentioned the spermicide Nonoxynol-9 by name.

We next asked about ways to prevent gonorrhea or "drop." This was not a leading question; we had reason to believe all healers thought that this illness is preventable. Fifty-seven (81 percent) gave fully correct answers, meaning two or more correct preventive means (not three because gonorrhea was given less emphasis than HIV/AIDS in the workshops);

ten gave correct answers (one correct preventive means); and two gave inadequate or incorrect answers. Use of herbs for prevention of gonorrhea—very widespread in South Africa—was counted neither as correct nor incorrect. Condom use was usually mentioned, as was sticking to one partner.

### *Circumcision Revisited*

We asked, "Do you believe that if a man is circumcised, it can help him avoid STDs?" This was of course a follow up to our earlier findings. Fully sixty-five (93 percent) said yes to the question. This is perhaps not a surprising answer among healers from circumcising societies, but it is for the thirty-one Swazi and Zulu respondents. No doubt, answers were influenced by the fact that most or all the workshop facilitators discussed circumcision in the context of the need to sterilize razors blades for traditional circumcision operations. Facilitators were also found to have made observations to the effect that the foreskin can carry STD germs that can facilitate HIV transmission.

But the question remains, do Swazi and Zulu healers really believe their answers to this question, or are they just trying to give what they believe from their training to be a correct answer? We posed this to the Swazi healer who helped train healers in the Swazi self-governing area KaNkwane. She said she thought Swazi healers *do* believe in the causal connection because many healers may have noticed differences in STD treatment outcomes between uncircumcised Swazis, circumcised Tsongas and others in kaNkwane, but they had never had an opportunity to discuss this openly until the issue was raised as a topic in her AIDS workshop. She felt that what she taught Swazi healers helped them confirm their own experience with their patients; and when one healer related his experience, this prompted others to reveal similar experience.

For those fifty-eight healers affirming a circumcision/STD connection,

TABLE 8.2 Why Does Circumcision of Men Help Prevent STD Infection? (multiple responses possible)

| *Cause* | *No. of Citations* |
|---|---|
| Foreskin stores dirt, STD germs | 52 |
| STDs more difficult to treat among uncircumcised men | 6 |
| Foreskin causes STDs | 5 |
| Foreskin rots | 3 |
| Uncircumcised men prone to STDs | 3 |
| Foreskin hard to clean, usually not washed | 1 |
| Total | 70 |

we asked what the connection is. The responses are seen in Table 8.2.

Healers from a circumcising tradition tend to have more to say on the subject and to give culturally sanctioned reasons, such as the Sotho who commented, "The foreskin is something that was meant to be removed like a child's first teeth, otherwise it causes sickness." Another Sotho said, "The wife of an uncircumcised man will die of pelvic inflammatory disease before the age of forty-five." Swazi and Zulu healers tended to state simply that the foreskin stores or retains germs and/or that STD treatment outcomes are poorer among uncircumcised men.

***Experience in Treating AIDS***

In answer to the question, "Have you treated any cases of AIDS or HIV?" eighteen healers (26 percent) said yes; forty-eight said no and four were not sure. The relatively low number answering yes was unsurprising as AIDS was still not widespread in South Africa. HIV seroprevelance rates appear to be highest in Natal, KwaZulu, and in the large cities. They also appear high in the Swazi self-governing area of KaNkwane.

Of the eighteen who claim to have treated one or more HIV/AIDS cases, sixteen said they knew what they were dealing with because their patients were tested for HIV/AIDS in a hospital. Seven specified that they have only treated these cases since their training in the AIDSCAP workshop; eleven said they encountered cases both before and after the workshop; and one said she had one case only before the workshop. Some additional comments were:

> "I treated a commercial sex worker and her partners. I had treated AIDS patients before the workshop but I didn't understand the symptoms or why they didn't respond to treatment. I've had more HIV patients since the workshop."
>
> "I might have previously (treated some) but I would not have known, really."
>
> "No, only STD patients, but they might have been HIV positive. I have sent some patients for HIV testing but I don't know if they went."
>
> "The patient was referred by the hospital."

We also asked those who have treated AIDS/HIV to describe generally what their treatment consisted of. All said they gave their patient herbs, usually to drink. Seven specified that they treated external sores with herbs, one mentioned herbal enema, and three said they gave their patients counseling, preventive advice, and/or love. Only one said she referred a patient to a hospital. One mentioned treating the patient's partner as well. Other comments included: "I gave three types of herbs: for energy, for cleansing the blood, and for fighting septic sores" and "I reconnected the patients with their ancestors."

TABLE 8.3 Type of Advice or Counselling Given to HIV/AIDS Patients

| | No. of Citations |
|---|---|
| Promoted positive attitude, acceptance of condition | 13 |
| Showed caring, love, under-standing, acceptance | 7 |
| Advised condom use | 8 |
| Reinforced family and social ties, involvement | 6 |
| Promoted abstinence, fidelity, partner reduction | 4 |
| Advice on maintaining health, diet, nutrition | 3 |
| Advice on partner testing, treatment | 2 |
| Religious/spiritual counselling | 3 |
| Biomedical referral | 2 |
| Total | 48 |

In case advice and counseling were not mentioned previously, we asked of the eighteen who had treated AIDS, "Please describe generally what *advice* and *counseling* you have given a person with AIDS or HIV. More than eighteen answered this, some thinking that the question meant what advice one would or might give.

We next asked whether AIDS can be cured, either by traditional or by "modern" treatment. Judging by healers' comments, the question was often interpreted to ask whether AIDS is curable in the future rather than curable right now. Others took the question to refer to treating or curing the opportunistic infections of AIDS, rather than AIDS itself. Still others took the question to refer to prevention rather than cure. In any case, thirty-two said yes; thirty said no; and eight said they didn't know.

A number of healers mentioned preventive measures such as condom usage and marital fidelity. More than two healers said that AIDS is not curable, "unless we combine knowledge with traditional healers all over the world." Other comments include:

"Not right now. Healers need to consult their ancestors."

"No, not now, when healers don't want to share herbal information."

"Healers will be able to cure it in the future."

"The doctors can confirm the HIV tests and the healers give (herbal) treatment."

"Only the symptoms can be treated."

"By God's help only."

For those answering yes, we asked how AIDS can be cured. Thirty-seven mentioned herbal treatment, or consulting or beseeching the ancestor spirits; eleven said this will be possible in the future through traditional-biomedical cooperation; and seven said both traditional and biomedical healers can now treat symptoms or opportunistic infections. At least one mentioned condoms. Again we see that many healers took the question to refer to hoped-for cures in the future, while some took it to mean prevention in the present.

### *Sexual Behavior*

We asked healers to estimate the average age at which boys and girls usually begin to experiment with sex. The mean, median, and mode clustered around age 13.5 for boys and around 11 for girls. There were no significant differences in answers by ethnolinguistic group or by rural/urban residence. These estimates are close to those given in the November 1992 workshop survey (means of 14.2 for boys and 12 for girls). During that workshop, healers made comments to the effect that in former times, elders took boys to the bush to educate them about proper sexual behavior. This included instruction in "thigh sex" or other intercourse where there is no penetration, intended for youth and the unmarried. In the present survey we asked healers if any people in their area practice thigh sex or other nonpenetrative intercourse. Only thirteen (19 percent) said yes, usually with the qualification that the practice has become increasingly rare; forty-two said no, and fifteen did not know. In some urban areas such as Capetown, healers commented that the practice is "unknown" among younger people. A number of healers in the predominantly rural Tsonga "homeland" commented that people were no longer interested in thigh sex (*mantanga*), one noting, "even the youngest want penetrative sexual intercourse."

Thigh sex was reported to be common only in the Swazi self-governing area of KaNkwane, where healers sometimes encourage the practice when a wife is menstruating. Note the potential that might be exploited for promoting safer sex, at least with this group. Additional comments include:

> "No, not those who grew up in Soweto, but maybe those who grew up in the Homelands."
>
> "People around here are no longer interested in the practice"
>
> "Women and men practice it only if they are being treated (for STDs)."
>
> "No, (people here) think it's like playing next to a dish of food when you're hungry."
>
> "Very few, but per the traditional healer's recommendation."

We also asked what types of sexual behavior are forbidden, or considered bad or dangerous in the healer's area and tradition. With multiple responses possible, the results are shown in Table 8.4.

Taboos surrounding intercourse with widows and women who have

TABLE 8.4 Types of Sexual Behavior Traditionally Considered Forbidden or Dangerous (multiple responses)

| | *No. of Citations* |
|---|---|
| Intercourse with a widow (prior to cleansing) | 57 |
| Homosexuality | 34 |
| Intercourse during menstruation | 27 |
| Intercourse with woman who has aborted/miscarried | 19 |
| Commercial sex | 16 |
| Miscelleneous | 10 |
| Total | 163 |

aborted or miscarried were mentioned most often, reflecting the widespread belief in Africa that death is a mystically polluting force that can adversely effect health. The importance of pollution-through-death-contact beliefs has already been mentioned in earlier chapters. Infrequent citations include anal intercourse, intercourse immediately after birth or during pregnancy, oral sex, and premarital penetrative sex. As noted, a question such as this is better explored in focus group discussion or in open-ended, in-depth interviews. Adultery was not mentioned, even though this is generally held to be taboo, dangerous-to-health, or at least disapproved of in Africa. Perhaps it was regarded as too obvious to mention.

We next asked if any men in the healer's area engage in homosexual behavior. Sixteen answered yes with certain qualifications; nine answered no, and forty-five did not know. This is another question that, based on experience in the 1992 workshop, yields more useful information when explored in group discussion or in-depth interviews. The consensus in group discussion then was that homosexuality, while it occurs among certain men—usually those deprived of female contact—is quite rare among black South Africans. Similar comments were found in the present survey. In addition, elite economic status and/or Western/white influence and was said to account for some homosexual experimentation among blacks, a belief we encountered in Liberia. Comments about "tsotsis" (urban criminals or tough show-offs) who experiment with homosexuality emerged for the first time:

"It's not very common, (only among) tsotsis, or young, smart men."

"It's very common among township criminals. . . . We know about this when they come to us for luck medicine."

"It's common because they get that information from video cassettes, books and television."

### *Training Impact*

We asked how healers felt generally about the usefulness of the AIDSCOM/AIDSCAP-supported workshop they had attended. All rated their workshop "very useful" (the highest category).[3] Healers were asked to describe the two most useful things they learned at their AIDS workshop. Results are seen in Table 8.5. Multiple responses were possible.

Miscellaneous answers included role-playing, the anatomy and physiology of genitalia, learning more about STDs, and tuberculosis. The popularity of the condom demonstration may be due to it having been an actual participatory demonstration—not just something spoken about—and because healers were given a new skill along with a dildo which they could use in educating their clients. As we see below, all healers reported having given condom demonstrations to not only clients but to essentially anyone in their communities with any potential interest. There is indirect evidence that this new skill along with the accompanying AIDS/STD knowledge has increased healers' status and improved or expanded their practices. Additional comments include:

> "I can now teach about AIDS. I can be open about the disease. It's no longer a secret."
>
> "I don't believe what I learned from television. (When I learned about AIDS) from my *gobela,* it's from the horse's mouth. In the workshop you can take time and have questions answered."
>
> "We can . . . touch, love HIV/AIDS patients. I have overcome fear and avoidance. I have now been given the power to love and help these patients."

We also asked if there were any things related to AIDS or STDs that should have been discussed in the workshop, but were not. Only eight (11 percent) answered yes. Several healers commented that they could

TABLE 8.5 Most Useful Things Learned at Workshop

| | *No. of Citations* |
|---|---|
| Condom demonstration | 62 |
| AIDS symptoms, prevention, transmission | 36 |
| Sexual behavior | 33 |
| Counselling, care, and support of patient | 17 |
| Sterilization of razors, protection of healer | 6 |
| Traditional AIDS treatment | 3 |
| Hygiene and cleanliness | 3 |
| Miscellaneous | 8 |
| Total | 168 |

always consult their local workshop facilitator (first-generation healer) if questions arose. Suggestions from those who saw room for improvement included:

> "General health education about diet and exercise and healthy lifestyle. Otherwise we healers will only give *timbita* (herb decoctions). We have some food taboos that hurt nutrition."
>
> "The relationship between mental illness and AIDS, septic sores, more information on STDs, and (pediatric AIDS)."
>
> "Community mobilization and the role of civics organizations."
>
> "The relationship between HIV and TB, HIV and epilepsy."
>
> "Information about traditional healers outside of South Africa—their treatments for AIDS."
>
> "The role of social workers. Since the workshop, social workers refer patients to me."

Informal interviews suggest that AIDSCAP training has boosted the healer's reputation in the community and may have improved the healer's practice as measured by an increase in clients. However, some healers reported no change in client load due to prevailing poverty, high unemployment and a corresponding inability of clients to pay. Nevertheless, these healers—like others—proudly showed us the certificate of training issued at their workshop; virtually all had paid to have them framed.

Several reported that relations with local clinics and nurses had improved. While this is not always an unalloyed blessing (see section on KaNkwane below), it is usually a positive development for at least the patient. One trained healer in Alexandra township sent a patient of hers whose STD symptoms kept recurring to the local clinic for HIV testing. The clinic nurse was surprised to see a patient who had been referred and properly advised about HIV testing by a traditional healer. The clinic now refers patients to that healer.

### *Condoms and Condom Demonstrations*

We next asked if healers had tried to influence the sexual behavior of their patients by counseling them or giving them sex education, since the AIDS workshop. All said yes except for two healers who took the question to mean that they must have already had AIDS patients. The advice given was to avoid risky sex, remain faithful to one partner, use condoms, get tested for HIV, learn the dangers of STDs, and have existing STDs treated.

In response to another question, all healers reported that they had advised *friends, family or people in their community* (other than patients) about AIDS or STDs. Community people designated include young people, people at community meetings, healers' trainees (*amatwasa*), people at ANC meetings, civic society members, sports team members, healers who couldn't attend a workshop, healers at traditional gatherings such as graduations, traditional circumcisers or surgeons, friends on commuter trains, and people in nearby squatter camps. This, of course, is a most welcome finding. Regarding the advice given, healers mostly specified condom education, the means of prevention and the modes of transmitting AIDS, responsible sexual behavior, and "AIDS 101" as the basics were called in the first workshop.

The eight-year-old diviner complained, "I have a problem in that whoever I tell about AIDS or sex or STDs, they report it to my father and sometimes I'm seen as a little girl who knows too much about sex or is already involved with boys."

We next asked how healers felt about seeing a condom demonstration with a dildo, and we probed for whether such demonstrations were culturally acceptable or offensive. We asked this partly because at the Berlin international AIDS conference, a healer from the November 1992 workshop was asked publicly whether South African healers had been pressured into accepting dildos to use in condom demonstrations, since these might appear to offend African tradition. In the present survey *all* healers said they liked the demonstration and that the use of the dildo made it realistic. Most used adjectives such as useful or very useful. Furthermore, all healers had already given condom demonstrations to other healers, to patients and to others in their communities, using dildos in all cases with the exception of the few healers who had not yet received dildos.

The whole subject of condoms and dildos was discussed at the July 1993 workshop for "first generation" healers. Healers were emphatic in saying they wanted the lifelike "erect dildos with veins, preferably brown." The issue was in fact put to a formal vote. No one preferred to work in AIDS education without use of a dildo, or with a wooden dildo. It was thought to be dangerous to demonstrate condoms using bananas, fingers, or bottles.

There is a traditional mechanism for introducing new objects—that is, objects unfamiliar to the ancestor spirits—in a special corner of the healer's ritual house (*indumba*. This may become a ritual room in an urban area). The item is ritually presented to the ancestors and its use is explained. First- and second-generation informants reported that the dildo has been introduced in this way by healers that have them; dildos have thus been incorporated and added to the standard instruments of the healer.

One female healer reported at the workshop that the dildo has proven useful in diagnosis and discussion with male patients. She is able to indicate on the model exactly where there are sores or other symptoms, rather than try to describe them in vague, embarrassed terms. She implied that a patient showing his penis to a female healer would violate rules of decorum. She also said that women can empower themselves by telling their husbands that the dildo can be a substitute for their attentions: "It is AIDS-free and won't infect the wife with the diseases the husband carries back from his girlfriends." Spontaneous comments from the survey include:

> "I showed (the dildo) to my *amatwasa* (trainees) and to my son. They can now do (condom demonstrations) themselves."
>
> "The women especially were very shy but they became used to it in the end."[4] They realized their responsibility as healers is to teach patients (about AIDS).
>
> "The dildo makes it easy to show a patient how to use a condom."
>
> "It was useful although I'm not yet allowed to use it since I am *litwasa* (a trainee)."

Informal discussions also showed that both dildos and books we distributed that provide photographs of symptoms (*AIDS Atlas* or *Skin Manifestations of AIDS*) were highly valued by healers, partially perhaps as symbols of prestige and of cooperation with medical doctors.

We asked if healers have ever advised a patient to use a condom. All but one said yes. Circumstances cited refer to the prevention of HIV/AIDS as well as STDs and sometimes unwanted pregnancies. One healer volunteered the comment that a patient must use a condom if he wishes to have intercourse while taking herbal treatment for STDs.

We also asked if healers have ever shown a patient *how* to use a condom; fifty-six (93 percent) said they had. Virtually all said they used a dildo in demonstrating the condom, even in front of friends and in public gatherings. Among the four who had not, we were told, "No, I haven't seen an STD patient since the workshop" and "No one has consulted me yet." The other two appear to have been *amatwasa* (healers still undergoing initiation) who are prevented by custom from giving treatment until they have fully qualified as healers.

One healer interviewed detailed the advice he said he gives before he "issues a condom to a patient." He gave an extremely detailed description of correct advice regarding condoms to the point of proper hygienic disposal after use. Many healers specified that they demonstrated condoms for STD prevention. One noted, "I demonstrated this for my family; both my kids have had STDs."

Finally on this topic we asked, "Have you encountered any problems promoting or demonstrating condoms?" Only eighteen (26 percent) said yes and an additional two said "slightly" or "a little." Problems proved to be with the availability of condoms, not with audience reaction (only one Natal healer mentioned patient aversion to condoms). Several healers volunteered that they "like" or "enjoy" demonstrating condoms. Other volunteered comments are illuminating:

> "Some laugh at first. Some women were a bit shocked, but it was okay. . . . It's serious; we can't hide from this AIDS."
>
> "It's important to do this in private away from members of the opposite sex."
>
> "No (problem), my husband gave me permission."
>
> "Condoms are not available" (a considerable number of healers said this).
>
> "I warned them first, to prepare them."

### *Problems Dealing with National Organizations*

As a last survey item we asked what organizations of traditional healers (national, regional, or local) the healer has belonged to, beginning with any present organization and going backward in time. What stands out in the answers is the number of healers who have switched association membership recently or who have dropped out of associations altogether. In an informal discussion a group of urban healers estimated that only about 20 percent of all healers in the Johannesburg area are currently affiliated with formal healer organizations. They believe a greater number may have belonged to an organization at one time and then dropped out.

National and regional organizations appear to be unstable due to power struggles, politics, and rank-and-file healers resenting leaders who "start acting superior to us." One widely respected healer commented, "As soon as a leader starts talking about 'my people' he or she is going to cause a lot of resentment and that leader is on the way out." Another commented, "Formal associations breed jealousy among healers. No one is treated with respect in them." In the course of group and individual discussions during site visits, we compiled the following complaints made by healers trained in AIDS against healer associations that claim national membership. Many of the complaints have to do with the nature and behavior of association presidents. Keep in mind that most healers interviewed—and trained in AIDS—were women.

- association membership is not truly national. Membership lists may include false addresses for some members to make it appear that membership is national;

- presidents collect money to pay for legal services, funerals, and financial support upon the death of a spouse as well as other things of interest to healers, yet such funds are often not available for members when they are in need—in fact the funds often disappear;
- there are no traditional or agreed-upon mechanisms for conflict resolution within associations;
- association presidents tend to be men, and they "boss" members around, women in particular. They do not treat members with the respect they deserve;
- presidents of major associations may be non-South African in origin: they are "mainly interested in collecting money from healers in South Africa";
- presidents break the very moral behavioral codes they pretend their association upholds. Some have forced themselves sexually upon their female *amatwasa* (initiates-in-training). Some have seduced patients;
- some presidents have dubious credentials as *sangomas* (diviner-mediums), at least according to locally recognized criteria such as membership in a known *impande* (see below). If presidents did not undergo the formal process of *sangoma* initiation,[5] ". . . their behavior is not acceptable to the traditions and cultural beliefs of *sangomas*";
- many healers may be reluctant to join formal healer associations because they cannot read and write, or because they cannot speak English or African languages other than their own. Such healers may also be gullible and vulnerable and easy prey for a smooth-talking, would-be president.
- some presidents have tried to make paid membership in their associations a prerequisite for attending AIDSCAP-supported workshops, or specifically for receiving a training certificate. Others have tried to enlist first-generation healers to recruit local second-generation healers for their own association, collecting fees on their behalf. Loud complaints were voiced over this at a group meeting of second generation healers.

A columnist in *The Star* (Johannesburg) (August 5, 1993) could have been speaking about national healer associations when he wrote, "Presidentialism has been the curse of Africa precisely because it concentrates so much power in one person. . . ." South African healers are strongly egalitarian; they are deeply suspicious of any peer who claims superior status and tries to exercise authority over the rank-and-file. Although there is a traditional hierarchy of statuses, status differences are either between types of healers or they relate to seniority, meaning that today's trainee will become tomorrow's senior *gobela.* It is also true that formal associations are a historically recent attempt on the part of healers to exercise power in the larger state polity (Last 1986; MacCormack 1986). As such they are still in an inchoate and unstable developmental stage; they have not yet developed structures that ensure stability and continuity. Most seem bedeviled by problems of financial management.

Because of the foregoing, we decided to explore the possibility of AIDSCAP *not* formally dealing with national associations but instead with indigenous, existing associations of healers that seem to have existed in South Africa for many generations, namely *impandes.* This term is used or at least understood by virtually all black groups in South Africa; the Xhosa may use the term *ingcambu.* Ngubane (1981) describes them as *sangoma* networks without using a Bantu name.

According to my limited period of research in South Africa, an *impande* is a named network or association of *sangomas* that trace what might be called spiritual kinship ties through association with a *gobela* (initiator or trainer of diviner-mediums), a *gobela*'s initiator (*koko*) or a *gobela*'s initiator's initiator (*kokogasi* for females or *kokokhulu* for males). The term *impande* refers not only to people but to the medicines and distinctive rituals and ceremonies used by all who "descend" from the same *gobela.* Initiates (a term preferable to members) in the same *impande* refer to one another as sister or brother if they have been *sangomas* for roughly the same period of time. Those who are two or more "generations" of initiates above a *sangoma* are both addressed and referred to as *gogo* (grandmother) or *koko* (great-grandparent).

Like lineages, *impandes* may be subdivided or segmented into smaller groupings consisting of more restricted membership, depending on need or purpose. As *impandes* become too dispersed and too large, new *impande* groupings or segments develop, yet a sense of belonging together remains between members of the larger, older *impande.*

Members of an *impande* are known by special insignia, such as beads of a certain color or other decorative items that are worn. Names used to designate *impandes* may refer to a recent *gobela,* although a full name might actually consist of a succession of names of senior *gobelas*—one's lineage of initiators—as well as the places where initiation took place. An *impande* name may also refer to a class of spirits, such as *emandau* or *emanzawe* (believed to be the spirits of people from tribes other than one's own who were slain during the period of tribal warfare). The insignia of diviner-mediums possessed by *emandau* consist of a necklace of white and red beads from which is suspended a beaded object.

No one knows the exact size of an *impande* since written records are not kept and since new *impandes* or *impande* segments develop at a perhaps indefinable point of growth. Certainly they grow exponentially: a *gobela* may train or initiate as many as 100 to 200 healers in her lifetime. Her *amatwasa* may in turn train 100 to 200 others in their lifetimes, as may their *amatwasa*. Even if some *amatwasa*, upon becoming *gobela*s themselves, initiate far fewer numbers, an *impande* of several thousand members may easily develop within a generation.

The question arises: how feasible would it be for AIDSCAP or other donors to work with *impande*s rather than national healer associations in AIDS prevention? We note immediately that the former are indigenous, existing structures; foreign donors would not seem to be forcing healers to join formal associations in order to benefit from AIDS-related training—just because donors might be more comfortable dealing with formal, "national" associations. It would seem preferable to build upon a time-honored structure that already exists. We discovered several additional characteristics of *impande*s that would seem to recommend them further over national—and perhaps any formal—associations.

One is their multiethnic membership. It can be observed that *sangoma*s often apprentice under a *gobela* from a different ethnic group. *Sangoma*s are emphatic in insisting that it is one's ancestors and not oneself who chooses the *gobela*, but it can be observed that ancestors often guide would-be initiates to a *gobela* from a different ethnic group. We might refer to the mechanism that ensures *impande* multiethnicity as ethnic discordance in the initiation process, and it would doubtless be interesting to speculate as to why it developed in southern Africa. One result of the practice is that *sangoma*s have some intimate familiarity with another culture. This might be a factor of how a healer practicing in a plural society can attract clients from diverse ethnic groups, although a *sangoma* would never explain this feature of the initiation process in such terms. Nevertheless we saw that urban-based healers attract clients from diverse groups.

At a deeper, functionalist, analytic level, ethnic discordance in the initiation process might be seen as a functional mechanism that has developed to mitigate and reconcile ethnic divisiveness and strife in the broader society as it moves toward greater sociocultural integration. In any case the structure and function of *impande*s seem to make it unnecessary for AIDSCAP or other donors to issue criteria designed to ensure equal access by "tribe" to donor resources; South African healers are already adept practitioners of cultural pluralism.

*Impande* membership is also geographically dispersed. As noted, healers may train and be initiated in a different area of South Africa—even a neighboring country—and then return to practice at home. Moreover, healers seem to be at least as geographically mobile as the rest of South Africa. In these ways, initiates of an *impande* quickly spread all over the country and beyond. A *sangoma* can travel anywhere in the region and expect to see another *sangoma* wearing the beads characteristic of her *impande*. When this happens, the two greet each other joyfully and there is said to be an immediate sense of kinship and intimacy.

Another characteristic of *impandes* is that members are bound to each other by spiritual ties; they are forbidden by custom to squabble with each other but if this occurs, mechanisms exist for conflict resolution. A dispute is brought to the common *gobela* (*gogo, koko*), who, with the ancestors, serves as a kind of court of appeals that provides a spiritually sanctioned resolution for any conflict. *Impandes* are described as apolitical or above political concerns. Again the explanation lies with the ancestors: they are said to care nothing about politics. In the words of one *sangoma*, "The ancestors don't know who the ANC or Inkatha Freedom Party are; they have never heard of them."

*Impande* initiates meet on a regular basis, such as during ceremonies when newly initiated *sangomas* demonstrate their spiritual qualifications. Initiates are also expected to share healing information with one another and with their *gobela*, and to refer clients to one another. There is said to be mutual respect.

As already noted, second-generation training in the northeast Transvaal (Gazankulu) appears to have been especially successful. Here healers were recruited and trained through the N. E. Transvaal Tinyanga and Herbalists Association (NETTHA), a local as distinct from national association. We found that about 95 percent of NETTHA's membership belonged to the same *impande*. Most members formerly belonged to a larger formal association based in the Tsonga self-governing area of Gazankulu, but they became disillusioned with it for most of the reasons already cited as problems with national organizations. At the time of the evaluation NETTHA was trying to build upward, joining with local organizations in Venda, Lebowa, and elsewhere to form a truly regional, multiethnic organization for the northern Transvaal. The passage of time might show if it is better to build from regional associations-up than from Johannesburg-down.

It may prove useful to work with or through regional as distinct from national healer associations, if that is what healers in areas such as the northern Transvaal wish to do. However, paid membership in any association should not be a precondition for benefiting from AIDSCAP-supported training.

## Some General Problem Areas

### *Availability of Condoms*

In November 1992 the AIDS Programme of the Department of National Health and Population Development promised USAID and AIDSCOM/AIDSCAP that it would provide condoms for every traditional healer who became an AIDS educator and condom distributer through the AIDSCAP project. This has not happened. Lack of condom availability has become a major constraint to meeting the condom distribution objective of the traditional healer program. The government AIDS Programme was said to be having a great deal of trouble importing the quantity of condoms needed for its own program.

Our recommendation was that AIDSCAP-trained healers be linked up with a U.S. condom social-marketing program, as we suggested in Mozambique. Healers could buy condoms at a discounted, subsidized price and then pass the small price along to their clients.

***Problems in KaNkwane***

Healers in KaNkwane proved to not be as well trained in AIDS prevention as those in other areas surveyed. At first, this seemed to be an area of particular success because the KaNkwane Ministry of Health had provided a hospital venue for the AIDSCAP-supported healer workshop, and the first generation healer-trainer was made a member of the Themba Hospital Executive Committee on AIDS (she is the only nonbiomedically trained member). Moreover, shortly after our evaluation site visit, there was a two-day AIDS workshop for a very large group consisting of the KaNkwane Legislative Assembly, the senior staff of the assembly, and the chiefs and *indunas* (subchiefs) of the area. The AIDSCAP-trained healers were invited to help convey knowledge—or at least lend traditional sanction to the workshop.

Yet the evaluation survey found that KaNkwane healers were relatively weak in answering such knowledge questions as defining HIV and describing symptoms or means of transmission. In fact, a number of common misconceptions about HIV transmission were repeated, such as sharing toothbrushes. It appears that the well-intentioned participation of Themba hospital staff was at least part of the problem. Staff from the hospital apparently took advantage of healers being assembled for the purpose of learning biomedical concepts of AIDS, and expanded the curriculum to include tuberculosis and primary health care. A formal lecture was given by the hospital director about TB transmission and prevention; the message to healers was to beware sharing toothbrushes, kissing, sharing dishes, etc. This information apparently confused healers since they offered answers of this sort to describe modes of HIV transmission. Other junior hospital staff apparently took charge of teaching some of the fundamentals about AIDS, and some of their information was said to be inaccurate. Even with accurate information, the training agenda of the hospital took away time from learning about AIDS.

It was also reported that Themba staff lectured the healers rather than use culturally appropriate adult education principles. The first-generation healer of the area reported that AIDSCAP is considered "progressive" by healers because it provides adequate time to discuss things with healers, clarifies difficult points, encourages questions and answers, and organizes group discussions and various other forms of participation. Some hospital-run workshops for healers were said to have consisted of 200 or more participants. Healers told us that a speaker—especially one who is lecturing—cannot hold the attention of more than a few healers at a time. With so many participants there are numerous distractions such as people moving around and going in and out of the lecture area.

Still, Themba hospital should be commended for collaborating with traditional healers in KaNkwane for the past two or more years. It is hoped that any criticisms reported here will be used constructively.

### *Overdependence of Some HIV Patients*

One problem that has emerged with only a few healers but that might grow in the future is that of unrealistic demands and expectations on the part of some HIV/AIDS patients. In a few cases HIV or AIDS patients have attached themselves to AIDSCAP-trained healers and tried to manipulate them in such a way that healers have ended up boarding and feeding them. Part of the moral/ethical code of *sangomas* is that they are forbidden by their ancestor spirits to reject patients. In the words of one *sangoma*, "We always have to think about ancestors and community." Ancestors here refer to moral rules while community relates directly to the *sangoma*'s reputation, which also relates to business and livelihood. Some HIV-positive patients have seemingly tried to exploit the ancestor/community concerns of the *sangoma* by saying, as reported by one healer, "Look, you have this special training in AIDS, so you have to take care of me." Some patients even expect to be given pocket money for things like cigarettes.

As outlandish as this might seem to the outsider, we were told that if a *sangoma* turned away an AIDS patient who moaned and complained at her front door, and then died a few days later, it would seem to the whole community that the healer was not working with the ancestor spirits let alone fulfilling her responsibility as an AIDSCAP-trained healer. Some such healers were interested in discussing the limits of a healer's responsibility, considering that AIDSCAP training was in prevention rather than treatment (although care and counseling was part of the training). They also wished to discuss with AIDSCAP and other healers how certain people know how to "manipulate the system."

## Conclusions

One might expect that the training provided to the first generation of healers would become somewhat diluted in the second generation. Yet the second generation was found to be as well trained as the first.

Actually this should not be surprising. First, we know our method of selecting first-generation healers was not the best because we worked through national healer associations, which seemed to be our only entry point at the time. First-generation healers were probably better than AIDSCAP in selecting capable, motivated participants for second-generation training. Second, the organization of the workshop and much of the training was U.S.-designed, whereas second-generation training was in the hands of traditional healers themselves assisted in most cases by a (black) South African AIDSCAP facilitator with extraordinary skills and cultural sensitivity. Skilled in multicultural communication themselves, first- and second-generation healers remarked favorably about this facilitator's abilities to communicate effectively among diverse groups.

One change in curriculum made after the first workshop in 1992 was excluding a section on death and dying. This was the least favorite section according to the evaluation of the first workshop, although the cultural offensiveness of this topic did not emerge very well in the formal evaluation. In fact, *sangomas* believe that death is mystically polluting and therefore taboo for certain possessing spirits. The death of a client under a healer's care leads to legal culpability, especially if the client dies on the premises. Even a rumor of death is deleterious to a healer's reputation and practice. Naturally, this has implications for healers who may be caring for AIDS patients. Legal protection for the healer might be the only context in which death and dying would be a discussion topic acceptable to healers.

All *sangomas* consulted on the issue liked the idea of AIDSCAP working with *impandes*, most offering comments to the effect that the *impande* is a "natural" organization and that there is no conflict among fellow initiates. In view of the foregoing evidence and experience, it was recommended that AIDSCAP/South Africa discontinue recognizing or dealing with healers on the basis of their membership in formal, national organizations of healers. Instead, AIDSCAP should seek to identify and train motivated healers who are respected in their home communities. Experience including the present evaluation suggests that these healers need not be educated or even literate, but they should possess leadership skills and be able and willing to train other healers. AIDSCAP should encourage these healers to disseminate AIDS knowledge through their *impande*; if training extends beyond this (as it tends to), so much the better. Healers already know how best to share knowledge with their fellow *impande* initiates; indeed, there are already opportunities and mechanisms to do so.

By shifting focus from putative national organizations to *impandes*, donors such as AIDSCAP should be able to avoid many or most of the problems that constrained the program for its first seven months—resulting, for example, in falling short of the original training numbers.[6] Another consideration is that a number of black South Africans have criticized USAID-funded programs including AIDSCAP for working only through major NGOs, which are often white dominated. These critics suggest that USAID work instead with genuine community-based organizations (CBOs) with indigenous leadership. Although *impandes* cut across many communities they are nevertheless existing, indigenous grassroots organizations that have many features of CBOs at the local level.

We have found that *impandes* have cooperated fruitfully in some workshops and even in some formal associations, especially at the regional level. However, we need to discover more about the conditions for establishing a cooperative working relationship between two or more *impandes*.

It should be noted that the AIDSCAP traditional healer program is heavily focused on women. Working with and through *impandes* should further this since *impande* membership is primarily women, perhaps 80 to 85 percent. There are any number of reasons why emphasis on women is justified in South Africa, including their relative vulnerability to HIV infection, their subordinate status and inability to negotiate sexual relations, their role as childbearers and child-rearers, their role in family health care, and their disproportionate contribution to food production and hence to nutrition (Chin 1990; Karlander 1991; Krieger and Margo 1991; Schoepf 1991). There is also health program experience in Africa that suggests women may be more willing than men to change health-related behavior.

The question arises about the involvement of *non*-diviner-mediums, especially herbalists. Would they be excluded if donors work directly or indirectly with *impandes* rather than with formal organizations? Herbalists seem to lack organizational structure comparable to that of *sangomas*. Yet *sangomas* and a very few herbalists we were able to consult, reported that herbalists routinely work together with *sangomas* in order to include divination in the treatment of their clients. In this way they are associated with the cooperating *sangoma's impande*. Herbalists are often invited to initiate "graduations" and other *impande* gatherings. Some Christian "Zionist" (*amazioni, mazioni*) faith healers are also said to be associated with *impandes*, in fact, two Zionist healers were invited to and attended the AIDSCAP-supported workshop in the Capetown area. Still, the participation of herbalists could and perhaps should be monitored in the future, assuming AIDSCAP works with *impandes* in order to ensure their inclusion.

Other questions that must surely arise include: Can and do different *impandes* cooperate with one another? Can projects work with more than one *impande* in the same area? The answers seem to be yes to both. It has already happened. Of the thirty-four healers trained in Soweto and Orlando, six *impandes* were represented. These townships are ethnically heterogeneous but this alone does not ensure cooperation between *impandes*. We believe there are qualities inherent in *impandes* that contribute to such cooperation. We recall that healers themselves chose those who were trained and we note that the present evaluation shows that the training seems to have had the desired impact.

The position being recommended has already begun to be implemented in some areas by healers themselves. Second-generation healers in the Capetown area have organized themselves into an association of some 100 members from nine townships: Paarl, Stellenbosch, Ceres, Langa, Nyanga, Khayelitsha, KTC Squatters Settlement, and New Crossroads. The association consists of four cooperating *impandes*. There was a conscious decision *not* to form a Western-type formal association with a president presiding—some of the local leaders had already had negative experiences with a Johannesburg-based national association. Instead, Capetown healers decided to follow the *impande* structure in their new association. In descending order of status, this consists of "elders" or established *sangomas*, recently trained initiates, *amatwasa* (initiates-in-training), and herbalists. There is an executive committee consisting of two representatives from each category.

Because the AIDSCAP training was done with input from the national women's association Phambile, the name taken by the healers for their new organization is *Nompumelelo Phambile*, ("Progressing Under Phambile"). There are no fees to belong to the organization, and all decision making is by full consensus of its membership, as dictated by tradition. Although we are describing an association rather than an *impande*, it seems to stand as an example of an urban-based organization of cooperating *impandes* governed by consensus as well as the shared traditional values and mutual understandings that characterize *impandes*.

It should be noted that our recommendation is at odds with an official midterm evaluation of the AIDSCOM/AIDSCAP project that occurred in early 1993. It observes, "The sustainability of the traditional healer initiative depends on the ability of the project to work in a disciplined way with the traditional healer organizations. . ." (Nell and Shapiro 1993: 64–66). These evaluators unfortunately interviewed only five traditional healers; all were presidents of putative national associations. Only one of these healers had participated in an AIDSCOM/AIDSCAP workshop. There was not a single interview with a rank-and-file member of a healer's association, let alone a nonmember. It is not surprising that the evaluators' recommendation was for AIDSCAP to work *more* through the formal authority structure of national organizations—a recommendation bound to please association presidents.

It should also be noted that there is little or no tradition in southern Africa of healers organizing themselves beyond the local level, such as under a chief within a chieftaincy or under a *gobela*. It is to be expected that there will be power struggles, ethnic and other rivalries, and accusations of financial mismanagement and of leaders or followers acting "superior," within unfamiliar organizations that are based on urban-Western models.

We have seen evidence that leaders of national associations become threatened when more junior members attend workshops and become more knowledgeable than their leaders about AIDS prevention, and perhaps better able to organize a workshop. Part of the problem here is that some entrenched leaders regard themselves as too senior to attend an AIDS workshop in what they regard as a student role. Instead they send a hand-picked member of their association in their place, but then try to undermine this person later because he or she is viewed as a potential threat to the leader's authority.

## Recommendations Concerning Future Training

We sought to determine through formal and informal means how prepared second generation healers were to train a third generation of healers in HIV/AIDS and STD prevention. According to the formal evaluation, healers in all areas except KaNkwane possessed adequate accurate knowledge about HIV/AIDS and STD prevention to train others healers and indeed nonhealers in their communities. Many have already started to do the latter.

However, subjectively, most second-generation healers did not feel quite ready to hold a workshop entirely on their own. Most still preferred to have assistance from an AIDSCAP facilitator, from one of the health-related NGOs that work with AIDSCAP, or from one of the first-generation healers who are widely respected and adept in more formalized training. A few healers felt such help was not necessary, but most seemed to prefer to have some outside assistance for the first one or two workshops where they themselves are facilitators. Of course this only pertains to formal workshop-type sharing of their AIDS knowledge. Such outside facilitators seem to provide authority and prestige with healers as well as with NGO and government AIDS workers in the area. It would prove problematic if the wish (if not need) for an AIDSCAP facilitator were never outgrown, so to speak. Clearly, AIDSCAP could not send a facilitator to 630 third-generation workshops—even to their openings.

Several healers commented that if a facilitator is not able to communicate in more than one African language there needs to be somebody present who can translate. Thus, for a healer-trainer to hold a workshop solo (s)he ought to be multilingual, preferably in an Nguni language (Zulu, Swazi, Xhosa, Ndebele) and in siSotho.

A final and most important question facing the AIDSCAP traditional healers initiative is how much continuing contact and support should be provided those trained so far—the first and second generations—versus efforts to assist in the training of a third generation? This is at the top of the agenda for the next workshop for planning and assessment currently scheduled for late November 1993. The agenda for this workshop is being planned in advance in collaboration with the traditional healers Executive Steering Committee elected at Emaweni partly for this purpose.

## Notes

1. Some of the following material will appear in shortened form in Green, E. C., B. Zokwe, and J. D. Dupree, "The Experience of an AIDS Prevention Program Focused on South African Traditional Healers. *Social Science and Medicine* (in press). By mid-1993, AIDSCAP was the sole project funder.
2. She was found to be giving accurate AIDS preventive advice to age-mates as well as to adult clients.
3. One exception was the 8-year old diviner who rated it "moderately/somewhat useful" because her father wouldn't allow her to receive a dildo for condom demonstration purposes like the other workshop participants.
4. A traditional healer laughing with apparent embarrassment at the sight of a dildo was captured by a photographer at a second generation workshop in the Transvaal and published in the August 1993 issue of *Drum* magazine (p. 16) as part of a flattering article.
5. For a description of this process, see Green 1989b.
6. By September 1993, 1,510 healers had been trained, all but 28 by other healers.

# 9

# Summary and Conclusion

### A Summary of Epidemiology and the Potential Role of Healers

To summarize some salient facts discussed in Chapter 1, HIV is transmitted in three major ways in Africa: (1) through sexual intercourse, (2) through contaminated blood supplies (very rarely through sharing hypodermic syringes or through any sort of skin-piercing traditional healing practices), and (3) through perinatal mother-to-child transmission (pediatric AIDS). Prevention of HIV infection through contaminated blood supplies is a technical problem of screening. Prevention of "vertical" transmission lies at this stage in preventing the heterosexual infection of the mother in the first place. In any case, the second and third transition modes together account for less than 20 percent of HIV infection cases in Africa.

That leaves the first transmission mode, sexual intercourse, which accounts for over 80 percent of HIV cases. This appears to be largely because of the prevalence of other untreated or improperly treated sexually transmitted diseases which facilitate the transmission of HIV. Most standard STDs are curable as well as preventable. I have argued that health ministries, private organizations, and others must work collaboratively with traditional healers in order to either cure or prevent STDs or HIV infection.

The prevention of infection through sexual intercourse lies largely within the realm of behavior change. HIV is sexually transmitted in Africa through standard penile-vaginal intercourse, and the evidence shows that this occurs when one or both partners already have an STD, with or without genital lesions. As noted, lack of male circumcision and other conditions may also assist HIV transmission. The chances of becoming HIV infected through sexual intercourse are, as would be expected, greatly enhanced if one has many sexual partners, one's partner has had many other partners, and/or one's partner is in a high-risk category such as being a prostitute, a truck driver, or perhaps a soldier. Since

Africans seem to rarely engage in unsafe practices common in the industrialized West, such as anal sex, it would appear that if Africans did not suffer from other, standard STDs (and possibly if all men were circumcised), HIV infection rates in sub-Saharan Africa might be comparable to those found currently in North Africa and the Middle East, which are low by today's world standards.

## Some Tentative Conclusions About Locally Recognized STDs

Some tentative conclusions can be drawn from the ethnomedical findings presented in this book that relate to STDs. First, emic or indigenous nosological categories of illnesses related to sexual intercourse may not correspond with biomedical categories, and in fact are often broader. Symptoms relating to tuberculosis, (urinary) schistosomiasis, hernia, leprosy, diarrhea, or seizures might also be seen as sexually transmitted. But this does not mean that such conditions are necessarily *always* sexually transmitted, rather that they *can* be transmitted through at least certain types of sexual intercourse. This notion can best be understood in light of the prevailing belief in much traditional African thought that many illnesses can result from either sorcery or contamination, and that sexual intercourse provides one common point of contact for the medicine, spell or contamination causing or transmitting such illnesses. Another theme common to African health beliefs is that pathology in social relations leads to illness. Transgression of rules regarding sexual behavior (such as committing adultery) is obviously a common source of social strife. As pointed out by Pellow (1990:77), citing A. L. Epstein's work on Zambia, "... The African notion of sex includes mystical ideas, it carries magical potency, and to avoid supernatural dangers, one must observe taboos and respect social boundaries."

The foregoing offers an explanation of why STDs, including various related or unrelated conditions *emically* regarded as sexually transmitted, are widely regarded as being in the domain of traditional rather than biomedical treatment. Even if biomedical practitioners were thought to have potent treatments for the *symptoms* of "STDs," it is to traditional healers one must turn to treat the underlying cause of such conditions, conditions that may involve superhuman forces.

At the same time, there may be more naturalistic, impersonal explanations for illnesses related to sexual intercourse, such as those locally classified as *siki* in central Mozambique. With these, an unseen, impersonal agent of illness is simply passed from one partner to another through intercourse. There are also the examples of the Swazi illnesses *gcunsula* or *timbilapho*, which, for some healers at least, are seen as resulting from a man taking purifying herbal decoctions—or nowadays, pills—then resuming intercourse before his blood has been purified. The impurities which have accumulated in the man's body are believed to be passed through sperm to a sexual partner. Common to fidelity-protection, *siki* and passing-on-impurity illnesses is a single, basic, causal explanation that links several illnesses together with the result that they are understood and treated in essentially the same way.

Whatever the local beliefs or our interpretation of these, we see from the data I have presented as well as from a few other studies in geographically diverse parts of Africa that gonorrhea, syphilis, chancroid, and other common STDs are believed to be conditions that can be successfully treated by traditional medicines and practitioners. The corollary belief—among healers if not their clients—is that orthodox biomedical practitioners are less successful in treating these disorders.

Since biomedical treatment of common STDs usually entails the use of antibiotics that show rapid and marked results, how do we account for the widespread belief that traditional medicine is more effective in treating STD symptoms? There seem to be a number of possible reasons:

1. It is the nature of most common STDs that the symptoms go into latent stages whether or not there has been treatment. There may be sufficient cause and effect relationship between administration of traditional STD treatments and the apparent disappearance of symptoms that both healers and patients believe in the efficacy of the treatments.
2. Many STD patients may use modern and traditional therapies simultaneously, and nowadays this may include antibiotic self-treatment. If a patient recovers from his symptoms, anyone involved can take credit for the cure.
3. Patients treated by healers may disappear after treatment, not because they are cured but because they seek treatment elsewhere. The healer may assume he or she has cured the patient.
4. There is considerable antimicrobial resistance in many parts of Africa (especially in N. gonorrhoeae), meaning that "hospital medicine" may indeed be as ineffective as healers often characterize it. Even when antibiotics could be effective, patients may not take the full course for various reasons. It appears fairly common for Africans to take antibiotic pills *preventively,* i.e., one or two capsules before intercourse with a questionable partner.
5. Antibiotics are often not available in hospitals and clinics. This, in combination with antimicrobial resistance, means that traditional medicines might often be no less effective than a hospital visit.
6. We must always be open to the possibility that traditional STD medicines may be biomedically effective. Although the high and still-growing incidence of STDs would seem to belie this, it is

> possible that traditional medicines are effective but that patients repeatedly reinfect themselves. In other words, traditional treatment for STDs may have as high a failure rate as modern medicine in Mozambique for the same reasons: patient behavior, high prevalence levels of infections in the community, and lack of the technical means of protection against infections (e.g., condoms, spermicides).

On the other hand, it is possible that the supreme confidence that healers express in their STD medicines is at least in part a marketing and public relations strategy intended to impress clients. After all, one of the reasons African medicine works so well is because the therapist uses whatever means available to gain the implicit faith of his or her client.

Regarding the possibility that indigenous plant-, animal-,or mineral-derived medicines could be effective against some STDs, it has been well documented that traditional healers use medicines that are pharmacologically active and effective for some illnesses. A government botanist at Zimbabwe's National Herbarium reports that the bark of *Cassia abbreviata,* which is known to have antibiotic properties, is commonly grown around homesteads and typically used to treat gonorrhea. The botanist believes that preparations from this bark might actually be effective against gonorrhea (Mavi 1991). In fact, quite a number of poisonous plants have antibiotic properties at strong enough concentrations, but the patient would probably die before these concentrations were reached. The same may be true of animal-derived medicines. The Blister beetle is used in Zimbabwe as an STD treatment. The beetle is crushed up whole, or perhaps powdered, mixed in water with the powdered roots of *Carissa edulis,* and then drunk. It is toxic to the kidneys and patients sometimes die from this concoction (Gelfand et al. 1985:308).

Whatever the efficacy of particular treatments, it seems unlikely that vast numbers of traditional healers in widely separated areas of Africa comprising a great variety of natural environments are all using naturally occurring antibiotics, and even if so, that the dosages would be adequate to kill the infective microbes. Of course, more than one organic antibiotic could be in use and we saw that healers in South Africa may mix sulfa powder with traditional medicines in their STD decoctions and poultices.

## Should There Be a Role for Healers in STD Treatment?

Although any sort of collaborative programs involving traditional and Western-trained practitioners in Africa have been few and far between—at least before the AIDS pandemic—surveys of African healer attitudes and limited programmatic experience have consistently shown willingness on the part of traditional healers to learn more about orthodox biomedicine and to cooperate and collaborate with Western-trained practitioners (Messing 1976; Hall et al. 1977; Osborne et al. 1977; Rubel and Sargent 1979; Green and Makhubu 1985; Hoff and Maseko 1986; Warren 1986; Warren and Green 1988; Green 1989; Green and Monger 1989). As noted earlier, prestige and recognition appear to be fundamental incentives underlying healers' willingness to cooperate. Healers may well enjoy prestige in their local communities, but collaboration with physicians or government officials often bestows an additional respectability and recognition in the modern, urban sector that indigenous practitioners have come to value. This prestige, along with any skills acquired in Western medicine as a result of contacts with Western-trained practitioners, enables a healer to attract more clients and expand his or her practice. The relatively few healers who have participated in government sponsored training courses tend to display proudly and prominently any certificates or diplomas that testify to their training.

In spite of willingness and interest on the part of African healers, there are powerful obstacles in the way of establishing educational or other programs for traditional healers. These were discussed in Chapter 2 and need not be repeated here except to note that in addition to opposing a number of traditional practices on public health grounds, many Western-trained practitioners regard traditional healers as economic and prestige threats, with the result that the former often oppose measures—including proposed educational programs—that would result in sharing power and medical prerogatives with the latter. In short, the recent history of medical professionalism in Africa shows a tendency to recapitulate the longer history of medical professionalism in the West (Last 1986), which may be characterized as a struggle for consolidation of power by orthodox biomedical practitioners accompanied by efforts to legislate against or otherwise restrict the power of nonorthodox health practitioners. This helps explain why, years after the joint WHO/UNICEF resolutions at Alma Ata supporting the use of indigenous health practitioners in government-sponsored health programs, there has been little progress in this area, especially in Africa where physicians are outnumbered by indigenous practitioners probably more than in any other continent.

Where there have been educational programs aimed at "upgrading" the skills of traditional healers or birth attendants, the technologies transferred to indigenous practitioners have been of the most rudimentary kind, primarily homemade sugar/salt solution to prevent dehydration from infectious child diarrheal disease, or nonprescriptive contraceptives such as condoms. Some ministries of health have opposed allowing traditional healers to distribute packets of oral rehydration salts on the grounds that ORS is a medicine and only trained health care personnel should handle medicines. In any case, many or most such programs have emphasized preventive education and "appropriate referrals" (i.e., referrals from indigenous to Western-trained practitioners) rather than "technology transfer."

In order to contain the spread of STDs it would seem that at the very least indigenous practitioners—both healers and birth attendants—should be taught the rudiments of diagnosis of the major STDs. To fail to do so would to be to ignore the general importance of indigenous practitioners (i.e., their prestige, credibility, accessibility, and the cultural appropriateness of their diagnosis and healing methods) as well as the fact that in many parts of Africa, STD victims consult indigenous rather than Western-trained practitioners. With a biomedically correct diagnosis, indigenous healers might begin to refer STD cases to biomedical practitioners for appropriate antimicrobial treatment. They could also play an important role in educating their clients and the general public about the causes, symptoms, treatment, and prevention of STDs.

However, in making referrals to clinics and hospitals, indigenous practitioners would risk losing clients and forfeiting business, and perhaps losing prestige and credibility in the eyes of clients and others in the local community. A healer might well believe that to decline treating a client with a STD would be to lose that client to another traditional healer. And it must be remembered that many or most traditional healers believe that their own therapies are as good or better than Western biomedical therapies.

Perhaps a more "radical" approach is justified, one in which healers are involved in biomedical treatment of STDs. A number of complex issues arise if consideration is given to training traditional healers in antibiotic therapy. These are discussed in the next section.

## A Pilot STD Treatment Program Proposal in Mozambique

As part of our project in Mozambique, we proposed training and supervising a group a healers in the use of oral antibiotics on a pilot program basis. The proposal was as follows. Healers participating in the department's pilot program would be carefully selected in consultation with leaders of AMETRAMO or local associations of traditional healers. Specialists in STDs with large case loads would be sought. Additional selection criteria included interest on the healer's part in Western biomedicine as well as his/her reputation in the local community. The pilot program in Manica province would be carefully monitored to see if diagnosis and antibiotic treatment were carried out according to accepted public health standards. If that proved to be the case, the program could be replicated on a wider scale.

We recognized that we were proposing a "technology transfer" of one of the most demonstrably powerful of biomedical *materia medica*, namely antibiotics, to nonphysicians who already pose economic and prestige threats to medical professionals. On the other hand, antibiotics have already become available in markets and other outlets in Mozambique, as in Swaziland, South Africa, and many other parts of Africa. There is no reason to expect that trained and medically supervised traditional healers would be less responsible with antibiotics than the many laypeople who have begun to self-medicate.

Training healers in antibiotic therapy can be regarded as a radical measure warranted by the extreme nature of the problem of AIDS in a country like Mozambique. Just as it would be desirable to offer free health care to all citizens—as indeed the government tried to do—it would be desirable if only trained health personnel at the level of nurse or higher would administer antibiotics. But this is not possible in Mozambique for a variety of reasons.

Still, it is important to embark on the proposed program having thought of all important ramifications and possible consequences, the more important of which are presented in Table 9.1.

A possibility that has been discussed is to import a new drug for exclusive use in the proposed pilot projects, that is, an antibiotic not currently in use in Mozambique. Two such antibiotics have been discussed that can successfully treat both gonorrhea and chancroid after only one or two oral administrations. One is Augmentin, a compound of clavacycline and amoxycillin in a single pill. One advantage of a new drug is that the experimental pilot programs would not contribute to resistance to penicillin or tetracycline (penicillin has already been abandoned for treatment of gonorrhea, at least in Maputo).

It is recognized that the new oral antibiotics under consideration, if improperly used, would provoke resistance faster than drugs like penicillin, therefore we would need to emphasize correct use in our training. It is also recognized that Neisseria gonorrhoeae develops resistance to any antibiotic eventually, therefore it becomes a matter of delaying resistance to the extent possible and getting maximum usage out of whatever drug is used.

There could be another advantage to importing a new drug for exclusive use in the pilot programs. We could trace how this drug is used and where it goes much more easily if healers are the only ones officially receiving it. We might consider a kind of tracking study, a tool of market research used to track or trace the dissemination and distribution of a new product over time.

The new drug option would also keep the ministry's other STD programs somewhat separate from the pilot program. A disadvantage is

TABLE 9.1 Possible Disadvantages and Advantages of Training and Supervising Traditional Healers in Antibiotic Therapy for STDs

| *Disadvantages or Arguments* Against *Involving Traditional Healers in Antibiotic Therapy* | *Advantages or Arguments* For *Involving Traditional Healers in Antibiotic Therapy* |
|---|---|
| Accurate diagnosis of the various STDs prevalent in Africa, especially in the absence of laboratory tests, would be difficult. For example, herpes simplex lesions might be mistaken for lesions resulting from syphilis and might therefore be inappropriately treated with antibiotics. | Healers could treat common STDs with oral antibiotics in cases where there is no access to modern practitioners. Since standard STDs are major co-factors in the spread of AIDS in Africa, we can reduce the spread of AIDS by lowering the incidence of standard STDs such as gonorrhea & syphilis. This would also reduce PID, infertility, congenital blindness, and other sequelae of STDs. |
| It is hard enough to train, supply and supervise nurses and paramedical personnel in proper antibiotic use. Why add to the problem? Traditional healers are likely to misuse or over-use antibiotics, which would have various negative consequences. | Healers may not be easy to train and supervise in use of oral antibiotics, but they should become better at this than laymen who are already self-medicating with antibiotics—they should also be better than *un*trained, *un*supervised healers. |
| Healers should not be encouraged to adopt Western medicines. They are not competent to use them and we would be meddling with their traditional role. | Traditional healers in more economically-developed parts of Africa may already be adopting Western medicines. We may anticipate the same in Mozambique. |
| Allowing healers greater access to antibiotics might contribute to the growth of penicillin-resistant gonorrhea and other infections, assuming healers will misuse and over-use antibiotics. | Not allowing healers greater access to antibiotics might contribute even more to the growth of penicillin-resistant infections, because those who are totally untrained and unsupervised will misuse and over-use antibiotics to a greater extent than trained healers. |

(*Continues*)

| | |
|---|---|
| Access to antibiotics by healers and laymen and actual use of antibiotics may not (yet) be widespread in Mozambique, therefore arguments based on such assumptions are weak. If healers are already using antibiotics, this may only be happening in urban areas. | Access to antibiotics by healers and laymen will probably increase significantly over the next 2–3 years as private enterprise grows. Such is already the case in many parts of Africa. Therefore it is better to train certain healers properly and better ensure access to quality medicinal supplies than to turn a blind eye and leave the whole process to market forces. If the focus is on urban healers, these are easier to supervise and resupply than rural healers. |
| Why not just improve paramedical training in proper treatment of STDs? | There is widely-held belief in Africa that traditional medicine is more effective than Western medicine in treatment of STDs. Therefore there are cultural constraints to treating STDs in "modern" health facilities. These operate even in cities. We should recognize this and find some way to use healers in STD treatment, to take advantage of the fact that they already have many STD patients who are not motivated to visit hospitals or clinics. |
| Antibiotics are expensive. Who would pay for the pills healers would have to be supplied in vast quantities if we were to achieve the desired impact? Many African governments can't even afford to supply their own health facilities. | Healers, unlike government health workers, have their own sources of income. Many could afford to pay for oral antibiotics, a cost that could be passed along to their patients.<br><br>Healers could make wholesale, bulk purchases of antibiotics through the professional healer associations such as Ametramo. If these drugs were imported through the |

*(Continues)*

TABLE 9.1 (*Continued*)

| | |
|---|---|
| | Essential Drugs Program, wholesale costs could be kept at a minimum. |
| Unless we can trace and treat the various sexual partners of the STD patient, we can't have much impact. | Healers might be in a better position than hospitals to find and treat the partners of their patient. |
| If healers begin to use one type of Western treatment, why would it stop there? Demand for medicines would be impossible to satisfy. | Healers have been using ORS in many parts of Africa for 10 years or more, without any great demand for other medicines. |
| It is against the law for the non-medically trained to use antibiotics. | It is not against the law for doctors to refuse to serve in rural areas. In any case, laws can be amended to serve the public health. |

that the new drugs would be somewhat more expensive than standard antibiotics.

Whatever the financial costs of such programs, they would be much lower than those required to treat both AIDS and other STDs that have gone untreated or been inappropriately treated. Based on experience with healers elsewhere in Africa, and on a few discussions with healers in Mozambique, it is expected that traditional healers would be willing to pay for allopathic drugs, at least long enough to test their effectiveness with clients. The government could buy antibiotics in bulk under its Essential Drugs Programme and then sell specially designated supplies wholesale to traditional healers. If healers charge their clients more than the nominal fees required at modern health facilities—which they appear to do already even without antibiotics—clients are of course free to opt for clinic or hospital treatment instead.

True, there might well be nonfinancial costs and other problems associated with such a program. For one thing, accurate diagnosis of the various STDs prevalent in Africa, especially in the absence of laboratory tests, would be difficult. While it may be relatively easy to diagnose symptomatic gonorrhea sufferers by purulent discharge and pain in urination, the same cannot be said for asymptomatic gonorrhea victims or for syphilis in various active or latent stages. Genital sores and lesions from a variety of STDs may be difficult to distinguish from one another, making diagnosis and therefore appropriate treatment difficult. For example, to the inadequately trained, herpes simplex lesions might be mistaken for lesions resulting from syphilis and might therefore be inappropriately treated with antibiotics.

In fact, syphilis was considered in the Manica pilot program. Syphilis is easily cured with penicillin and it develops resistance to this drug relatively slowly. However, it is difficult to diagnose syphilis in the absence of laboratory tests. It can be confused with chancroid, herpes, and a variety of non-STD skin infections. Syphilis is also considerably less prevalent than gonorrhea.

Gonorrhea in its various phases can also be difficult to diagnose outside the laboratory. It is however quite easy to diagnose in men the acute phase which lasts for about a week and is apparent soon after initial infection. Men have a purulent, milky discharge. Based on preliminary research, healers who deal with STDs already make distinctions between types of genital discharges. By the second or third week, the infection travels through the urethra to the upper part of the testicle whereupon it causes pain and swelling. Again, our research suggests that the acute and secondary symptoms of gonorrhea appear to be regarded as separate diseases by healers. The only other STD symptoms likely to be confused with those of male gonorrhea symptoms in the acute phase would be those of chlamydia in 3 to 5 percent of the cases in men.

Kenya is one of a few countries experimenting with an STD-control approach known as syndrome-based treatment. Stephan Moses, a University of Manitoba technical adviser to the Kenya program, states the rationale: "We know (from the data) that in men with urethral discharge, about 60 percent is caused by gonorrhea and 10 percent to 15 percent by chlamydia. . . . We also know that more than half of the gonorrhea is resistant to penicillin alone (quoted in Finger 1992:7).

The program developed a flow chart for urethral discharge based on these findings. It assumes that men with thick, copious urethral discharge are likely to have gonorrhea.

> The flowchart recommends that all men with this symptom receive amoxycillin, a penicillin-based drug; Augmentin, whose active ingredient, clavulanic acid, makes the resistant gonococcal organism sensitive to penicillin; and probenecid, which makes the amoxycillin last longer in the bloodstream. (Finger 1992:7)[1]

Since this flowchart approach was introduced into three Nairobi clinics in 1991, some 1,500 patients a month have been treated for STDs. Dr. Moses observes that this is the cheapest effective regimen for penicillin-resistant gonorrhea—and he notes that it is a one-time treatment. "These algorithms could be used anywhere in Kenya where there is a health worker." (Finger 1992:7). My argument of course is: why not at least

TABLE 9.2 Flowchart for Syndrome-Based Treatment of Gonorrhea

| | | |
|---|---|---|
| *Urethral Discharge*<br>(Male) Gonorrhoea (GC)<br>Non-Gonococcal Urethritis (NGU), mainly caused by Chlamydia trachomatis | | *1st Line gon. Rx*<br>Amoxycillin 3 g stat + Augmentin 1 tablet stat 1 Probenecid 2 tablets stat |
| Thick, pus-like yellow discharge<br>1st line gonorrhea Rx | Scanty, thin discharge<br>Non-Gonooccal Urethritis Rx | (*If Penicillin Allergy*) use 2nd line Rx<br>*2nd Line gon. Rx*<br>Ciprofloxacin 250 mg stat |
| *Follow-up After 7 Days, if No Cure*<br>2nd line gonorrhea Rx<br>+<br>Non-Gonococcal Urethritis Rx | 1st line gonorrhea Rx<br>+<br>repeat Non-Gonococcal Urethritis Rx | *Non-Gonococcal Urethritis Rx*<br>Tetracycline 500 mg capsules QID for 7 days<br>*If Pregnant*<br>Erythromycin 500 mg QID for 7 days |
| *Follow-up After 7 Days, if No Cure*<br>Refer for Gram stain/culture | | |

SOURCE: Based on Kenyan Ministry of Health. Finger 1992:7

experiment with involving traditional healers in syndrome-based treatment, since they already see most of the STD cases?

It is recognized that treatment of single STD patients is a losing battle unless we can trace and treat the various sexual partners of the patient. Hospitals have a difficult time doing this, and it is possible that healers might be in a better position to find and treat the partners of their patient. It would seem, for example, that the partners would be more physically accessible to a healer situated in or near the patient's community, compared to a hospital or health center.

As for cost, the antibiotic currently in use in Mozambique for gonorrhea costs MT400–450 (about U.S.$ 0.20) for a full course of treatment, which is two pills daily for seven days. The cost of clavocycline/amoxycillin was not determined during our discussions in Mozambique, dependent as it is on several factors including size of order. But even if it cost five or ten times the price of the current pill, it would still be less than the MT5,000 that our very preliminary data seem to indicate people are willing to pay for traditional gonorrhea treatment.

Our tentative conclusion for a future pilot program was as follows. In order to: (1) keep a collaborative program simple; (2) maximize its chances for success; and (3) minimize a variety of health risks and potential program problems, our recommendation was to deal only with gonorrhea in its acute phase in men—at least during a program's initial phase. A selected group of healers who already see and treat STD cases would be trained to recognize in men the thick, milky, abundant discharge of acute gonorrhea, which is something they seem to already recognize easily and probably distinguish from other conditions. Healers would be trained to administer the clavocycline/amoxycillin oral antibiotic as treatment. An important feature of the program is that healers would ask the gonorrhea patient to name all of his recent sexual partners. These would then be brought to the healer and treated with the same oral antibiotic regardless of whether or not they presented symptoms (the same procedure followed in Mozambique's hospitals).

A program such as this may appear to be a radical intervention inasmuch as it may not have been tried elsewhere and because it carries with it certain risks. However, Mozambicans are already at risk for AIDS infection due to the high prevalence of standard STDS, aided by protracted civil war and vast social upheaval. In other words, the problem is extreme, therefore a radical solution is justified.

After much discussion of the foregoing proposal with several key ministry officials, it was agreed that we should not begin initial efforts of intersectoral collaboration with the transfer of antibiotic technology, even in a restricted pilot project involving a small number of healers. The one argument I could not really take issue with is that such a controversial element should not be included in the first year or two of an inaugural collaborative program. It was simply not politic, in effect, to give detractors of such programs ammunition to mount stronger opposition. Instead, we agreed to begin with AIDS and STD preventive education and to think about a syndrome-based antibiotic treatment program involving traditional healers during the second or third project year.

## Future Prospects

I have argued that traditional healers *could* have a significant impact in the following areas that directly or indirectly address the known and suspected AIDS risk factors: (1) referring STD cases or—with proper biomedical collaboration—treating cases themselves; (2) identifying, locating, and accessing the sexual partners of clients infected with STDs for the purpose of treatment of referral; (3) preventing the emergence of new STDs through the promotion of "barrier" birth control devices as well as spermicides; (4) influencing sexual behavior in the direction of faithful, single-partner relationships; (5) influencing people to adopt safe, nonpenetrative sexual practices, such as thigh sex, as an alternative to penetrative sex; (6) providing appropriate counseling and otherwise assisting in meeting the psychosocial needs of clients with HIV or AIDS as well as their family, friends, and local community; and (possibly) persuading African men to become circumcised in hospitals—assuming enough evidence accumulates to confirm this as a significant risk factor—

particularly those men from societies where circumcision is not traditionally practiced. Clearly, no other biomedical or other practitioner appears to be even a close second in potential of this sort. Yet to realize traditional healers' potential in impacting the spread of HIV and other STD infection, there must be collaboration with biomedical practitioners and their supporting institutions and organizations, and collaboration must take certain forms.

To many, the logic of poorly financed, understaffed African health ministries working collaboratively rather than competitively with indigenous healers seems unassailable. Yet the experience of the last fifteen years has shown that collaborative programs are very difficult to initiate and, once started, are fragile and prone to discontinuation of support. Skeptics of programs involving healers may present some strong arguments against working with or "encouraging" traditional healers in any way, some of which were outlined in Chapter 2. Others, in their enthusiasm, may want to move collaborative programs along too far, too quickly, as in the case of those who argue that ministries of health should attempt to transform traditional healers into civil servants.

What are the prospects for the development of viable collaborative programs focusing on AIDS, STDs, and family planning on a wide scale in Africa? The history of the allopathic medical profession in wealthier countries—especially the United States—has been one of consolidating a monopoly of power and stamping out competition from homeopaths, naturopaths, osteopaths, chiropractors, herbalists, and any other "heterodox," competing health care systems (cf. Cassidy, Baer, and Becker 1985). If this provides any clue to prospects for physicians sharing economic and political power in Africa, the outlook is not hopeful, especially since indigenous practitioners outnumber physicians by hundreds to one. While it seems unlikely that physicians will share power with healers voluntarily, it might be possible for healers to assert political power through their newly formed professional associations in such a way that health ministries, foreign donors, and private health organizations have no choice but to recognize and collaborate with indigenous practitioners. African governments may eventually have to adopt a stronger human resource development orientation that realistically assesses all available humanpower and develops policies and health service delivery programs in light of this.

The goal of cooperation and intersectoral collaboration has not been, and obviously should not be, the displacement or replacement of modern biomedicine with traditional medicine. It should be partly the preservation of medical pluralism, that is, the availability of more than one system of medical therapy that most Africans currently and of necessity rely on. It should also be, following the arguments and directives of the late King Sobhoza II of Swaziland, the eventual development of a synchretistic system that can combine the best features of biomedicine and traditional medicine in order to best serve human needs. Perhaps synchretism can never develop very far due to a basic incompatibility between the two paradigms of illness and the supporting worldviews, but projects to date suggest that intersectoral cooperation can be achieved and there is no reason to suppose that cooperation cannot be extended to all areas of public health concern, including AIDS, STDs, and other infectious diseases and nutrition, child immunization, and alcoholism, for example.

Any form and degree of intersectoral collaboration would be better than none. I have suggested several forms of how collaboration might take place in AIDS, STD, and family-planning programs based on my experience in several countries. Approaches that seem more "radical" and for which we have little precedent, such as healers' participating in syndrome-based treatment with oral antibiotics, probably ought to be limited in scope due to political and health-risk considerations. They should also be attempted initially on a pilot basis and carefully monitored and evaluated. There are risks in such approaches, but the health payoffs in reduced HIV and STD incidence reduction are potentially great and I believe the danger posed by AIDS in many parts of Africa justify taking such risks.

It should be clear that there is no technological "fix" to the AIDS problem in the form of condoms, yet condom procurement and promotion have consumed a disproportional amount of financial and human resources in the struggle against AIDS in Africa. On the other hand, I hope I have not presented collaboration with indigenous healers as a panacea, nor traditional healers as the only cadre or local group able to help in AIDS/STD control and prevention efforts. The potential for all local groups who are or could be powerful opinion influencers and/or effective service deliverers should also be explored and developed, including business and industry, national and local women's organizations, churches and church-related organizations, and councils of chiefs and other local and traditional leaders

Finally, I have not advocated collaborative programs with African healers in STD reduction to the exclusion of the promotion of condoms or other changes in behavior that help slow the spread of HIV/AIDS. It has been my experience that the very groups that are most inclined to oppose an AIDS campaign that involves condom promotion and frank discussion of sexual behavior are the ones with the best grassroots outreach and the most credibility and authority to assist such efforts. In addition to healers, these include church and religious leaders—both orthodox and synchretistic—as well as traditional political leaders. All AIDS prevention programs in Africa ought to make special effort to involve these three groups, on their own terms if necessary. With religious groups in particular, this might mean little or no promotion of condoms on their part, at least officially or initially. There is still much churches can do, for example, reinforce traditional behavior such as premarital chastity and marital fidelity. They can also promote abstinence or at least partner reduction, and possibly safer sexual practices. They can assist in counseling and HIV testing, and they can even help in treatment of existing STDs. Moreover, whatever a church's official position on condoms, experience in countries like Uganda has shown that as their AIDS programs develop and progress, they actually desensitize themselves regarding condoms and open discussion of sexual behavior. In other words, as long as an organization is involved in AIDS education, the subject of condoms will emerge and discussion of condoms becomes inevitable, as does referral to condom outlets—even if priests and imams do not wish to distribute condoms themselves.

Churches and other indigenous, nongovernmental organizations have been denied their share of foreign donor support for AIDS prevention unless they have agreed to actively promote condoms, an official or unofficial policy that has been counterproductive to say the least.

### *The Care and Counseling of AIDS Patients*

To the extent that all preventive efforts fail to prevent HIV infection and at a later stage, AIDS, what of Africa's countless thousands of HIV/AIDS sufferers? In their review of African AIDS-related literature, Caldwell et al. 1993:10–11) note the high and growing demand for treatment of opportunistic infections as well as the need for "social counseling and psychic support." In addition to any positive effects their medicines might have on opportunistic infections, traditional healers are clearly in a key position to provide emotional, psychological, spiritual, and—as we saw in South Africa—even material support to these sufferers who are at least as stigmatized in Africa as their counterparts are in America and for whom there is even less help available from Western biomedicine and social services. Healers can relieve private and government health services in their burden of treating the growing number of AIDS, ARC, and HIV-positive patients. Traditional healers can provide more personal and culturally appropriate care for the sick and dying than can biomedical institutional services, and traditional medicines may have some effect in easing the symptoms of opportunistic infections.

It seems appropriate to conclude this book by sharing some findings from interviews with two urban traditional healers in Tanzania, where AIDS has been well established for a number of years. The interviews and observations were made in April 1993 in two indigenous healer clinics in Dar es Salaam that specialize in the treatment of STDs and AIDS. The first was selected randomly from a newspaper advertisement, the other referred by a Tanzanian working in AIDS prevention.

The first herbal clinic was a clean, attractive establishment with a screen door to keep out insects. It was run by two herbalists who have gone into partnership together. One worked for several years on the police force (forensics division) and was actually sent by USAID to the United States on an educational trip (after retirement he returned to his earlier calling as traditional healer). There were five assistants, four of them women, dressed in crisp, attractive uniforms. The male assistant works with herbs; for example, he compounds herbal powders into tablets with a tablet-press machine. The women take care of correspondence, keep records, cook, clean up, and generally help out. They assist when a woman patient has to be examined and feels embarrassed by being alone with the male herbalist. There are health education posters on the wall as well as a color picture of the Pope.

According to apparently well-kept records, some 50 to 80 patients a day visit the clinic. In December 1992, there was a total of 249 patients: 49 had "gonorrhea," 13 had "syphilis," and another high category (listed under "staflacocus infections") was also said to contain a number of patients who had become infected through sexual intercourse.

Ndugu (meaning Comrade or Mr.) M. told me that HIV is not really an illness; it is more a predisposition to a range of illnesses. With HIV infection, a patient can get skin diseases, fungal infections, sores in the mouth, and other symptoms, all of which can be treated with herbs. However, such a patient will remain HIV positive. Regarding AIDS counseling, Ndugu M. advises that HIV-positive or full AIDS patients try to avoid high fevers, especially malaria since it could "finish a patient off." This requires keeping mosquitoes away from the patient. The patient should also avoid contracting STDs. Ndugu M. uses a traditional medicine, which he said has the effect of multiplying white blood cells (see next note on same point). He gives his patients massage to help circulation, specifically to help medicines pass via the blood through dry, wrinkled skin. He also gives medicines to eliminate toxins from the body—to "cleanse and purify" the body's system. He also tries to keep the patient hydrated with plenty of fluids.

Regarding diet, Ndugu M. recommends that HIV patients eat a lot of fruits and vegetables, take all necessary vitamins, drink milk, and eat less starchy foods. He advises his patients to avoid alcohol and smoking. They are also to avoid sexual intercourse not only because it will spread the disease but because patients would "waste their survival energy." He further advises avoiding alcohol and sex for patients with standard STDs and urges such patients to bring their sexual partners to the clinic so that they can be treated as well. The herbalist's partner, Ndugu B., observed that unlike government hospitals, the traditional healer has a business incentive to identify and treat all sexual partners of an STD patient, because more patients means more business. He said that STD patients at the nearby hospital (Muhimbili Medical Center, Tanzania's top referral hospital) are simply written out a slip that instructs them where to go for their course of injections. No one there takes the responsibility—or even cares—whether the patient will go out and become reinfected or infect new partners.

The second clinic I visited had been operating since 1982. It is run by Mrs. N., who said she worked as a hospital nurse for fourteen years before returning to her earlier calling as an herbalist. She presently uses only medicines derived from herbs or minerals. Mrs. N. sees about 150 patients a week, of whom roughly half are STD and HIV/AIDS patients; in fact she specializes in the latter. For her HIV/AIDS patients, she recommends a high protein diet along with plenty of vegetables, especially wild greens. She also recommends seafoods, and eating a lot of fruit and spices, believing that spices are good for the nerves and stimulate the appetite. There should be no smoking or alcohol consumption. She also recommends exercise, especially social-type hobbies or sports such as netball and dancing. Mrs. N. said that such activities are in part to help patients overcome depression and morbid thoughts. She emphasized the importance of "encouraging" AIDS patients.

She noted that homosexuality is fairly common along Tanzania's coastal area. Part of her AIDS advice is that men not have sex with each other. She does not recommend condom use. Mrs. N. is a Muslim but expressed what she told me were her personal views about condoms.

Mrs. N believed that her herbs for AIDS symptoms can prolong and improve the life of an AIDS patient. Other treatments, such as massage, can also help. She administers massages using a linament made of cloves. She said patients like a massage because it relieves pain, especially in the lower limbs. But she also emphasized that massage is very important psychologically: most people wish to have no physical contact with AIDS patients, so receiving a massage is very reassuring to them. It is a form of acceptance. This same point was made by an AIDS patient at the healer workshop in South Africa.

We might ask ourselves who else in Africa is providing a service comparable to this, and who else is capable of providing it on a large scale? And to what extent could this service be replicated, possibly improved, and given emphasis in both AIDS prevention and effective STD treatment if financial and other resources were directed toward this end?

## Notes

1. A more detailed chart based on the "syndromic approach" was published in a recent Population Reports (Lande 1993).

# References


Ademuwagun, Z. A. "The Relevance of Yoruba Medicine Men in Public Health Practice in Nigeria." *in* Warren, D. M. et al. (eds.), *African Therapeutic Systems*, Waltham, Mass.: Crossroads Press, 1979, pp. 153–157.

Adikwu, M. U., "Could the Law Governing the Use of 'Prescription Only' Medicines Be Extended to Traditional Medicines?" *Tropical Doctor*, Vol. 22(3), July 1992, p. 122.

Althaus, F. A., "Reproductive Tract Infections and Women's Health." *International Family Planning Perspectives*, 17(4):145–150, 1991.

Asuni, T. "The Dilemma of Traditional Healing with Special Reference to Nigeria." *Social Science & Medicine*, 1979, Vol. 13, pp. 33–39.

Asuzu, M.C., N. A. Rotowa, and I. O. Ajayi, "The Use of Mail Reminders in STD Contact Tracing in Ibadan, Nigeria." *East African Medical Journal* 67(2):75–78, 1990.

Bailey, Allen, "Powerful Medicine" (film in the series The Nature of Things, supported by the National Cancer Inst., USAID, et al.), 1986.

Baku, E. S. K., "The Nazareth Healing Complex." *Contact*, (Christian Medical Commission, World Council of Churches) 103, p. 3, June 1988.

Bannerman, R. H., J. Burton, and C. Wen-Chieh, *Traditional Medicine and Health Care Coverage*, Geneva: WHO, 1983.

Barnett, T. and P. Blaikie, *AIDS in Africa: Its Present and Future Impact*. New York: The Guilford Press, 1992.

Barton, T., "Sexually Related Health and Disease in Africa: A Brief Overview." Paper presented at the Southwestern Anthropological Association 59th Annual Meeting, Monterey, Ca., March 25, 1988.

Barton, T., *Sexuality and Health in Sub-Saharan Africa: An Annotated Bibliography*. Research Triangle, N.C. Family Health International/AIDSTECH, 1989.

Bassett, M. T., and M. Mhloyi, "Women and AIDS in Zimbabwe: The Making of an Epidemic." *International Journal of Health Services*, 21(1):143–156, 1991.

Beinart, William, "Worker Consciousness, Ethnic Particularism and Nationalism: The Experience of a South African Migrant," *in Politics, Class and Nationalism in South Africa*, ed. S. Marks and S. Trapido, pp. 286–309, New York, 1987.

Benson, P., "Spermicides and STDs." *Outlook*, 6(2):7–8, 1988.

Bentley, M., G. H. Pelto, W. L. Straus et al., "Rapid Ethnographic Assessment: Applications in a Diarrhea Management Program." *Social Sci. & Med.*, 27, 1:107–116, 1988.

Berkley, S., "Parenteral Transmission of HIV in Africa." *AIDS* 5 (suppl 1):S87–S92, 1991.

Bibeau, G. et al., *Traditional Medicine in Zaire.* Ottowa, Canada: International Development Research Centre, p. 13, 1980.

Biggar, R. J., "The AIDS Problem in Africa." *Lancet,* pp.79–82, January 11, 1986.

Biggar, R. J., "Preventing AIDS Now. Treating Other Sexually Transmitted Diseases Could Help." *British Medical Journal,* November 9, 1991; 303(6811): 1150–1151.

Bird, K. D., "The Use of Spermicide Containing Nonoxynol-9 in the Prevention of HIV Infection." *AIDS,* July 5(7):791–796, 1991.

Boerma, J. T. and M. S. Baya, "Maternal and Child Health in an Ethnomedical Perspective: Traditional and Modern Medicine in Coastal Kenya." *Health Policy and Planning* 5(4):347–357, 1990.

Bongaarts, J., P. Reining, P. Way, and F. Conant, "The Relationship between Male Circumcision and HIV Infection in African Populations." *AIDS,* Vol. 3, No. 6, pp. 373–377, 1989.

Booth, A. R., "'European Courts Protect Women and Witches': Colonial Law Courts as Redistributors of Power in Swaziland 1920–1950." *Journal of Southern African Studies,* Vol. 18, No. 2, June 1992, pp. 254–270.

Brokensha, D., "Overview: Social Factors in the Transmission and Control of African AIDS." *in* Miller, N. and R. Rockwell (eds) *AIDS in Africa: The Social and Policy Impact.* Lewiston, N.Y.: Edwin Mellen Press, 1988.

Bryant, Published posthumously in 1966. Material on STDs was first published in the *Annals of the Natal Museum,* vol. II, No. 1, 1909.

Caldwell, J. and P. Caldwell, *Cultural Forces Tending to Sustain High Fertility in Tropical Africa,* The World Bank, PHN Technical Note 85-16, October 1985.

Caldwell, J. and P. Caldwell, "The Cultural Context of High Fertility in Sub-Saharan Africa." *Population and Development Review,* 13:3, 1987, pp. 409–437.

Caldwell, J., P. Caldwell, E. M. Ankrah, J. K. Anarfi, D. K. Agyeman, K. Awusabo-Asare, and I. O. Orubuloye, "African Families and AIDS: Context, Reactions and Potential Interventions." *Health Transition Review,* Vol. 3, Supp. Issue, 1993, pp. 1–16.

Caldwell, J., P. Caldwell, and P. Quiggin, "The Social Context of AIDS in Sub-Saharan Africa." *Population and Development Review* 15, No. 2:185–234, 1989.

Caldwell, J., P. Caldwell, and P. Quiggin, "The African Sexual System: Reply to Le Blanc et al." *Population and Development Review* 17, No. 3:506–515, 1991.

Cameron, D. W., J. N. Simonsen, L. J. D'Costa et al., "Female to Male Transmission of Human Immunodeficiency Virus Type 1: Risk Factors for Seroconversion in Men." *Lancet,* 2(8660):403–407, August 19, 1989.

Cassidy, C., H. Baer, and B. Becker, "Selected References on Professionalized Heterodox Health Systems in English-Speaking Countries." *Medical Anthropology Quarterly,* Vol. 17, No. 1, 1985, pp. 10–18.

Cates, W. "Sexually Transmitted Diseases and Contraceptive Choice." *Outlook,* 6(2):2–6, 1988.

CDA (The Community Development Association) et al., *Strengthening Civil Society and Community Development in Southern Africa,* Workshop, Maputo, April 1992, p. 39.

CDC (Centers for Disease Control), MMWR (Morbidity and Mortality Weekly

Report): "Condoms for Prevention of Sexually Transmitted Diseases." *Journal of American Medical Association,* 259 (13) 1988: 1925–1927.

CDSC (Communicable Disease Surveillance Centre), AIDS Dialogue, No. 14, January 1991:9.

Chavunduka, G. L., "ZINATHA: The Organization of Traditional Medicine in Zimbabwe." *in* M. Last and G. L. Chavunduka, eds., *The Professionalization of African Medicine,* Manchester (UK): Manchester Universutty Press, 1986, pp. 29–49.

Chin, J., "Current and Future Dimensions of the HIV/AIDS Pandemic in Women and Children." *Lancet,* 1990 July 28; 336(8709): 221–224.

Chirwa, B. U. and E. Sivile, "Enlisting the Support of Traditional Healers in the Zambian AIDS Education Campaign." *AIDS Health Promotion Exchange* (2):1: 7–10, 1989a.

Chirwa, B. U. and E. Sivile, "Enlisting the Support of Traditional Healers in an AIDS Education Campaign in Zambia." *International Quarterly of Community Health Education* 9(3):221–229, 1989b.

Chiwuzie, J. et al., "Traditional Practitioners Are Here to Stay." *World Health Forum* 8(2), 1987, pp. 240–244.

Compton, J. L., "Strategies and Methods for the Access, Integration, and Utilization of Indigenous Knowledge in Agriculture and Rural Development." *in* D. M. Warren, L. J. Slikkerveer, and S. O. Titiloa, eds., *Indigenous Knowledge Systems: Implications for Agriculture and International Development.* Ames: Technology and Social Change Program, Iowa State University, 1989.

DeJong, J., *Traditional Medicine in Sub-Saharan Africa.* Washington, D.C.: The World Bank, Population and Human Resources Department, *Working Papers* WPS 735, July 1991.

Dupree, J. D., "Frequently Asked Questions about HIV/AIDS: Suggested Responses." Braamfontein (S. Africa): AIDSCOM Project, 1992.

Dyson, T. and M. Murphy, "The Onset of Fertility Transition." *Pop.Devel. Rev.,* September 1985.

Egboh, Michael, personal comm., March 1988.

*Epidemiological Comments* 20(3) March 1993.

Erwin, J. O., "Reproductive Tract Infections among Women in Ado-Ekiti, Nigeria: Symptoms Recognition, Perceived Causes and Treatment Choices." *Health Transition Review,* Vol. 3, Supp. Issue, 1993, pp. 135–149.

Fassin, D. and E. Fassin, "Traditional Medicine and the Stakes of Legitimation in Senegal." *Social Science & Medicine,* 27 (4): 353–357, 1988.

Fennell, W. M., "A Perspective on AIDS" (letter), *South African Medical J.,* 79(10):626, 1991.

Fink, A. J., "Circumcision and Heterosexual Transmission of HIV Infection to Men" (letter). New England Journal of Medicine. 316 (24): 1546–1547, June 11, 1987.

Freeman, M., ed.,"Recognition and Registration of Traditional Healers: Possibilties and Problems." Conference Proceedings. Johannesburg: Centre for Health Policy, University of Witwatersrand. April 1992.

Freeman, M. and M. Motsei, "Is There a Role for Traditional Healers in Health

Care in South Africa?" The Center for the Study of Health Policy, Department of Community Health, University of the Witwatersrand, Paper No. 20, Johannesburg, March 1990.

FHI (Family Health International), "Sexually Transmitted Diseases: Priorities Outlined for Africa." *Network,* 8:1, Autumn 1986, 4–5.

Finnegan, W., *A Complicated War.* Berkeley: University of California Press, 1992.

Frank, Odile, *Demand for Fertility Control in Sub-Saharan Africa,* The World Bank, PHN Technical Note 85-2O, November 1985.

Furnivall, J. S., *Colonial Policy and Practice.* New York: New York University Press, 1948.

van der Geest, S., "The Illegal Distribution of Western Medicines in Developing Countries: Pharmacists, Drug Peddlers, Injection Doctors and Others." *Medical Anthropology* 6 (4): 197–219, 1982.

Gelfand, M., S. Mavi, R. B. Drummond, and B. Ndemera, *The Traditional Medical Practitioner in Zimbabwe.* Harare: Mambo Press, 1985.

Georges, A. J. et al., "Epidemiologie des Infections a VIH en Afrique," *Rev. Prat,* 40 (23): 2131–2135, 1990.

Gluckman, M., *Custom and Conflict in Africa.* New York: Barnes and Noble, 1956.

Goldberg, H. I., N. C. Lee, M. W. Oberle, and H. B. Peterson, "Knowledge about Condoms and Their Use in Less-Developed Countries during a Period of Rising AIDS Prevalence." *Bulletin of the World Health Organization,* 67(1):85–91, 1989.

Goliber, T. J., "Sub-Saharan Africa: Population Pressures on Development." *Population Bulletin,* Population Reference Bureau, Inc., Vol. 4O, No. 1, February 1985.

Good, C. M., "The Community in African Primary Health Care: Problems of Strengthening Participation and a Proposed Complementary Strategy," paper presented to the Takemi Program in International Health, Harvard School of Public Health, Boston, Mass., June 1987 (1987a).

Good, C. M., *Ethnomedical Systems in Africa. Patterns of Traditional Medicine in Rural and Urban Kenya.* New York: Guilford Press, 1987b.

Good, C. M., "Traditional Healers and AIDS Management in Africa." *In* N. Miller and R. Rockwell, eds. *AIDS in Africa: The Social Impact.* New York: Mellon Press, 1988.

van der Graaf, M. and R. Diepersloot, "Transmission of Human Immunodeficiency Virus (HIV/HTLV-III/LAV): A Review." *Infection* 14: 203–211, 1986.

le Grand, A. and P. Wondergem, *Herbal Medicine and Health Promotion.* Amsterdam: Royal Tropical Institute, 1990.

Green, E. C., "A Modern Appalachian Folk Healer." *Appalachian Journal,* 6 (1):2–15, 1978.

Green, E. C., "Roles for African Traditional Healers in Mental Health Care." *Medical Anthropology,* Vol. 4, No. 4, pp. 489–522, 1980.

Green, E. C. "U.S. Population Policy, Development and the Rural Poor of Africa." *Journal of Modern African Studies,* Vol. 20, No. 1, pp. 45–67, 1982.

Green, E. C., "Factors Relating to the Presence and Use of Sanitary Facilities in Rural Swaziland." *Tropical and Geographical Medicine,* Vol. 37, No. 1, 1985a.

Green, E. C., "Traditional Healers, Mothers and Childhood Diarrheal Disease in Swaziland: The Interface of Anthropology and Health Education." *Social Science and Medicine,* Vol. 2O, No. 3, pp. 277–285, 1985b.

Green, E. C., "Collaborative Programs for Traditional Healers In Primary Health Care and Family Planning in Africa." *in* C. Fyfe and U. Maclean, eds., *African Medicine in the Modern World,* University of Edinburgh, Centre of African Studies, Seminar Proceedings No. 27, December 1986, pp. 115–144.

Green, E. C., "Beliefs and Behavior Related to Water in Rural Swaziland." *International Journal of Water Resources Development,* Vol. 2, No. 4, pp. 29–42, 1987a.

Green, E. C., "The Integration of Modern and Traditional Health Sectors in Swaziland," *in* R. Wulff and S. Fiske, eds., *Anthropological Praxis,* Boulder: Westview Press, 1987b, pp. 87–97.

Green, E. C., "AIDS in Africa: An Agenda for Behavioral Scientists." *in* N. Miller and R. Rockwell, eds., *AIDS in Africa: The Social and Policy Impact.* New York: Mellen Press, pp. 175–196, 1988a.

Green, E. C., "Can Collaborative Programs Between Biomedical and African Indigenous Health Practitioners Succeed?" *Soc. Sci. & Med.,* Vol. 27, No. 11, pp. 1125–1130, 1988b.

Green, E. C., *A Survey of Health, Fertility and Human Reproductive Knowledge and Attitudes among Nigerian Traditional Healers.* Washington, D.C., The Futures Group, p. 22, February 1989a.

Green, E. C., "Mystical Black Power: The Calling to Diviner-Mediumship in Southern Africa." *in* C. S. McClain, ed., *Women as Healers: Cross-Cultural Perspectives.* N.J.: Rutgers University Press, pp. 186–200, 1989b.

Green, E. C., "Assessing the Impact of Development Education for Rural Women's Organizations and Traditional Leaders in Swaziland." USAID/Swaziland and Management Services International, Washington, D.C., December 31, 1990.

Green, E. C., "The Anthropology of Sexually Transmitted Diseases in Liberia." *Social Science and Medicine,* Vol. 35, 1457–1468, 1992a.

Green, E. C., "Evaluating the Response of Swazi Traditional Leaders to Development Workshops." *Human Organization,* Vol. 53, No. 4, 379–388, 1992b.

Green, E. C., "Sexually Transmitted Disease, Ethnomedicine and Health Policy in Africa." *Social Science and Medicine,* 35(2):121–130, 1992c.

Green, E. C., "Women's Groups and Income Generation in Swaziland." *Practicing Anthropolgy,* Vol. 14, No. 4, 1992d, pp. 19–23.

Green, E. C. and A. Conde, "AIDS and Condoms in the Dominican Republic: Evaluation of an AIDS Education Campaign." *in* R. Kulstad, ed., *AIDS 1988: AAAS Symposium Papers.* Washington, D.C.: American Association for the Advancement of Science Press, 1988, pp. 275–288.

Green, E. C. and A. Jurg, *Traditional Health Beliefs and Practices Related to Child Diarrheal and Sexually Transmitted Diseases.* USAID and the Academy for Educational Development, Washington, D.C., December 1991.

Green, E. C., A. Jurg, and A. Dgedge, "Sexually Transmitted Diseases, AIDS and Traditional Healers in Mozambique." *Medical Anthropology,* Vol. 15, No. 3, Spring 1993, pp. 261–281.

Green, E. C. and L. Makhubu, "Traditional Healers in Swaziland: Toward Improved Cooperation Between the Traditional and Modern Health Sectors." *Social Science and Medicine*, Vol. 18, No. 12, pp. 1071–1074, 1984.

Green, E. C. and H. Monger, *AIDs and Other Sexually Transmitted Diseases in Liberia: Results of a Qualitative Study* Washington, D.C.: The Futures Group, March 1989.

Green, E. C., J. Williamson, and P. Nimpuno-Parente, *Evaluation of the Children and War Program, (PRITECH evaluation).* Maputo: Save The Children/USA and USAID. Mozambique, July 1992.

Green, E. C. and B. Zokwe, "Evaluation of the 'Second Generation' of South African Traditional Healers Trained in HIV/AIDS Prevention and Management." Arlington, Va.: Family Health International, August 1993.

Green, E. C., B. Zokwe, and J. D. Dupree, *The Role of South African Traditional Healers in HIV/AIDS Prevention and Management*. Arlington, Va.: Family Health International, AIDSCAP Project, December 1992.

Greenblatt, R. M., S. A. Lukehart, F. A. Plummer, T. C. Quinn, C. W. Critchlow, R. L. Ashley, L. J. D'Costa, J. O. Ndinya-Achola, L. Corey, and A. R. Ronald, "Genital Ulceration as a Risk Factor for Human Immunodeficiency Virus Infection." *AIDS*, 2(1): 47–50, 1988.

Guinness, Frank, personal comm., December 1990.

Hall, Clarence, ed., "Report of the First National Workshop on Traditional Medicine and Its Role in the Development of Primary Health Care in Zambia," sponsored by Ministry of Health/UNICEF/WHO, May 9–13, 1977.

Hammond-Tooke, W. D., *Boundaries and Belief: The Structure of a Sotho Worldview.* Johannesburg: Witwatersrand University Press, 1981.

Hanlon, J., *Mozambique: Who Calls the Shots?* Bloomington: University of Indiana Press, 1990.

Haram, L., "Tswana Medicine in Interaction with Biomedicine." *Social Science and Medicine*, 33(2):167–175, 1991.

Helitzer-Allen, D. and H. Allen, "Focused Ethnographic Study of Sexually Transmitted Illnesses in Malawi." Arlington, Va.: Family Health Internationl/AIDSCAP Project, 1992.

Herman, E., "Theme: Traditional Healers." *Technical Literature Update on Diarrhea*, Vol. VII, No. 1, 1992, pp. 1–7.

Hoff, W. "Training Traditional Healers to Assist in the Control of Childhood Diseases in Swaziland." Paper presented at the National Council of International Health Annual Meeting, Washington, D.C., June 10–12, 1986.

Hoff, W. and D. N. Maseko, "Nurses and Traditional Healers Join Hands." *World Health Forum*, Vol. 7, pp. 412–416, 1986.

Hogel, J. and A. Prins, "Prospects for Collaborating with Traditional Healers in Africa." Arlington, Virginia: PRITECH Project (Management Sciences for Health), April 1991.

Hogel, J. et al., "Indigenous Knowledge and Management of Childhood Diarrhoeal Diseases." Arlington, Va.: Management Sciences for Health (PRITECH Project) August 1991.

Holmberg, S. D., C. R. Horsburgh, J. W. Ward, and H. W. Jaffe, "AIDS Commentary. Biologic Factors in the Sexual Transmission of Human Immunodeficiency virus." *Journal of Infectious Disease* 162(1):274, 1990.

Holmes, K. K., "Gonococcal Infections." *in* E. Braunwald et al., eds., *Harrison's Principles of Internal Medicine.* (11th ed.), pp. 578–579, New York: McGraw-Hill, 1987.

Hrdy, D. B., "Cultural Practices Contributing to the Transmission of Human Immunodeficiency Virus in Africa." *Review of Infectious Diseases,* 9(16):1109–1119, 1987.

Hunt, C. W., "Migrant Labor and Sexually Transmitted Disease: AIDS in Africa." *Journal of Health and Social Behavior,* 30(4): 353–373, 1989.

Huntington, D., "AIDS-Africa Ethnographic Component: Liberia." SOMARC Trip Report. Washington, D.C.: The Futures Group, 1988.

Imperato, P. J., "Traditional Medical Practitioners among the Bambara of Mali and Their Role in the Modern Health-Care Delivery System." *Rural Africana,* Vol. 26, pp. 41–54.

Ingstad, B., "The Cultural Construction of AIDS and Its Consequences for Prevention in Botswana." *Medical Anthropology Quarterly* 4(1):28–40, 1990.

Janzen, J., "Health, Religion, and Medicine in Central and Southern African Traditions." *in* L. Sulllivan, ed., *Caring and Curing: Health and Medicine in World Religious Traditions.* New York: MacMillan, 1989a, pp. 225–254.

Janzen, J., "Strategies of Health Seeking and Structures of Social Support in Central and Southern Africa." *in* J. Caldwell, J. et al., eds., *What We Know about Health Transition: The Cultural, Social and Behavioural Determinants of Health.* Proceedings of an International Workshop, Canberra (Australia), May 1989b.

Jessamine, P. G., F. A. Plummer, J. O. Ndinya-Achola, M. A. Wainberg, I. Wamola et al., "Human Immunodeficiency Virus, Genital Ulcers and the Male Foreskin: Synergism in HIV-1 Transmission." *Scandinavian J. of Infectious Diseases* (Supplementum). 69:181–186, 1990

de Jong, J., "Cooperaço Gradual Entre a Medicina Tradicional e a Medicina Moderna e Mecanismos da sua Interligaço com a Saüde Mental em Moçambique." Maputo, Mozambique: Department of Traditional Medicine, October 1990.

Jurg, A., T. Tomas, and J. de Jong, "Fornecedores e utentes de cuidados modernos ou tradicionais de saüde em Maputo, Moçambique: opinioes e preferencias mutuas em Moçambique." Maputo: Instituto Nacional de Saüde, GEMT, pp. 4–5, July 1991.

Jurg, A., T. Tomas, and J. Pividal, "Antimalarial Activity of Some Plant Remedies in Use in Marracuene, Southern Mozambique," *Journal of Ethnopharmacology,* 33, 1991.

Kaijage, F. J. "The AIDS Crisis in the Kagera Region, Tanzania, from an historial perspective." *in* J. Z. J. Killewo, G. K. Lwihula, A. Sandstrom, and L. Dahlgren, eds., *Behavioural and Epidemiological Aspects of AIDS Research in Tanzania.* Proceedings from a workshop. Dar es Salaam, 6–8 December, 1989.

Karlander, O. "Women and Children Living in the Shadow of AIDS." *Interface,* 1991; 8(2):10–11.

Katz, S. S. and S. H. Katz, "The Evolving Role of Traditional Medicine in Kenya." *African Urban Studies,* 1981, 9:1–12.

Kikhela, N., B. Bibeau, and E. Corin, "Africa's Two Medical Systems: Options for Pplanners." *World Health Forum,* 1981; 21:96–99.

Krieger, N. and G. Margo, "Women and AIDS: Introduction." *International Journal of Health Services,* 21(1):127–130, 1991.

Kreiss, J., M. Carael, and A. Meheus, "Role of Sexually Transmitted Diseases in Transmitting Human Immunodeficiency Virus." *Genitourin Med.,* 64, pp. 1–2, 1988.

Laga, M., A. T. Kamanga, M. Kivuvu et al., "Non-Ulcerative Sexually Transmitted Diseases as Risk Factors for HIV-1 Transmission in Women: Results from a Cohort Study." *AIDS* 7:95–102, 1993.

Lambo, T. A. "Experience with a Program in Nigeria." *in* R. Williams and L. Ozarin, eds., *Community Mental Health: An International Perspective,* San Francisco: Jossey-Bass, Inc., 1967, pp. 97–110.

Lambo, T. A. "Services for the Mentally Handicapped in Africa." *Royal Society of Health Journal,* Vol. 93, 1973, pp. 20–23.

Lamptey, P., Interview in *Africa Report,* July–August 1992, pp. 27–29.

Lamptey, P. and G. Goodridge, "Condom Issues in AIDS Prevention in Africa." *AIDS* 5 (suppl. 1) 1991, pp. 183–191.

Lande, R., "Controlling Sexually Transmitted Diseases." *Population Reports* Series L, No. 9, June 1993.

Langhoff, E. and W. A. Haseltine, "Dendritic Leukocytes in HIV-1 Infection." Paper presented at AAAS Annual Meeting, Boston, February 6, 1993.

Last, M. "The Professionalization of African Medicine: Ambiguities and Definitions," *in* M. Last amd G. L. Chavunduka, eds., *The Professionalization of African Medicine,* Manchester (UK): Manchester University Press, 1986, pp.1–19.

Le Blanc, M., D. Meintel, and V. Piche, "The African Sexual System: Comment on Caldwell et al." *Population and Development Review,* Vol. 17, No. 3, 1991, pp. 497–505.

Lewis, J., B. Janowitz, and M. Potts, "Methodological Issues in Collecting Data from Traditional Birth Attendants." *Int. J. Gynaecol. Obstet.,* 23:291–303, 1985.

Liljestrand, J., S. Bergstrom, F. Nieuwanhuis, and B. Hederstedt, "Syphilis in Pregnant Women in Mozambique." *Genitourinary Medicine, 61* (6):355–358, December 1985.

MacCormack, C., "The Articulation of Western and Traditional Systems of Health Care," *in* M. Last and G. L. Chavunduka, eds., *The Professionalization of African Medicine,* Manchester (UK): Manchester University Press, 1986, pp. 151–162.

Malinowski, B., *Magic, Science and Religion, and Other Essays.* Boston: Beacon Press, 1948.

Mann, J. M., J. Chin, P. Piot, and T. Quinn, "The International Epidemiology of AIDS." *Scientific American,* October, pp. 82–89, 1988.

Marx, J. L., "Circumcision May Protect Against the AIDS Virus (news)" *Science,* August 4, 1989; 245(4917): 470–461.

Masango, G. I. and K. G. Pallangyo, "Characterization of Tanzanian Outpatients Presenting with Sexually Transmitted Diseases." *E. African Med. J. 64* (1):31–6, 1987.

Masango, G. I. and M. J. Rakolojane, "Sexually Transmitted Diseases Baseline Survey," Mbabane: Family Life Association of Swaziland, July 1987.

Matthe, D., "Ethnomedical Science and African Medical Practice." *Medicine and Law*, 7:517–521, 1989.

Mavi, S., (Div. of Botany, National Herbarium, Zimbabwe), personal communication January 1991.

Mbura, J. S., H. N. Mgaya, and H. K. Heggenhougen, "The Use of Oral Herbal Medicine by Women Attending Antenatal Clinics in Urban and Rural Tanga District in Tanzania." *East African Medical Journal*, 62(8):540–550, August 1985.

McClure, G., "Introduction," *in* D. M. Warren, L. J. Slikkerveer, and S. O. Titiloa, eds., *Indigenous Knowledge Systems: Implications for Agriculture and International Development*. Ames: Technology and Social Change Prog., Iowa State University, 1989.

McLean, P., *Swaziland: Perceptions and Attitudes of Men and Women Towards Family Planning*. Family Life Association, December 1990.

Mefane, C., and M. Toung-Mve, "Syphilis in Pregnant Women in Libreville (Gabon)." *Bull. Soc. Patho. Exot. Filiales*, 80 (2): 162–170, 1987.

Meheus, A. and A. De Schryver, "Sexually Transmitted Diseases in the Third World." *in* J. Harris and S. Forster, eds., *Recent Advances in Sexually Transmitted Diseases and AIDS*. Edinburgh: Churchill Livingstone 1991.

Messing, S.D., "Traditional Healing and the New Health Center in Ethiopia." *The Conch*, 8, pp. 52–64, 1976.

Mhalu, F. S., "The Interrelationship Between HIV Infection and Other Sexually Transmitted Diseases." *E. African Med. J.*, 67 (7): 512–517, 1990.

MHSW (Ministry of Health and Social Welfare, Liberia), "Liberian National AIDs Guidelines and Policy." Monrovia: nd (1987?).

Moodie, T. Dunbar and W. Beinart, "Migrancy and Male Sexuality in the South African Gold Mines." *Journal of Southern African Studies*, 14(2):228–256, 1988.

Msamango, G. I. and K. J. Pallangyo, "Characterization of Tanzanian Outpatients Presenting with Sexually Transmitted Diseases." *E. African Med. Journal* 64 (1): 31–36, 1987.

Mshana and D. Scheinman, "Observing and Clinically Evaluating AIDS Patients Treated with an Herbal Regimen." Dar es Salaam: Department of Traditional Medicine, Muhimbili Medical Center, May 9, 1991.

Mshiu, E. N., personal communication, April 6, 1993.

Murdock, G. P. *Africa: Its People and Their Culture History*. New York: McGraw-Hill, 1959.

Murphy, E., *History of African Civilization*. New York: Dell Pulishing Company. 1972.

Musara, T. M., "Interview with a Traditional Healer." *in* M. A. Mercer and S. Scott, eds., *Tradition and Transition: NGOs Respond to AIDS in Africa*. Baltimore: The Johns Hopkins University School of Public Health and Hygiene, 1991.

Nell & Shapiro Consulting, "Evaluation of AIDSCOM/AIDSCAP/South Africa." Cc. (no date), p. 64, pp. 35–36.

N'Galy, B. and R. W. Ryder, "Epidemiology of HIV Infection in Africa." *Journal of Acquired Immune Deficiency Syndrome,* 1(6):551–558, 1988.

Ngubane, H., "Aspects of Clinical Practice and Traditional Organization of Indigenous Healers in South Africa." *Social Science and Medicine,* 15B, 1981, 361-365.

Ngubane. H., *Body and Mind in Zulu Medicine.* London: Academic Press, 1977.

Nhlengethwa, T. and L. Perez, "Report of the Training of Trainers Course for the Traditional Healers Organization in HIV/AIDS Prevention." Mbabane, Swaziland: Project HOPE/FLAS HIV/AIDS Prevention project, May 1991.

Nimpson, M., Chairman, National AIDS Program, Ministry of Health and Social Welfare (Liberia), personal communication, May 1988.

Nordstrom, Carolyn, USAID Monthly Progress Reports, Maputo, 1991.

Nsubuga, P., R. Mugerwa, J. Nsibambi, N. Sewankambo, E. Katabira, and S. Berkley, "The Association of Genital Ulcer Disease and HIV Infection at a Dermatology-STD Clinic in Uganda." *Journal of Acquired Immune Deficiency Syndrome,* 1990, 3(10): 1002–1005.

Oates, J. K., "Circumcision and Heterosexual Transmission of HIV Infection to Men." (letter) *New England Journal of Medicine,* 316 (24):1546, June 11, 1987.

O'Connor, P., M. T. Leshabari, and G. Lwihula, "Ethnographic Study of the Truck Stop Environment in Tanzania." Arlington, Va.: Family Health International (AISCAP Project), 1992.

O'Farrell, N. and D. Barlow, "Use of Nonoxynol-9" (letter), *LANCET,* July 18, 340(8812):179, 1992.

O'Farrell, N. and I. Windsor, "Sexual Behavior in HIV-1-seropositive Zulu Men and Women in Durban, South Africa" (letter). *J. of Acquired Immune Deficiency Syndromes,* 4(12):1258, 1991.

O'Reilly, K. R., "Sexual Behaviour, Perceptions of Infertility and Family Planning in Sub-Saharan Africa." *African Journal of Sexually Transmitted Diseases,* 1986 October, 2(2):4–9, 80.

Orley, J., "Indigenous Concepts of Disease and Their Interaction with Scientific Medicine." *in* E. E. Sabben-Clare, D. J. Bradley, and K. Kirkwood, eds., *Health in Tropical Africa During the Colonial Period,* based on the proceedings of a symposium held at New College, Oxford, March 12–23, 1977, Oxford: Clarendon Press, 1980, pp. 127–135.

Orubuloye, I. O., J. C. Caldwell, and P. Caldwell, "Sexual Networking in the Ekiti District of Nigeria." *Studies in Family Planning,* 22(2):61–73, 1991.

Osborne, O. et al., *Continuities between the Practices of Traditional and Scientific Botswana Health Care Practitioners,* African American Scholars, Inc., Washington, D.C., 1977.

Osoba A. O., "Sexually Transmitted Diseases in Tropical Africa." *British Journal of Venereal Disease* 57(2):89–94, 1981.

Pateguane, J. L., "Tuberculos pulmonar e alguns factores culturais ao abandono do tratamento." Trabalho Proposto as IV Jornadas de Saude, 1983.

Pela, A. O. and J. J. Platt, "AIDS in Africa: Emerging Trends." *Social Science and Medicine,* 28(1): 1–8, 1989.

Pellow, D. "Sexuality in Africa," *Trends in History,* 4(4) 1990: 71–96.

Pepin, J., F. A. Plumber, R. C. Brunham, P. Piot, D. W. Cameron, and A. R. Ronald, "The Interaction of HIV and Other Sexually Transmitted Diseases: An Opportunity for Intervention" *AIDS* 3:3–9, 1989.

Pepin, J., M. Quigley, J. Todd, I. Gaye, M. Janneh, E. Van Dyck, P. Piot, and H. Whittle, "Association between HIV-2 Infection and Genital Ulcer Diseases among Male Sexually Transmitted Disease Patients in The Gambia." *AIDS,* 6(5):489–493, 1992.

Pheterson, G., ed., *A Vindication of the Rights of Whores.* Seattle: Seal Press, 1989.

Pillsbury, B., "Policy and Evaluation Perspectives on Traditional Health Practitioners in National Health Care Systems." *Soc. Sci. & Med.,* 16, pp. 1825–1834, 1982.

Piot, P. and J. Harris, "The Epidemiology of HIV/AIDS in Africa." *in* P. Lamptey and P. Piot, eds.,*The Handbook for AIDS Prevention in Africa.* Durham, N.C.: Family Health International, 1990:1–19.

Piot, P. and S. Hira, "Control and Prevention of Sexually Transmitted Diseases." *in* P. Lamptey and P. Piot, eds., *The Handbook for AIDS Prevention in Africa.* Durham, N.C.: Family Health International, 1990: 83–104.

Piot, P. and R. Tezzo, "The Epidemiology of HIV and Other Sexually Transmitted Infections in the Developing World." *Scand. J. Infect. Disease. Suppl.,* 69: 89–97; 1990.

Piot, P., Quinn, T. C., H. Taelman, F. M. Feinsod, K. B. Minlangu, O. Wobin, N. Mbendi, P. Mazebo, K. Ndangi, W. Stevens et al., "Acquired Immunodeficiency Syndrome in a Heterosexual Population in Zaire," *Lancet,* 2(8394):65–69, July 14, 1984.

Platt, R., P. A. Rice, and W. M. McCormack, "Risk of Acquiring Gonorrhea and Prevalence of Abnormal Adnexal Findings among Women Recently Exposed to Gonorrhea." *JAMA,* 250:3205–3309, 1983.

Plummer, F. A., S. Moses, and J. O. Ndinya-Achola, "Factors Affecting Female to Male Transmission of HIV-1: Implications of Transmission and Dynamics for Prevention." *Network Newsletter,* August 2(2):6–9, 1991.

Plummer, F. A. et al., "Postpartum Upper Genital Tract Infection in Nairobi, Kenya." *Journal of Infectious Diseases,* 156(1):92–98, 1987.

Prual, A., S. Chacko, and D. Koch-Weser, "Sexual Behavior, AIDS and Poverty in Sub-Saharan Africa." *International Journal of STD and AIDS,* 2 (1): 1–9, 1991.

Quinn, T. C., "AIDS in Africa: Evidence for Heterosexual Transmission of the Human Immunodeficiency Virus." *New York State Journal of Medicine,* May 1987: 286–289.

Ramstedt, K., G. Hallhagen, B. I. Lundin, C. Hakansson, G. Johannisson, G. B. Lowhagen, G. Norkrans, and J. Giesecke, "Contact Tracing for Human Iimmunodeficiency Virus (HIV) Infection." *Sexually Transmitted Disease,* 17(1): 37–41, 1990.

Rosenberg, M., "Contraception and STDs." *IPPF Medical Bulletin,* 25(5):3–4, 1991.

Rosenberg, M., A. Davidson, J. Chen, F. Judson, and J. Douglas, "Barrier Contraceptives and Sexually-Transmitted Disease in Women: A Comparison of Female-Dependent Mothers and Condoms," *AJPH,* Vol. 82, No. 5 (May 1992): 669–674.

Rosenbert, M. J. et al., "Sexually Transmitted Diseases in Sub-Saharan Africa. A Priority List Based on FHI's International Meeting." *Lancet*, pp. 152–153, July 19, 1986.

Rubel, A. and C. Sargent, "Parallel Medical Systems: Papers from a Workshop on 'the healing process.'" *Soc. Sci. & Med.*, 13B, 1979.

Runganga, A., M. Pitts, and J. McMaster, "The Use of Herbal and Other Agents to Enhance Sexual Experience." *Social Science and Medicine*, Vol. 35(8): 1037–1042.

Ryder, R. et al., "Community Surveillance for HIV Infection in Zaire," paper presented to the Third International Conference on AIDS, Washington, D.C., June 1–5, 1987.

Sajiwandani, J. and K. Baboo, "Sexually Transmitted Diseases in Zambia." *Journal of the Royal Society of Health, 107* 5:183–186.

SATHC (the South African Traditional Healers Council) *Information Folder* (nd).

Scheinman, D., W. Mrisho, F. Mberesero, A. Chaze, and R. Nesje, "Treating HIV Disease with Traditional Medicine in Tanga Region, Tanzania. A Preliminary Report." Amsterdam: IX International Conference on AIDS and III STD World Congress. July 19, 1992a.

Scheinman, D., R. Nesje, E. Ulrich, and E. Malangalia, "Treating HIV with Traditional Medicine," *AIDS and Society* 3 (3):5, 1992b.

Scheinman, D., personal communication, April 26, 1993.

Schoepf, B.,"Epidemiologists, Social Scientists, and the Structure of Medical Research on AIDS in Africa." *Social Science and Medicine*, 1991; 33(7):791–793;

Schultz, K. F., W. Cates, Jr., and P. R. O'Mara, "Pregnancy Loss, Infant Death, and Suffering: Legacy of Syphilis and Gonorrhoea in Africa." *Genitourinary Medicine, 63* (5):320–325, October 1987.

Serwadda, D., "Church of Uganda AIDS KAP Survey" (draft). Kampala: Makerere Medical School, November 1992a.

Serwadda, D., "Islamic Medical Association AIDS KAP Survey" (draft). Kampala: Makerere Medical School, April 1992b.

Serwadda, D., M. J. Wawer, S. D. Musgrave, N. K. Sewankambo, J. E. Kaplan, and R. H. Gray, "HIV Risk Factors in Three Geographic Strata of Rural Rakai District, Uganda." *AIDS*, 6(9):983–989, 1992.

*Siyavuma* (traditional healer's newsletter) 5(1):7 Jan./Feb. 1990.

Skeet, M., "Community Health Workers: Promoters or Inhibitors of Primary Health Care?" *World Health Forum*, Vol. 5, pp. 291–295, 1984.

de Sousa, J. F., "Traditional Beliefs and Practices Related to Childhood Diarrhoeal Disease in a High-Density Suburb of Maputo." B.A. Thesis. Harare: Department of Sociology, University of Zimbabwe, 1991.

Spielberg, F., "Knowledge, Attitudes and Practices Concerning the AIDS Epidemic in Four Local Samples: A Pilot Study." McLean, Va.: Institute of International Research. October 1987.

Staugaard, F., "Role of Traditional Health Workers in Prevention and Control of AIDS in Africa." *Tropical Doctor* 21(1):22–24, 1991.

Subah-Bellah Associates, *Qualitative Exploration of Attitudes Toward Family Planning and Contraception among Liberian Adults*. Monrovia, April 1988.

Swantz, L., *The Medicine Man among the Zaramo of Dar es Salaam*. Uddevalla (Sweden): Scandanavian Inst. of African Studies, 1990.

Taylor, C., "Implications for the Delivery of Health Care." *Social Science and Medicine*, 13B, 77–84, 1979.

Textor, R. B. *A Cross-Cultural Summary*. New Haven: HRAF Press, 1967.

Tice, J, S. Allen, A. Serufilira, P. Van de Perre, J. Ziegler, and S. Hulley, "Impact of HIV Testing on Condoms/Spermicide Use among HIV Discordant Couples in Africa." International Conference on AIDS. 1990 June 20–23; 6(3):262 (abstract no. S.C.694).

Tomas, Taju, personal communication, December 1990.

Ulin, P., "The Traditional Healer of Botswana in a Changing Society." *Rural Africana*, 1974, 26:123–130.

Ulrich, E., M. Waziri, R. Nesja, and D. Scheinman, "Treating AIDS Patients with a Combination of Traditional Herbs and Modern Drugs in Tanga, Tanzania." Dar es Salaam: Department of Traditional Medicine, Muhimbili Medical Center, February 1991.

United Nations, *World Population Monitoring*, 1989. New York: UN, Department of International Economic and Social Affairs, pp. 162–163, 1990.

USAID and NIAID, "Anthropological Perspectives on AIDS in Africa: Priorities for Intervention and Research: Executive Summary. Washington, D.C. January 7–8, 1988.

Van de Perre, P. et al., "Seroepidemiological Study on Sexually Transmitted Diseases and Hepatitis B in African Promiscuous Heterosexuals in Relation to HTLV-III Infection." *Eur. J. Epidemiol*, 3(1): 14–18. March 1987.

van de Walle, E., "The Social Impact of AIDS in Sub-Saharan Africa." *Milbank Quarterly*, 1990; 68 Supplement 1:10.

Velimirovic, B., "Traditional Medicine is Not Primary Health Care: A Polemic." *Curare*, Vol. 7(1) 1984:61–79.

Velimirovic, B. and H. Velimirovic, "The Utilization of Traditional Medicine and its Practitioners in Health," *in* B. Velimirovic, ed., *Modern Medicine and Medical Anthropology in the United States–Mexico Border Population*. Washington, D.C.: Pan American Health Organization, 1978, pp. 172–185.

Ventevogel, P., *Aborofodee* (Whiteman's Things): Effects of Training Programme for Indigenous Healers in the Techiman Disctrict, Ghana. Master's Thesis, Free University of Amsterdam, The Netherlands, November 1992.

Voeller, B., "Spermicides for Controlling the Spread of HIV" (letter), *AIDS*, March, 6(3):341–342, 1992.

Waite, G., "The Politics of Disease: The AIDS Virus and Africa," *in* N. Miller and R. Rockwell, eds., *AIDS in Africa: the Social and Policy Impact*. Lewiston, N.Y.: Edwin Mellen Press, 1988.

Wallace, A. F. C., "Revitalization Movements," *American Anthropologist* 58:264–281, 1956.

Ward, H. and S. Day, "Prostitution," *in* J. Harris and S. Forster, eds., *Recent Advances in Sexually-Transmitted Diseases and AIDS*. Edinburgh: Churchill Livingstone 1991.

Warren, D. M., "Disease, Medicine and Religion among the Techiman-Bono of

Ghana: A Study in Culture Change." Unpublished doctoral dissertation, Indiana University, 1974.

Warren, D. M., "The Role of Emic Analysis in Medical Anthropology: The Case of the Bono of Ghana." *in* D. M. Warren, Z. Ademuwagun, J. Ayoade, and I. Harrison, eds., *African Therapeutic Systems,* Los Angeles: Crossroads Press for the African Studies Association, 1979.

Warren, D. M., "The Techiman-Bono Ethnomedical System," *in* P. S. Yoder, ed., *African Health and Healing Systems: Proceedings of a Symposium.* Los Angeles: Crossroads Press, 1982, pp. 39, 85–106.

Warren, D. M., "The Expanding Role of Indigenous Healers in Ghana's National Health Delivery System." *in* C. Fyfe and U. Maclean, eds., *African Medicine in the Modern World,* University of Edinburgh, Centre of African Studies, Seminar Proceedings No. 27, December 1986, pp. 73–86.

Warren, D. M., "Utilizing Indigenous Healers in National Health Delivery Systems: The Ghanian Experiment," *in* J. van Willigen, B. Rylko-Bauer, and A. McElroy, eds., *Making our Research Useful: Case Studies in the Utilization of Anthropological Knowledge,* 1989, pp. 159–178.

Warren, D. M. and E. C. Green, "Linking Allopathic and Indigenous African Health Delivery Systems: An Assessment of Collaborative Efforts During the 1980s," *in* D. M. Warren and L. J. Slikkerveer, eds., *Proceedings of the International Conference on Ethnomedical Systems In Sub-Saharan Africa,* University of Leiden and The African Studies Centre (The Netherlands) Press (forthcoming 1993).

Warren, D. M., L. J. Slikkerveer, and S. O. Titiloa, *Indigenous Knowledge Systems: Implications for Agriculture and International development.* Ames: Technology and Social Change Prog., Iowa State University 1989.

Warren, D. M. et al., "Ghanaian National Policy toward Indigenous Healers. The Case of the Primary Health Training for Indigenous Healers (PRHETIH) Program." *Social Science and Medicine,* Vol. 16, pp. 1873–1881, 1982.

Wasserheit, J. N. "Epidemiological Synergy: Interrelationships between HIV Infection and Other STDs" *in* L. Chen, J. Sepulveda, and S. Segal, eds., *AIDS and Women's Health: Science for Policy and Action,* New York: Plenum Press, 1992a.

Wasserheit, J. N., "Epidemiological Synergy: Interrelationships between Human Immunodeficiency Virus Infection and Other Sexually Transmitted Diseases." *Sexually Transmitted Diseases,* March–April, pp. 61–77, 1992b.

Welgemode, N. C., A. Mahaffey, and J. Van den Ende, "Prevalence of Neisseria Gonorrhoeae Infection in Patients Attending an Antenatal Clinic." *South African Medical Journal,* 69 (1):32–4, January 1986.

WHO, *Traditional Birth Attendants.* (Offset Publication no. 44) Geneva, 1979.

WHO, *Report on the Consultation on Approaches for Policy Development for Traditional Health Practitioners, Including Traditional Birth Attendants.* Geneva, 1985.

WHO, Special Programme on AIDS. Strategies and Structure, Projected Needs. Geneva, March 1987:II-3-4.

WHO, *Report of a WHO Informal Consultation on Traditional Medicine and AIDS: In Vitro Screening for Anti-HIV Activity.* Global Programme on AIDS and Traditional Medicine Programme. Geneva: 6–8 February 1989.

WHO, *Prevention of Sexual Transmission of Human Immunodeficiency Virus.* Geneva: WHO 1990a.

WHO, "Report on the Consultation on AIDS and Traditional Medicine: Prospects for Involving Traditional Health Practitioners." Traditional Medicine Programme and Global Programme on AIDS. Francistown, Botswana, July 23–27, 1990b.

WHO, *Traditional Healers as Community Health Workers: A Review of Projects Using Traditional Healers as Community Health Workers.* Geneva: WHO 1990b.

Wilson, K. B., "Cults of Violence and Counterviolence in Mozambique." Refugee Studies Centre, Oxford University, June 1992, p. 11.

Wondergem, P., K. A. Senah, and E. K. Glover, *Ghana: An Assessment of the Relevance of Herbal Drugs in PHC and Some Suggestions for Strengthening PHC.* October 1989, Department of Sociology, University of Ghana, Lagon.

WRI (World Resources Institute), *Biodiversity Prospecting,* WRI, May 1993.

Yoder, R. A., "Are People Willing and Able to Pay for Health Services?" *Soc. Sci. & Med.,* 29(1):35–42, 1989.

de Zalduondo, B. O., G. I. Msamanga, and L. C. Chen, "AIDS in Africa: Diversity in the Global Pandemic." Daedalus (Summer) 118(3), 1989:165–204.

# Index